W0106452

CHORION VILLUS
— SAMPLING —

CHORION VILLUS
— SAMPLING —

Edited by

D. T. Y. Liu, E. M. Symonds

and

M. S. Golbus

SPRINGER-SCIENCE+BUSINESS MEDIA, B.V.

© 1987 Springer Science+Business Media Dordrecht
Originally published by Chapman and Hall in 1987
Softcover reprint of the hardcover 1st edition 1987

ISBN 978-0-412-27910-2

All rights reserved. No part of this book may be reprinted, or reproduced or utilized in any form or by any electronic, mechanical or other means, now known or hereafter invented, including photocopying and recording, or in any information storage and retrieval system, without permission in writing from the publisher

British Library Cataloguing in Publication Data

Chorion villus sampling.
1. Prenatal diagnosis
I. Liu D. T. Y. II. Symonds, E. M.
III. Golbus, Mitchell S.
618.2'2 RG628

ISBN 978-0-412-27910-2 ISBN 978-1-4899-3362-1 (eBook)
DOI 10.1007/978-1-4899-3362-1

Contents

Foreword

The reduction of childhood handicap and serious genetic disease is an aim worthy of us all. Increasing knowledge about genetics and about the molecular pathology of inherited disease should provide many families at risk of handicapped children with the benefit of being forewarned, so that they can consider reproductive options. Genetic counselling is the cornerstone of such disease prevention and it is high time that this important service is made more generally available. At present the public are largely denied this knowledge, and so often reproach the medical profession when they learn too late of the help that might have been made available to them.

The most important adjunct of genetic counselling is undoubtedly prenatal diagnosis, which allows the couple at risk of fetal abnormality the opportunity of confirming the normality of their future offspring. Many thousands of couples now have healthy children only because the availability of a prenatal test enabled them to plan a pregnancy. In a comparatively small proportion of prenatal diagnoses the couple learn that their fetus is affected, and that they have to consider the option of termination. Invariably the diagnosis is made in the second trimester of pregnancy which means a late abortion and all its associated trauma and distress. The possibility of an early diagnosis in the first trimester is much more acceptable to the couple, and this explains the current widespread interest in developing first trimester diagnosis by chorion villus sampling (CVS).

The editors of this volume are to be congratulated in choosing a team of experts to produce such a valuable account of this important development. Progress has been dramatic when one considers that it has only been four years since Kazy and his colleagues (1982) re-awakened interest in the possibility of early prenatal diagnosis by reporting successful CVS under the guidance of endoscopy and ultrasound in a substantial series of cases. A year later Simoni indicated the potential for the diagnosis of fetal chromosome aberrations by showing that chromosome preparations could be made directly from rapidly dividing cytotrophoblast in chorion samples. Since then many pregnancies at high risk of metabolic disorders, chromosome abnormalities and disorders detected by DNA analysis have been tested successfully. This progress is covered clearly and comprehensively in the following pages, which not only indicate the current state of CVS, but detail the outstanding questions and concerns which at present limit the widespread application of the procedure. Chief among these is the question of safety, and an important contribution is made in chapter 16 by Jackson, who has co-ordinated an international collaborative effort to document a worldwide experience of over 13 000 CVS diagnoses, the first 6500 of which have been analyzed in some detail. This suggests that the excess fetal loss due to the procedure in experienced hands may be 0.5–1.5%, which is not too different from published data on amniocentesis. However, a reliable assessment of early and late complications can only be achieved by mounting appropriately controlled trials, and a compelling case is made for randomized trials of CVS versus amniocentesis by Chalmers in chapter 17. The ethics of offering CVS to couples at low risk of fetal abnormality (for increased maternal age, for example) outside the limits of a properly organized randomized trial are certainly debatable.

Experts in prenatal diagnosis will be interested to read the chapters on sampling techniques and laboratory methods. The introduction of the transabdominal approach to CVS shows particular promise in view of its increased patient acceptability and simplicity. It can be undertaken in the ultrasound room, and the avoidance of the transcervical route should reduce any risk of infection and allow greater flexibility at the time of sampling. An important problem for the laboratory is the difficulty in determining the significance of the fortunately rare cases of chromosomal mosaicism (such as normal/trisomy 2, 16 or 20) in trophoblast. The abnormal cell line noted in the trophoblast frequently cannot be confirmed in tissues obtained from the aborted fetus, and continuing pregnancies have been found to be normal on delivery. Until the origin and nature of such mosaicism is further clarified, it would seem wise to confirm findings of mosaicism in chorion by amniocentesis before attempting an interpretation.

If, as is likely, CVS proves to be the important advance that is suggested by the contributions to this volume, its widespread application will require considerable reorganization of obstetric and genetic services. The key is communication about the procedure, not only to the family doctors and obstetricians providing antenatal care, but also to the public, who need to know that the best time to consider prenatal diagnosis is before pregnancy and after genetic counselling. Whether this counselling is best done at combined genetics/obstetric clinics or at pre-pregnancy clinics will have to be determined, but it is already clear that the antenatal clinic is not the appropriate place. Debate on these and other issues relating to first trimester prenatal diagnosis is to be encouraged. It is to be hoped that this book will reach a wider audience than those with a professional interest in prenatal diagnostic services, because it has a most important message about a new technology which could substantially reduce the burden of disease in the community.

September 1986 *M. A. Ferguson-Smith*

Contributors

Stephen R. Barnes
University of Nottingham, Dept. of Genetics, University Park, Nottingham, UK.

Iain Chalmers, MB BS MSc DCH FFCM FRCOG
Director, National Perinatal Epidemiology Unit, Radcliffe Infirmary, Oxford, UK.

Dulcie V. Coleman
Cytogenetics Unit, Dept. of Experimental Pathology, St. Mary's Hospital Medical School, London, UK.

A. C. Crompton, MD FRCSEd FRCOG
St. James's University Hospital, Beckett St., Leeds, UK.

B. H. Czepulkowski
Cytogenetics Unit, Medical Oncology Unit, 45–47 Little Britain, London, UK.

M. Dommergues
Clinique Universitaire Port Royal, 123 Boulevard Port Royal, Paris, France.

Y. Dumez
Clinique Universitaire Port Royal, 123 Boulevard Port Royal, Paris, France.

John W. Eddy, FRCS FRCOG
Essex County Hospital, Colchester, UK.

A. H. Fensom
Paediatric Research Unit, United Medical and Dental Schools of Guy's and St. Thomas' Hospitals, Guy's Hospital, London, UK.

J. S. Fitzsimmons, MB BCh FRCP(E) DCH
Dept. of Clinical Genetics, City Hospital, Hucknall Rd., Nottingham, UK.

Mitchell S. Golbus, MD
Dept. of Obstetrics, Gynecology and Reproductive Sciences, and of Pediatrics, University of California, San Francisco, USA.

Christine Gosden, BSc PhD
MRC Clinical and Population Cytogenetics Unit, Western General Hospital, Crewe Rd., Edinburgh, UK.

J. Groves, DCR DMV
Superintendent Radiographer, Ultrasound Dept., St. James's University Hospital, Beckett St., Leeds, UK.

Björn Gustavii
Dept. of Obstetrics and Gynecology, University Hospital, S-221 85 LUND, Sweden.

Niels Hahnemann
Dept. of Obstetrics and Gynecology, Aalborg Hospital, Aalborg, Denmark.

Peter S. Harper
Section of Medical Genetics, University of Wales College of Medicine, Heath Park, Cardiff, UK.

D. E. Heaton
Cytogenetics Unit, Dept. of Experimental Pathology, St. Mary's Hospital Medical School, London, UK.

John B. Henderson, BA MSc
Health Economics Research Unit, Dept. of Community Medicine, University of Aberdeen, Foresterhill, Aberdeen, UK.

W. Allen Hogge, MD
Dept. of Obstetrics and Gynecology, School of Medicine, University of Virginia, Charlottesville, Virginia, USA.

David H. Horwell, MB FRCSEd MRCOG
Consultant Obstetrician, Luton and Dunstable Hospital, Luton, UK

Henry C. Irving, MB BS DMRD FRCR
Dept. of Radiology, St. James's University Hospital, Beckett St., Leeds, UK.

Laird G. Jackson
Division of Medical Genetics, Jefferson Medical College, Philadelphia, Pennsylvania, USA.

Peter M. Johnson, MA PhD MRCPath
Pregnancy Immunology Group, Dept. of Immunology, University of Liverpool, P.O. Box 147, Liverpool, UK.

Lyndal Kearney, BSc
Harris Birthright Research Centre for Fetal Medicine, King's College School of Medicine and Dentistry, Denmark Hill, London, UK.

R. J. Lilford, MRCP MRCOG PhD
Dept. of Obstetrics and Gynaecology, St. James's University Hospital, Beckett St., Leeds, UK.

G. Linton
St. James's University Hospital, Beckett St., Leeds, UK.

David T. Y. Liu, MD FRCOG
Dept. of Obstetrics, City Hospital, Hucknall Rd., Nottingham, UK.

M. K. Mason, MD FRCPath
St. James's University Hospital, Beckett St., Leeds, UK.

I. Z. MacKenzie, MA MD MRCOG
Nuffield Dept. of Obstetrics and Gynaecology, John Radcliffe Infirmary, Oxford, UK.

W. E. MacKenzie, MRCOG
Dept. of Obstetrics and Gynaecology, Birmingham Maternity Hospital, Queen Elizabeth Medical Centre, Edgbaston, Birmingham, UK.

D. J. Maxwell, MB BS MRCOG MRACOG
Senior Registrar and Lecturer, Dept. of Obstetrics and Gynaecology, Chenies Mews, University College Hospital, Gower St., London, UK.

Christina F. McKenzie
Harris Birthright Research Centre for Fetal Medicine, King's College School of Medicine and Dentistry, Denmark Hill, London, UK.

Bernadette Modell
Dept. of Obstetrics and Gynaecology, University College Hospital, London UK.

J. R. Newton, MD FRCOG
Dept. of Obstetrics and Gynaecology, Birmingham Maternity Hospital, Queen Elizabeth Medical Centre, Birmingham, UK.

Kypros H. Nicolaides
Harris Birthright Research Centre for Fetal Medicine, King's College School of Medicine and Dentistry, Denmark Hill, London, UK.

C. D. Ockleford, BSc PhD
Dept. of Anatomy, University of Leicester Medical School, University Rd., Leicester, UK.

J. M. Old, PhD
National Haemoglobinopathy Reference Service, Nuffield Dept. of Clinical Medicine, John Radcliffe Infirmary, Oxford, UK.

R. Quaife BSc MPhil PhD DipRCPath
Dept. of Cytogenetics, Molecular Genetics Section, City Hospital, Hucknall Rd., Nottingham, UK.

R. E. Richardson, MSc ARCS
Dept. of Medical Physics, City Hospital, Hucknall Rd., Nottingham, UK.

A. Roberts
Dept. of Obstetrics, University of Wales College of Medicine, Heath Park, Cardiff, UK.

Charles H. Rodeck, BSc MRCOG
Professor, Inst. of Obstetrics and Gynaecology, Queen Charlotte's Maternity Hospital, Goldhawk Rd, London, UK.

D. Ian Rushton, FRCPath
Dept. of Pathology, University of Birmingham Medical School, and Dept. of Pathology, Birmingham Maternity Hospital, Queen Elizabeth Medical Centre, Birmingham, UK.

Steen Smidt-Jensen
Dept. of Obstetrics and Gynecology, Section of Clinical Genetics, Rigshospitalet, Copenhagen, Denmark.

E. Malcolm Symonds, MD FRCOG
Chairman, Dept. of Obstetrics and Gynaecology, Queen's Medical Centre, University Hospital, Nottingham, UK.

A. Stanley Tyms, PhD
Division of Virology, Dept. of Medical Microbiology, St. Mary's Hospital Medical School, London, UK.

M. Upadhyaya, PhD
Senior Scientific Officer, Section of Medical Genetics, University of Wales College of Medicine, Heath Park, Cardiff, UK.

Humphry Ward, MA FRCOG
Consultant Obstetrician and Gynaecologist, University College Hospital, 88–96 Chienes Mews, London, UK.

Richard C. Warren
Harris Birthright Research Centre for Fetal Medicine, King's College Medical School, Denmark Hill, London, UK.

H. Williams
Section of Medical Genetics, University of Wales College of Medicine, Heath Park, Cardiff, UK.

Section I

STRUCTURE AND FUNCTION

1

Embryology and physiopathology of early pregnancy trophoblast

—— D. Ian Rushton ——

Chorion villus sampling provides the promise of the prenatal diagnosis of certain chromosomal, genetic and metabolic disorders before the end of the first trimester, thus allowing termination at an earlier gestation than is currently possible with most other prenatal diagnostic techniques. It is intended to limit this discussion of the normal and abnormal placenta to the first twelve to fourteen weeks of pregnancy.

During the first trimester rapid changes occur affecting the development, growth and maturation of the tissues of both the embryo and placenta. The vast majority of the biological wastage associated with reproduction also occurs during this period though much passes unnoticed by mother and doctor alike (Miller *et al.*, 1980; Whittaker *et al.*, 1983). Though the greater part of this wastage occurs prior to the gestation at which villus sampling is currently carried out, some abnormal pregnancies destined to abort spontaneously will inevitably be encountered in any population subject to villus sampling. Indeed even with current techniques carried out at about the sixteenth week of pregnancy, it is known there is a significant loss of chromosomally abnormal conceptuses that are not terminated because of parental refusal after intra-uterine diagnosis (Hook, 1978). The same is almost certainly true of spontaneous abortions of different aetiologies with normal karyotypes. Certain characteristic patterns of villous pathology have been described in the placentae of spontaneous abortions (Rushton, 1978; 1984) but, as will become apparent, these changes mimic or are closely allied to those occurring in the normal placenta in the junctional zone between the chorion frondosum and chorion laeve. It is therefore of paramount importance that tissue samples should be obtained from appropriate areas within the placenta since it is not a homogeneous structure. The risk of obtaining villi from the junctional zone is greatest when the placenta is approached from the lateral margin parallel to the chorionic plate (i.e. the usual situation using the transcervical route) and is least if the approach is at 90 degrees to the chorionic plate (i.e. the usual situation using the transabdominal route) (Fig. 1.1).

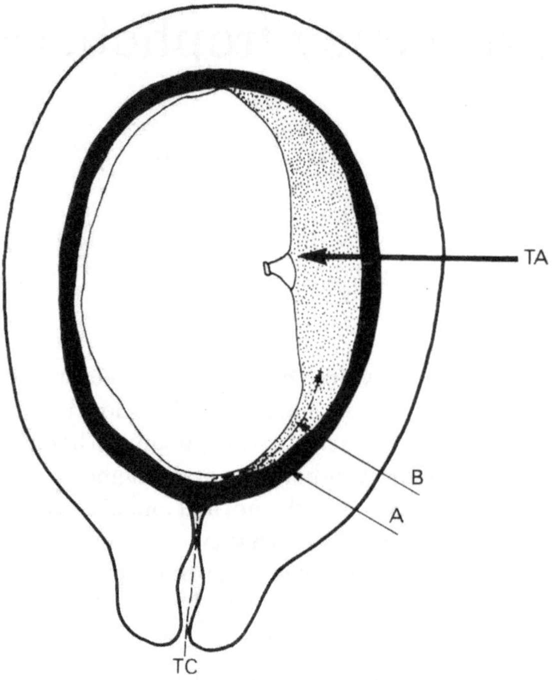

Figure 1.1 Diagrammatic representation of uterus at 10–12 weeks gestation. A – zone of villi showing microscopic hydatidiform change. B – zone of villi showing stromal fibrosis. TA – transabdominal route for sampling. TC – transcervical route for sampling.

1.1 NORMAL DEVELOPMENT

Fertilization generally occurs either in the fimbrial end of the fallopian tube or within the peritoneal cavity. Within three days the fertilized ovum consists of about 60 cells of which approximately 10% are destined to form the embryo while 90% will form the trophoblast (Wynn, 1975). During the next two days the conceptus completes its journey along the tube and enters the uterine cavity, where in a normal woman the secretory endometrium will be approximately 0.5 cm in thickness, the conceptus being only 0.2 mm in diameter.

On entering the uterine cavity implantation is not immediate, but once commenced is very rapid since the morula will be completely buried within the endometrium by about the 12th day (Hertig and Rock, 1941). It is during the phase of implantation that the greatest loss of fertilized ova occurs (Witschi, 1970). The process of implantation is associated with decidualization of the endometrium; this is initially a local process but eventually extends to involve the entire endometrium. In the early weeks of pregnancy there is substantially more decidua than placenta. The decidua is divided into three parts:

1. Decidua basalis which lies between the ovum and myometrium and becomes incorporated into the placental bed and is the area involved in the development of the placental site reaction.
2. Decidua capsularis which surrounds the rest of the ovum.
3. Decidua parietalis which lines the remainder of the uterine cavity.

As the conceptus expands the latter two parts of the decidua come together and eventually fuse obliterating the uterine cavity by about the end of the fourth month of pregnancy.

The most common site of implantation is the upper posterior wall of the uterine cavity. The process of implantation occurs as the result of proteolytic destruction of the endometrium by trophoblastic cells at the embryonic pole of the blastocyst. Concurrent differentiation of the trophoblast into cytotrophoblast, adjacent to the inner cell mass of the embryo and syncytial trophoblast on the maternal aspect is followed by progressive invasion of the endometrium by the syncytial trophoblast, while the endometrium surrounding the anembryonic pole of the blastocyst closes over the surface of the conceptus to envelope it by the 12th day. Vacuoles form within the syncytium and these eventually fuse to form lacunae into which maternal venous blood flows as the endometrial veins are penetrated. It is two to three days later that arterial blood begins to circulate within this labarynthine mass of lacunae. Initially these changes in the syncytium may involve the entire surface of the conceptus but they eventually become polarized on the maternal surface of the blastocyst. To ensure appropriate organization of the maternal blood supply the syncytial trophoblast extends along the intimal surface of the spiral arteries in the future placental bed and partially replaces the endothelium. Communication with the decidual veins allows the establishment of a primitive utero-placental circulation (Robertson, 1976). This previllous stage of development is followed by the differentiation and maturation of true functional villi.

Primary villi form as the result of growth and penetration of cytotrophoblastic columns into the syncytium. They contain neither stromal elements nor blood vessels. Secondary villi form as the result of either extension of the extra-embryonic mesoderm into this cytotrophoblastic core or by delamination of cells from the inner aspect of the cytotrophoblast.

From the end of the second week tertiary villi evolve with the development of primitive vascular channels within the stromal core. Primary angiogenesis may occur as the result of specialized differentiation of cells within the trophoblast or from the stromal cells, a problem that remains unresolved among embryologists (Hertig, 1935; Cibils, 1968; Dempsey, 1972). The result is the formation of a discontinuous network of vessels. These fuse and eventually join the vascular networks of the yolk sac and embryo to form the embryonic circulation within the placenta. Further villous growth proceeds by trophoblastic budding and extension of the villous core and its vascular network into the new branches, rather than by further local angiogenesis and fusion with the established embryonic circulation.

During the stages of villous development the cytotrophoblast, which was initially separated from the maternal tissues by the syncytial trophoblast, penetrates the myometrium and comes into direct contact with maternal tissues. As this layer of cytotrophoblast growing from each anchoring villus extends circumferentially within the decidua it fuses with similar tissue from adjacent villi to form the trophoblastic shell. From about the sixteenth day the primitive villi progressively give rise to branch villi which eventually become organized into the cotyledonary structure of the more mature placenta (Wigglesworth, 1967). Whether or not one stem villus and its blood supply forms the core of a single cotyledon is disputed (Gruenwald, 1975).

Thus by the end of the fifth week of pregnancy the basic components of the normal placenta are established. The villi on the embryonic pole continue to grow forming the chorion frondosum while those on the anembryonic pole atrophy to form the chorion laeve. The mechanisms leading to atrophy of these villi are uncertain though it is generally held that the poorer blood supply and nutritive capability of the decidua capsularis are important factors. However the morphology of the villi at the junctional zone between the chorion frondosum and chorion laeve suggests that failure to establish an embryonic circulation within them may be another controlling influence. The villi nearest the chorion frondosum are usually fibrotic and avascular or contain obliterated vessels (Fig. 1.2), a pattern normally associated with cessation of an established embryonic or fetal circulation whereas those further from the margin have an attenuated trophoblast and an hydropic or hydatidiform avascular stroma (Fig. 1.3), a pattern typical of the villi of an anembryonic blighted ovum (Rushton, 1984). Thus the organization of the embryonic and subsequently fetal circulation may play a vital role in determining placental size and shape. Whatever the mechanisms concerned the degeneration of the villi attached to the decidua capsularis is usually complete by the end of the third month of pregnancy, though remnants of these degenerate villi may still be identified microscopically at the margins of full-term placentae.

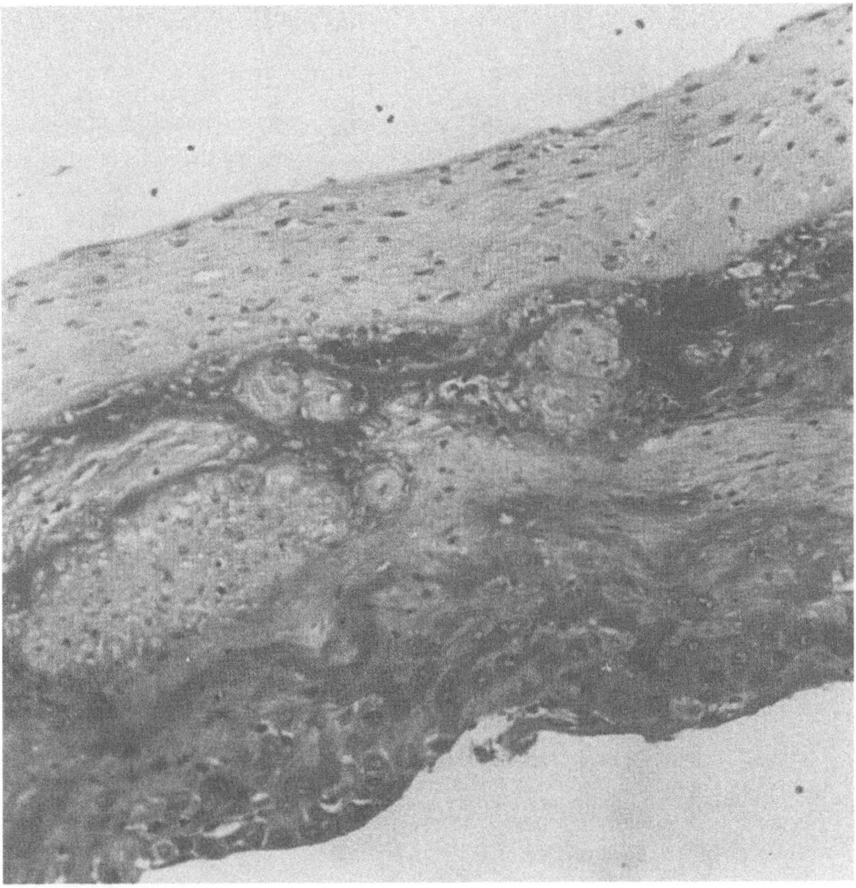

Figure 1.2 Marginal villi of normal 12 week placenta from zone B – villi showing stromal fibrosis (Haematoxylin and Eosin × 150).

Thus by the time chorion villus sampling is likely to be performed the placenta is far from being a homogeneous organ. The villi at the centre of the future cotyledons will be growing vigorously and will have a well-developed fetal capillary network (Fig. 1.4) while those at the margins will still be undergoing degenerative or regressive changes. It is reasonable to suppose the villi at the centre of cotyledons will have the greatest growth potential when sampled. There is, of course, the possibility that the risk of fetomaternal haemorrhage may be greater from these vascularized villi but any approach to the placenta parallel to the chorionic plate, as is likely if the cervical route of sampling is used, may carry a higher risk of decidual haemorrhage and placental separation. In addition, since the vagina and cervix are not sterile, infection might be introduced by this route.

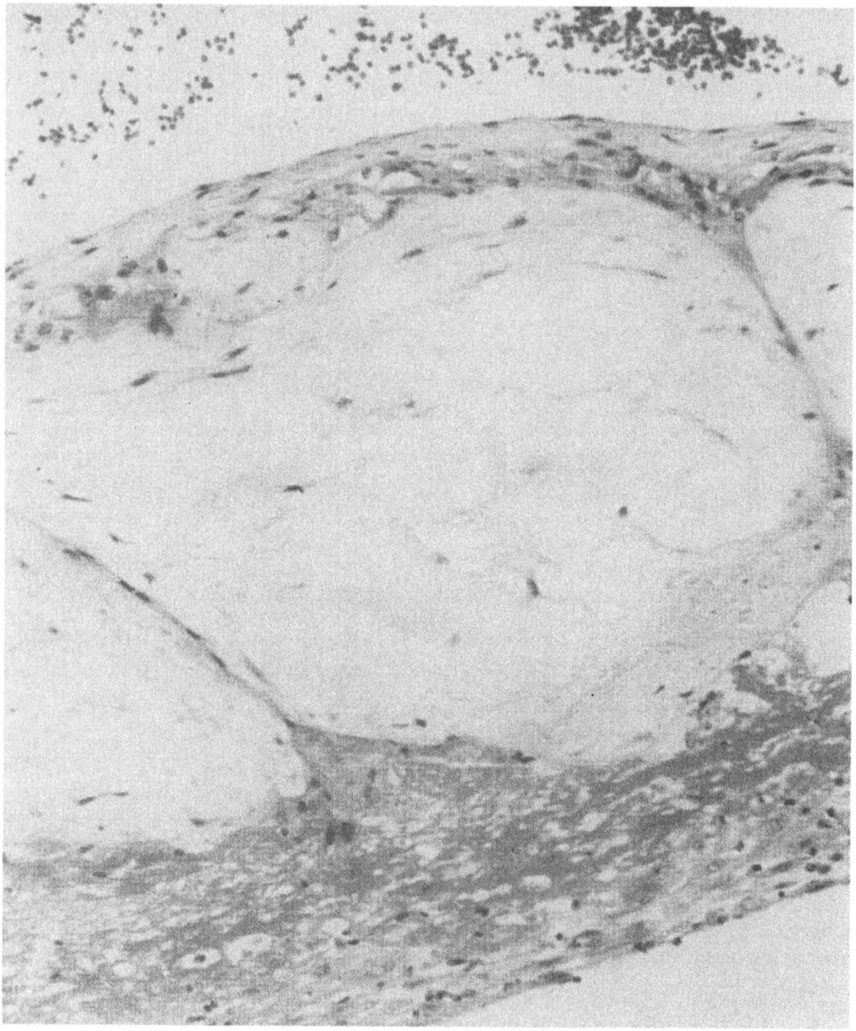

Figure 1.3 Marginal villi of normal 12 week placenta from zone A – villi showing microscopic hydatidiform change. Note absence of trophoblast (Haematoxylin and Eosin × 150).

Placental growth is rapid and until about the 16th week of pregnancy placental weight exceeds that of the embryo and fetus. At the beginning of the second month of pregnancy the placenta weighs about 5 g compared to an embryonic weight of 0.5 g. At the end of the third month (Fig. 1.5) the placenta may weigh 80 g and the embryo 25 g. At 16 weeks the weights are similar, i.e. about 135 g (Boyd and Hamilton, 1970). There is, however, a

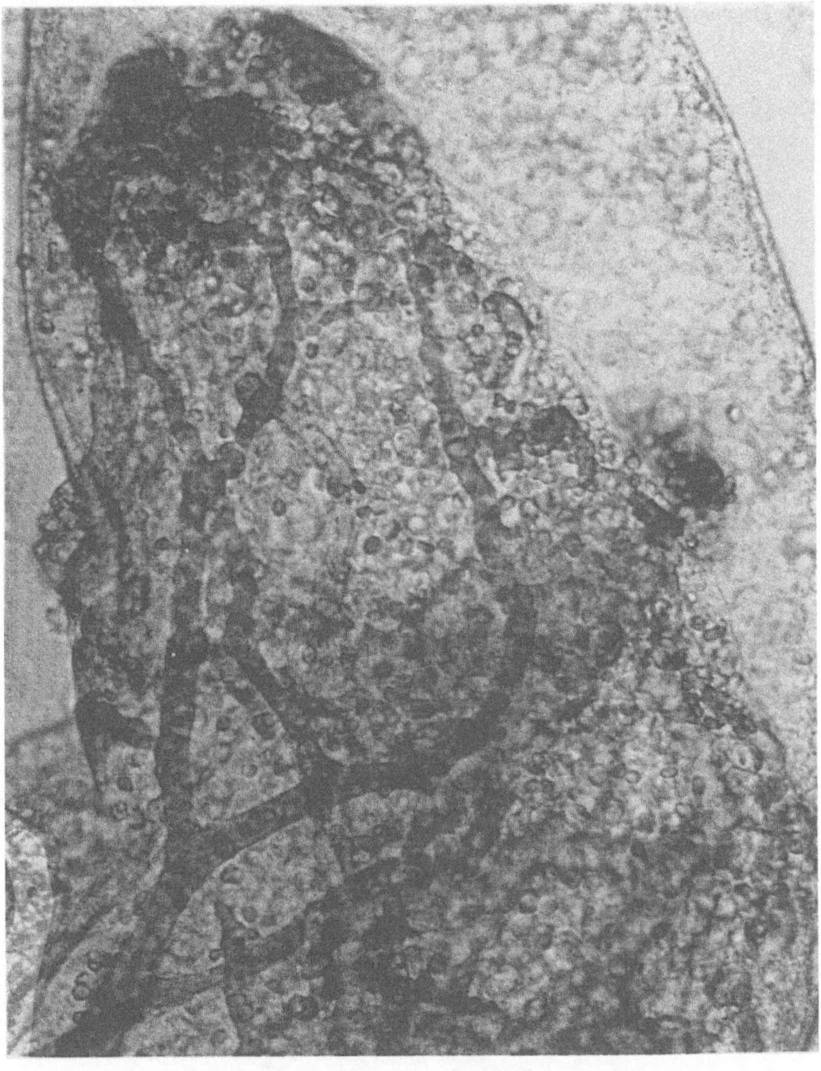

Figure 1.4 Vascular plexus in ten-week villus from the centre of the placenta (× 100).

wide variation in the weights of both embryo and placenta during this period some of which reflects natural variation. However, some may reflect our inability to be certain of the time of conception and to identify pathology in early pregnancy. During the first three months the size of the placenta increases from a microscopic structure to an organ which may measure 9 cm in diameter.

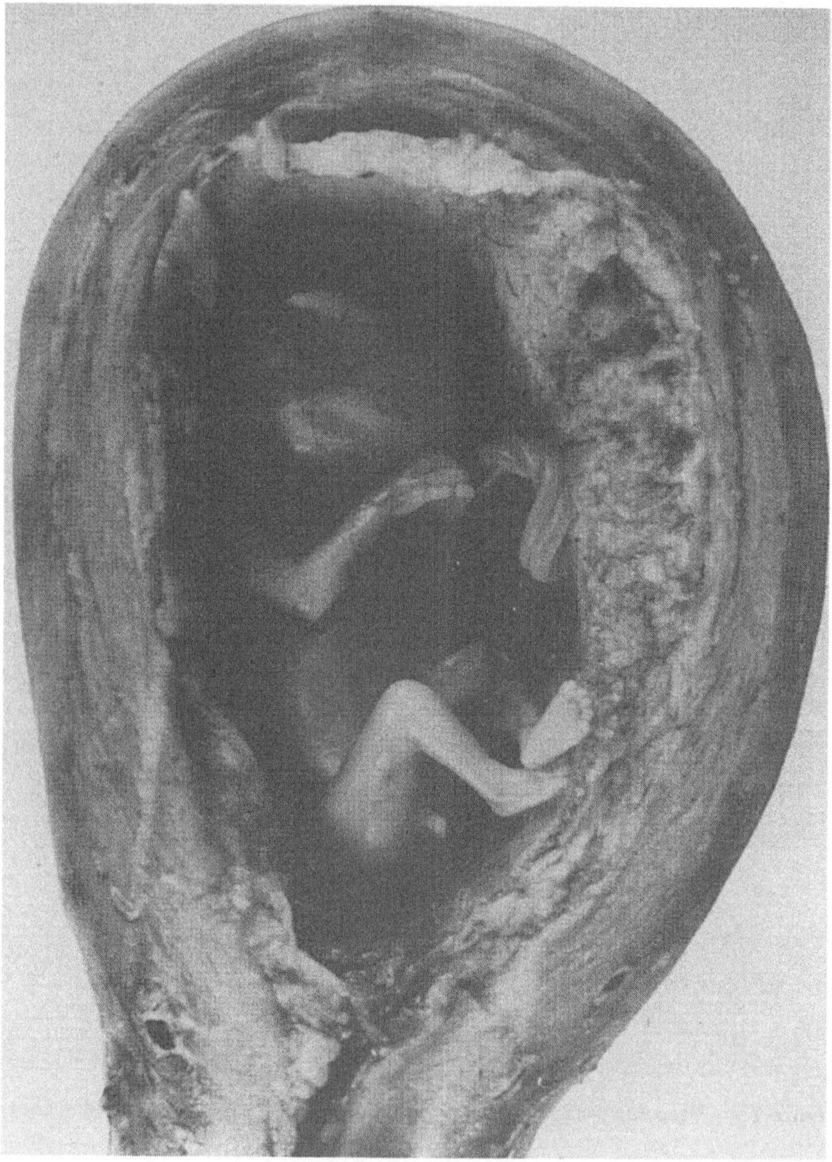

Figure 1.5 12 week pregnancy in utero emphasizing the relative sizes of the fetus and placenta (× 1.3).

1.2 PATHOLOGY

Since early pregnancy failure is the commonest complication of pregnancy any attempt at routine unselected chorion villus sampling will inevitably result in a significant proportion of specimens from pregnancies already destined to abort spontaneously. Many of these will be so-called blighted ova in which there is no, or at most minimal, evidence of embryogenesis. Today, such pregnancies may be identified ultrasonically (Robinson, 1975) and chorion villus sampling avoided.

There are few pathological lesions likely to be encountered in villus samples and it is of note that sampling of the placenta was recommended as a possible method of the assessment of the quality of the conceptus about 20 years ago (Alvarez, 1964; Aladjem, 1966). The latter author considered the following features to be pathological: hypoplasia of the syncytium; oedema and vacuolation of the villous stroma; avascularity of the villi. These have their counterparts at the edge of the normal placenta as described above.

Histological examination of sampled villi is frequently impossible as the whole sample is required for diagnostic tests so that the following pathological descriptions will be confined to the appearances of villi under the dissecting microscope, though the histological manifestations of these appearances will be given.

There are four pathological patterns that are likely to be encountered.

1. Villi showing hydropic or microscopic hydatidiform change.
2. Villi showing vascular obliteration and stromal fibrosis.
3. A mixed pattern of (1) and (2).
4. Villi showing either true or partial molar degeneration.

As has been emphasized, villi of types (1), (2) and (3) may be encountered in both normal and abnormal placentae depending on the site of sampling.

Type (1) villi (Fig. 1.6) are avascular and resemble a hydatidiform mole in miniature. Microscopy shows the villi to have attenuated trophoblast and an oedematous or cystic relatively acellular stroma. Type (2) (Fig. 1.7) are irregular in shape but characteristically stringy rather than swollen as above. They may be matted together by deposits of inter-villous fibrin. Microscopy reveals a bilaminar or attenuated trophoblast with a fibrotic sometimes densely collagenized stroma in which vascular remnants may be identified. There may be deposits of calcium and iron salts on the trophoblastic membrane or within the villous stroma. Type (4) villi (Fig. 1.8) will usually be from partial moles since true moles should be identified ultrasonically by 12 weeks gestation. Partial molar degeneration results in both molar and non-molar villi, with individual branches of single-stem villus showing both forms. Indeed the cystic dilatation of the villi may appear to be segmental.

Minor forms may be indistinguishable from type (1) villi. Microscopy

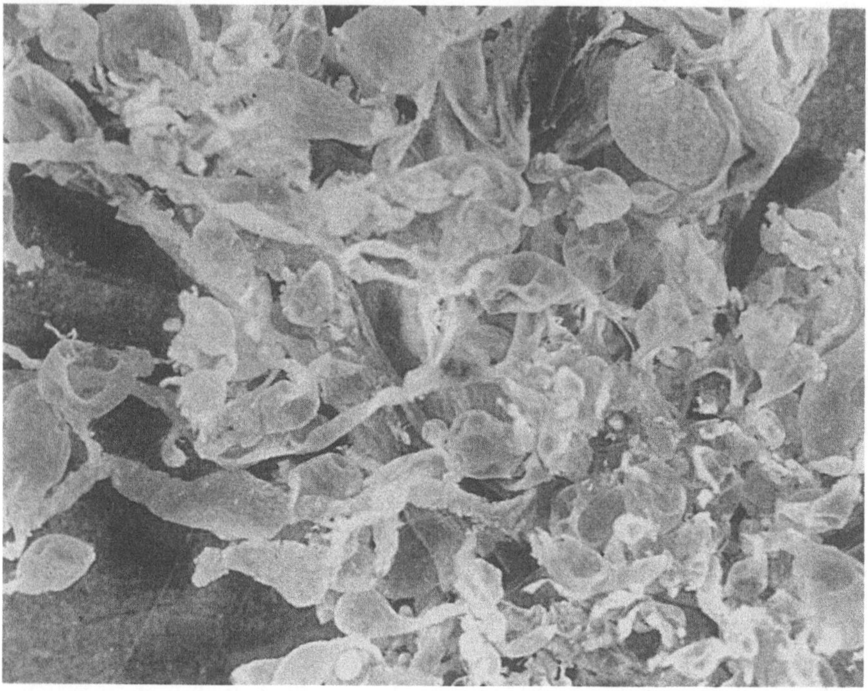

Figure 1.6 Villi from an anembryonic blighted ovum aborted at nine weeks gestation showing diffuse microscopic hydatidiform change (× 5).

shows a variable proportion of villi which are swollen often with a cystic central cavity lined by endothelial like cells. Around the cavity the stroma may contain vascular channels. There is usually no evidence of trophoblastic hyperplasia.

True moles show a much more uniform involvement of the villi and there is frequently some degree of trophoblastic hyperplasia. Vascular channels are rarely visible and are almost certainly discontinuous since embryonic or fetal development does not occur.

Though infection may occur in early pregnancy it is unlikely to be recognized under the dissecting microscope. To date little if anything is known of the morphological features of metabolic disorders which might affect the early placenta. Indeed knowledge is only likely to be gained once villus sampling becomes an established procedure.

1.3 SUMMARY

The development of the villous system of the human placenta is associated with both growth and degeneration of villi. Even in those areas where there is

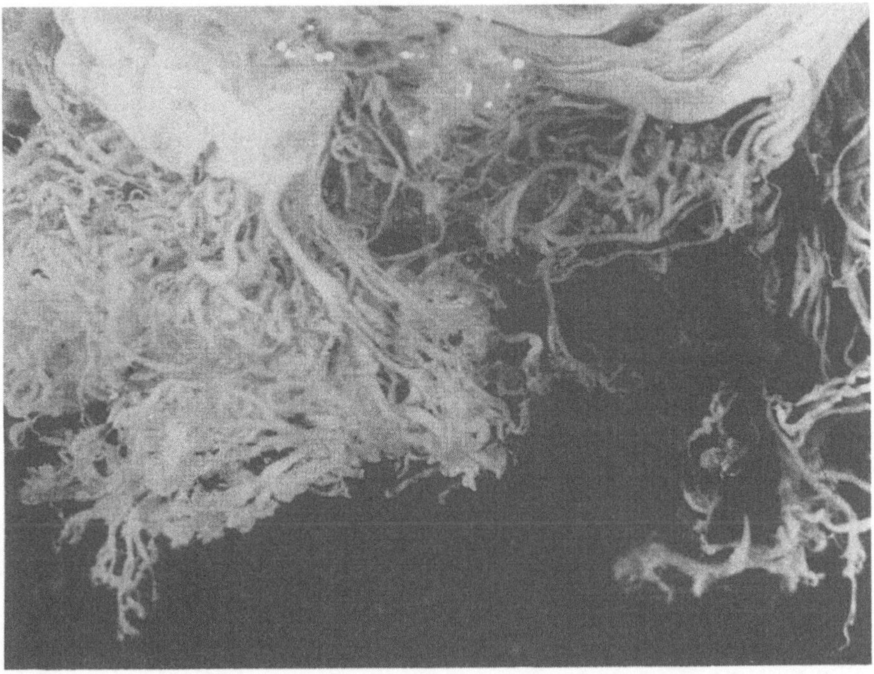

Figure 1.7 Villi from a macerated abortus with the typical stringy appearance associated with cessation of the fetal circulation (× 5).

active growth the morphology will be modified by age. It is therefore of paramount importance in interpreting the value of this relatively new technique to ascertain the quality of the villi that are obtained, as well as their quantity. The site of biopsy will probably greatly influence the success rate recorded. On a simplistic anatomical approach it would seem likely that villi from the centre of the placenta obtained via a transabdominal route will provide the best results. Whether or not the risk associated with this technique will be comparable to those of the transcervical approach remains to be evaluated.

It is, however, essential that the monitoring of these techniques takes into account not only the clinical methodology and chromosome constitution of pregnancies that fail subsequent to sampling, but also includes descriptions of the morphology of the conceptus, since at the gestation at which most chorion villus samples will be taken less than half of all spontaneous abortions will have a chromosomal abnormality. While the aetiology of the remainder remains obscure it should be remembered that the interrelationship between chromosomal and anatomical abnormalities of the fetus and the process of spontaneous abortion is by no means clear.

As well as providing an earlier method of prenatal diagnosis which may be

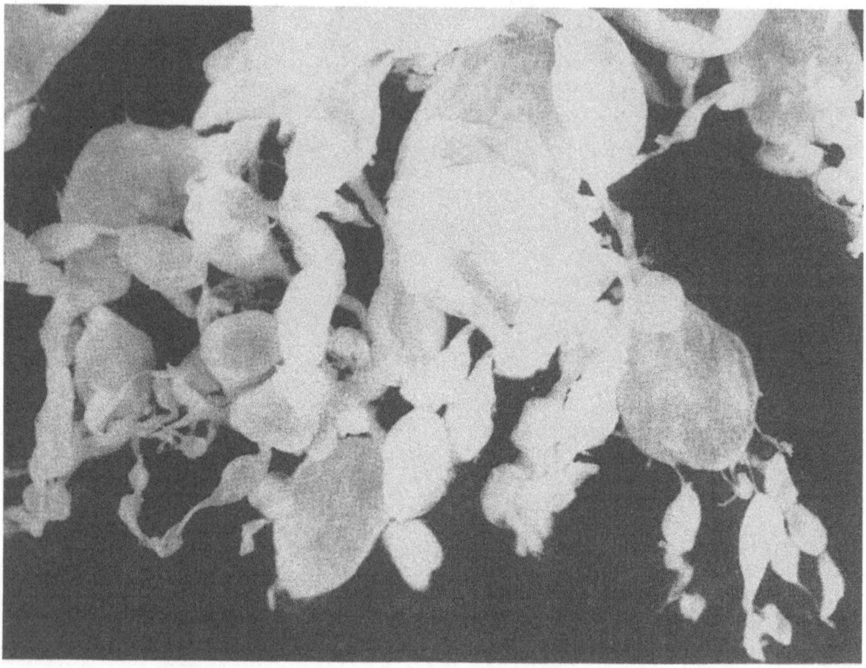

Figure 1.8 Villi from a triploid conceptus with partial molar degeneration. The irregular segmented appearance of the cystic villi is characteristic (× 5).

more acceptable to patients, chorion villus sampling may also provide an insight into one of the major routes by which the process of natural selection influences human reproduction.

REFERENCES

Aladjem, S. (1966) Perinatal evaluation and prognosis of the premature fetus and newborn infant through phase contrast microscopy of the placenta. *Am. J. Obstet. Gynaecol.*, **95**, 935–42.

Alvarez, H. (1964) Morphology and physiopathology of the human placenta. *Obstet. Gynaecol.*, **23**, 813–25.

Boyd, S. D. and Hamilton, W. J. (1970) *The Human Placenta*, W. Heffer and Sons, Cambridge. p. 79.

Cibils, L. A. (1968) Growth of the placental villi in the first trimester. *J. Reprod. Med.*, **1**, 377–87.

Dempsey, E. W. (1972) The development of capillaries in the villi of early human placentas. *Am. J. Anat.*, **134**, 221–38.

Gruenwald, P. (1975) Lobular architecture of primate placenta. In *The Placenta and its Maternal Supply Line. Effects of Insufficiency on the Fetus* (ed. P. Gruenwald), Medical and Technical Publishing, Lancaster. pp. 35–55.

Hertig, A. T. (1935) Angiogenesis in the early human chorion and in the primary placenta of the Macaque monkey. *Contributions to Embryology*, Carnegie Institute **25**, 37–81.

Hertig, A. T. and Rock, J. (1941) Two human ova of the pre-villous stage having an ovulation age of about eleven and twelve days respectively. *Contributions to Embryology*, Carnegie Institute **29**, 127–6.

Hook, E. B. (1978) Spontaneous deaths of fetuses with chromosomal abnormalities diagnosed prenatally. *New Eng. J. Med.*, **299**, 1036–8.

Miller, J. F., Williamson, E., Glue, J., Gordon, Y. B., Grudzinskas, J. G. and Sykes, A. (1980) Fetal loss after implantation. A prospective study. *Lancet*, **ii**, 554–6.

Robertson, W. B. (1976) Ulteroplacental vasculature. *J. Clin. Path.*, **29**. Supplement (Royal College of Pathologists), **10**, 9–17.

Robinson, H. P. (1975) Diagnosis of early pregnancy failure by sonar. *Br. J. Obstet. Gynaecol.*, **82**, 849–57.

Rushton, D. I. (1978) Simplified classification of spontaneous abortions. *J. Med. Genet.*, **15**, 1–9.

Rushton, D. I. (1984) The classification and mechanisms of spontaneous abortion. *Perspect. Pediatr. Path.*, **8**, 269–87.

Whittaker, P. G., Taylor, A. and Lind, T. (1983) Unsuspected pregnancy loss in healthy women. *Lancet*, **i**, 1126–7.

Wigglesworth, J. S. (1967) Vascular organisation of the human placenta. *Nature*, **216**, 1120–1.

Witschi, E. (1970) Teratogenic effects from overripeness of the egg. In *Congenital Malformations: Proceedings of the Third International Conference, Amsterdam* (eds F. C. Fraser and V. A. McKusick), Excerpta Medica, New York. pp. 157–69.

Wynn, R. M. (1975) Development and ultrastructural adaptions of the human placenta. *Euro. J. Gynaecol. Reprod. Biol.* **5**, 3–21.

2

Fine structure of chorionic tissue in health and disease

—— C. D. Ockleford ——

2.1 INTRODUCTION

Ultrastructural and cell biological methods allow a comparatively detailed picture of the cytoplasmic organization of chorionic tissue (Martin and Spicer, 1973; Clint *et al.*, 1979). However understanding of that organization is by no means complete (Sideri *et al.*, 1980; Jones and Ockleford, 1985). It is the purpose of this essay to briefly review the ultrastructure of the tissue, to indicate the progress of research on some remarkable organelles and to indicate a possible role for diagnostic ultrastructure in the analysis of chorion samples.

2.2 OBSERVATIONS

The first trimester chorionic vesicle is a layer bounded internally by the amnion and umbilical cord and externally by the decidual layers – the decidua basalis and the decidua capsularis. The chorionic tissue is 'fetal' in embryological origin. The epithelial cells, the cytotrophoblast and syncytiotrophoblast, form a continuous layer which covers a branching vascular connective tissue core. This arrangement is similar to that in the gut where the enterocyte epithelium invests the lamina propria which is the connective tissue core of the intestinal villus (Ockleford and Wakely, 1982). The epithelium in the first trimester consists of a basal lamina upon which a nearly continuous monolayer of cytotrophoblast cells lies. By term, this layer has been reduced in importance to only a few cells. These may be activated to repair injury (Clint *et al.*, 1979) or in cases of ischaemia (Fox and Jones, 1983) but otherwise are not as mitotically active as in the first trimester.

Overlying the cytotrophoblast cells is the unique feature of the tissue, the syncytiotrophoblast. By term, this is of the order of 10 m^2 in surface area (Aherne and Dunnill, 1966; Mayhew *et al.*, 1984). It is a true syncytium probably qualifying as the continuous cytoplasm with the largest surface area in the human body. The cytoplasm of the syncytium is obviously different in ultrastructural appearance from that of the cellular trophoblast despite the fact that it has been established that the syncytium derives from the underlying cytotrophoblast in development (Galton, 1962; Enders, 1965; Boyd and Hamilton, 1966). The cytotrophoblast has the morphology of a relatively uncommitted stem cell whereas the complexity of the syncytium results from the accumulation of organelles required for its multifunctional capacity as a 'lung', 'excretory organ', 'endocrine gland' and 'gut'.

The ultrastructural organization of the epithelium is indicated on the line diagram (Fig. 2.1) which has been adapted from a previous publication (Dearden and Ockleford, 1983). The syncytium encloses a variety of more or less ubiquitous organelles such as nuclei, mitochondria and lysosomes. In addition there are organelles related to more tissue-specific functions such as membrane-bounded granules involved in peptide hormone secretion (Sideri *et al.*, 1980) and non-membrane-bounded lipidic inclusions which are presumptive steroid hormone or its precursor (Wislocki and Dempsey, 1955). There are also microvilli which may be involved in uptake at the maternal oriented surface of the tissue (Ockleford and Clode, 1983), and vasculosyncytial membranes which are very thin dome-like regions thought to facilitate gas transport (Fox, 1978). Of the organellar components which are being characterized at present some deserve individual attention.

Coated vesicles which are micropinocytic vesicles (Fig. 2.2) are found as a rich population in the surface layers of the syncytiotrophoblast (Ockleford, 1976; Ockleford and Whyte, 1977; Ockleford *et al.*, 1977). They have so far been shown to take up transferrin, ferritin and IgG into the placenta by receptor mediated endocytosis (Chin-Tarng Lin, 1980; Ockleford and Clint, 1980; Booth and Wilson, 1981; King, 1982; Pearse, 1982) but may also be responsible for the uptake of other proteins and particles. They consist of a polygonal lattice of a structural protein called clathrin which invests the cytoplasmic surface of a phospholipid bilayer and a dense glycocalyx on its inner surface. The protein clathrin is thought to be present as a physiological subunit in the form of a trimer 'the triskelion' (Ungewickell and Branton, 1981). The specific receptors for the ligands mentioned above probably extend into the glycocalyx layer and become linked to clathrin to form a membrane complex (Ockleford, 1982; Fine and Ockleford, 1984). Extensive work on the IgG Fc receptor of syncytiotrophoblast has resulted in its characterization and isolation (Gitlin and Gitlin, 1976; McNabb *et al.*, 1976; Matre, 1977; Niezgodka *et al.*, 1980). Recent evidence (Dearden and Ockleford, 1982) indicates the possible involvement of a receptosome

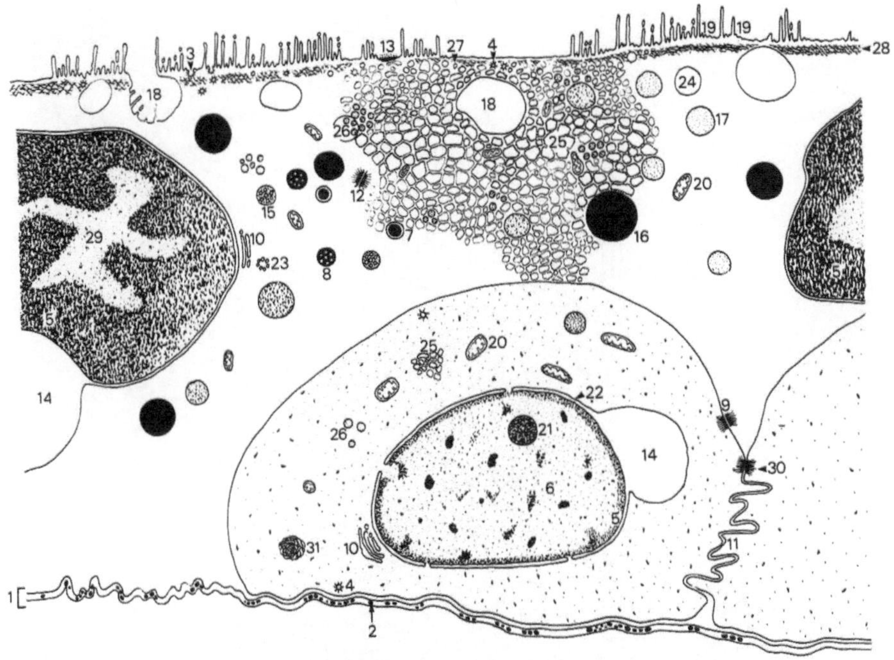

Figure 2.1 This schematic illustration indicates a portion of the trophoblastic epithelium which invests the chorionic villus tree.

Key

1. Basal lamina
2. Calcium containing granule
3. Coated pit
4. Coated micropinocytic vesicle
5. Condensed chromatin
6. Cytotrophoblast nucleus
7. Dense body
8. Dense multivesicular body
9. Desmosome
10. Golgi apparatus
11. Interdigitating microvilli
12. Intrasyncytial desmosome
13. Iron-binding organelle
14. Juxtanuclear vacuole
15. Light multivesicular body
16. Lipid droplet
17. Lysosome
18. Macropinocytic vesicle
19. Microvilli
20. Mitochondrion
21. Nucleolus
22. Nuclear envelope
23. Pre-multivesicular body
24. Receptosome-like organelle
25. Rough endoplasmic reticulum
26. Secretory granules
27. Smooth micropinocytic vesicle
28. Syncytioskeletal layer (microtubules, microfilaments and intermediate filaments)
29. Syncytiotrophoblast nuclei
30. Tonofilaments
31. Nematosome

(Modified after Figure 6 of Dearden and Ockleford, 1983.)

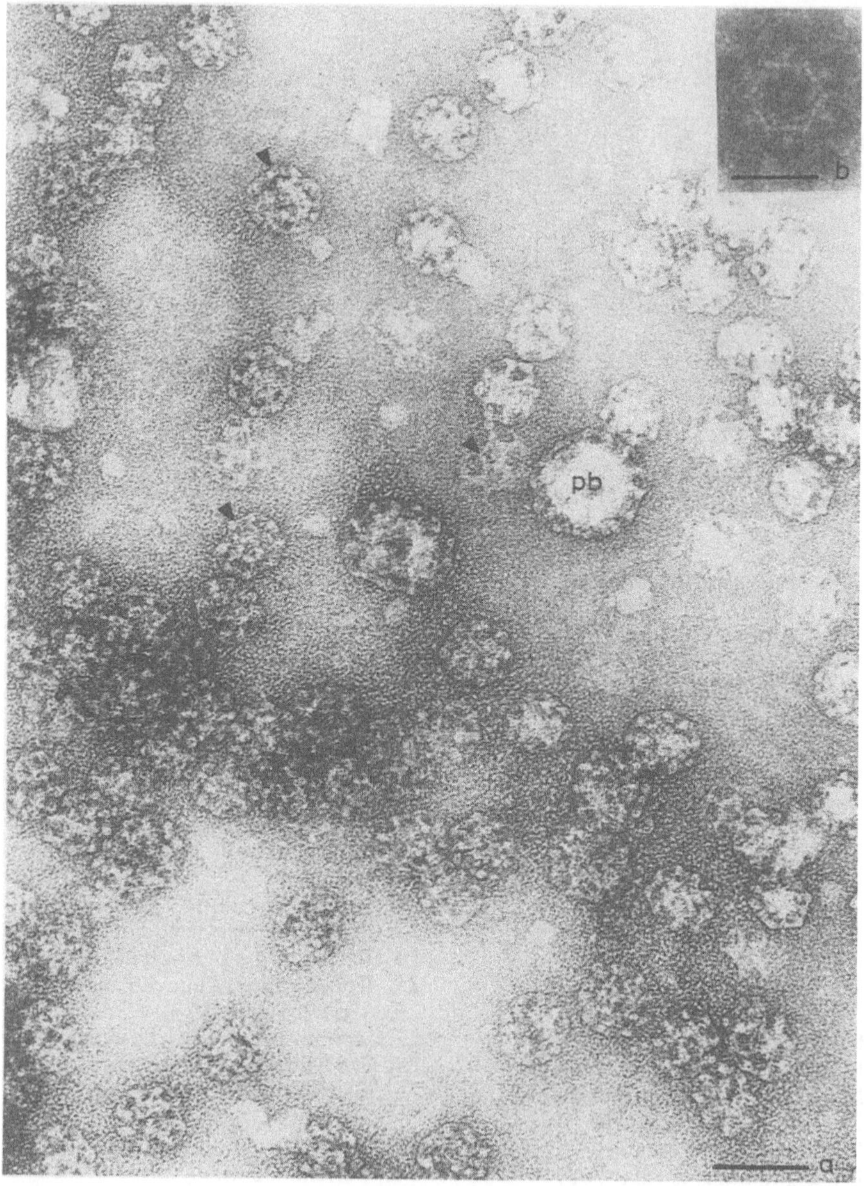

Figure 2.2 The electron micrograph (a) reveals a population of coated vesicles isolated from human placenta and negatively stained with 1% uranyl acetate. The polygonal lattice of clathrin (arrowheads) invests the cytoplasmic surface of the vesicles (pb). Such images can be reinforced to show hexagonal and pentagonal facets using the Markham rotation method as shown in the inset (b). (With permission from Dearden and Ockleford, 1983.) Scale = 75 nm.

(Willingham and Pastan, 1980) compartment which may receive the receptor-bound ligand from coated vesicles.

Polymeric proteins of the placenta appear to play an important role in defining the morphology of the villous tree. Arrays of f-actin, tubulin in the form of microtubules and intermediate filament proteins such as prekeratin and vimentin (Ockleford *et al.*, 1981) are disposed in the cytoplasm of trophoblast, mesenchymal and endothelial cells in such a way that they may provide or contribute to a structural basis for the high degree of anisometry in the tissue (Fig. 2.3). This work has led to the definition of a syncytioskeletal

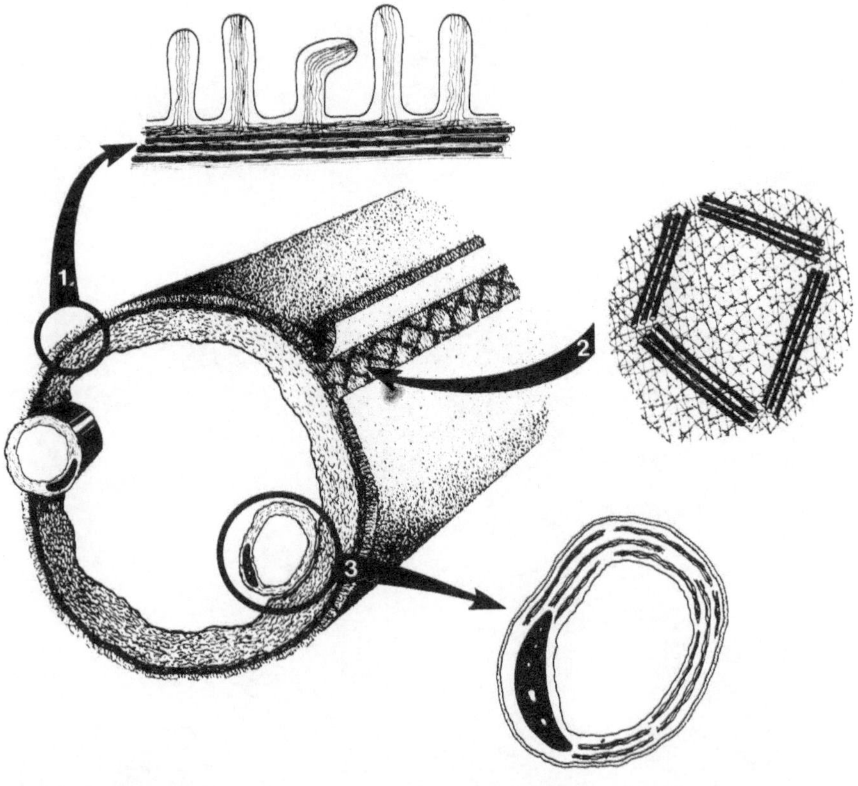

Figure 2.3 This illustration is reproduced from Ockleford, Wakely and Badley (1981) with permission of the copyright holders. It shows the positions where actin, tubulin, intermediate filament proteins and fibronectin are found in the chorionic villus. (1) A section through the syncytioskeletal layer reveals a mesh of f-actin part of which passes superficially into microvilli. (2) Is a plan view of the syncytioskeletal layer showing a more open arrangement of microtubules. (3) Is a transverse section through a fetal capillary. The wavy circumferential tresses in the cytoplasm of the endothelial cells represent intermediate filaments of vimentin. The outer layer of the capillary is the basal lamina which although thinner than the trophoblastic epithelial basal lamina shows greater anti-fibronectin fluorescence.

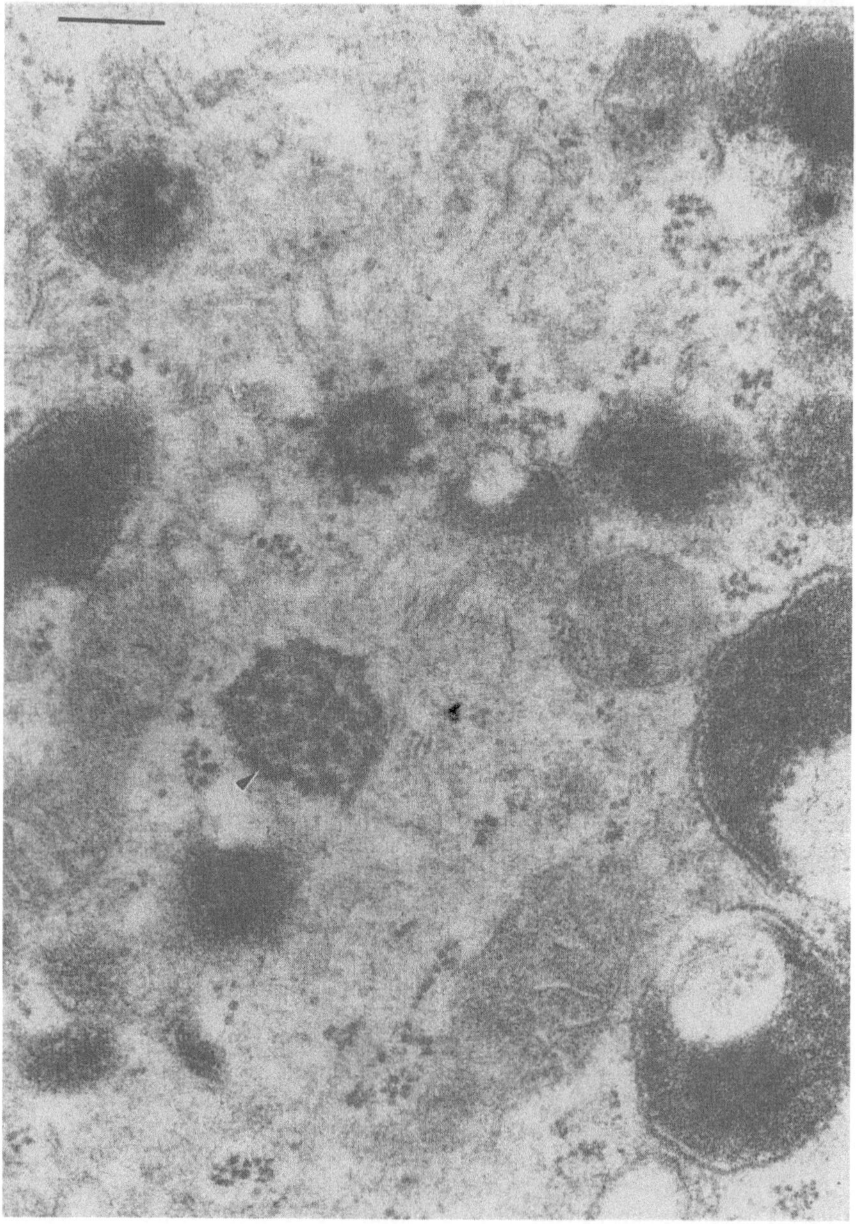

Figure 2.4 This transmission electron micrograph shows a portion of cytotrophoblast cytoplasm. Of particular interest is the nematosome (arrowhead). This organelle has recently been described in human placenta but its function is as yet undefined. The structure is a large cytoplasmic nucleolus-like organelle. Very similar

layer underlying the maternal-oriented syncytial surface analogous to the terminal web in cellular absorptive epithelia.

Most recently Jones and Ockleford (1985) have drawn attention to a relatively large organelle in the cytotrophoblast of the placenta. Up to 1.3 μm in diameter this organelle is probably present in several copies per term placental cytotrophoblast cell (Fig. 2.4). It is less common in the first trimester. At present its function is undefined. Suggestions so far put forward include the possibility that the organelle is a storage form of morphic or other forms of ribonucleoprotein.

2.3 DIAGNOSTIC POTENTIAL

Up to the present no extensive results of attempts to use diagnostic ultrastructural methods on chorion sampling have been published. There is, however, an extensive ultrastructural pathology literature relating to first trimester and term trophoblast tissue (e.g. Fox, 1978). There is no obvious reason why the techniques applied successfully for ultrastructural diagnosis of other organs' pathologies should not meet with the same success using early chorion.

Four interesting areas can be identified.

1. Diseases of the chorion.
2. Connective tissue disorders.
3. Infectious diseases.
4. Inborn errors of metabolism.

1 Diseases of chorion

Examples of diseases of chorion which may be detected using diagnostic ultrastructural methods include hydatidiform mole, invasive mole and choriocarcinoma. Both transmission, and scanning electron microscopy (Ockleford and Clode, 1983) can be useful in this context. The incidence of these diseases varies geographically being of greatest importance in certain far-eastern countries where, for example, hydatidiform mole is three times more common than it is in Britain (Elston, 1983).

2 Connective tissue disorders

The connective tissue core of the healthy first trimester chorionic villus examined ultrastructurally can be used to demonstrate the typical normal

---

organelles have been identified in oocytes, yolk sac, placental and neuronal cells in a variety of mammalian species. (Micrograph reproduced with permission from Jones and Ockleford, 1985.) The centriole with its nine-triplet microtubule organization is surrounded by nine satellite bodies. Scale = 400 nm.

extracellular matrix structures. These include the 64 nm period banding of collagen fibres. Conditions where ordered extracellular matrix structure is lost, for example lathyrism; dermatosparaxis; procollagen *N*-protease deficiency; lysyl hydroxylase deficiency; spondylo-epiphyseal dysplasia and scurvy (Byers *et al.*, 1978; Williams *et al.*, 1974; Bailey *et al.*, 1974; Levene *et al.*, 1977; Olsen, 1980) may be identified. These diseases with the possible exception of scurvy secondary to alcoholism are extremely rare in the West.

3 Infectious diseases

A number of infectious diseases contracted during the first trimester of pregnancy can have teratogenic effects on the developing fetus which are far more severe than their usual postnatal effects. Evidence that such agents have reached the conceptus may be obtained ultrastructurally by visualizing them. We have performed experiments which model this situation. We incubated *in vitro* trophoblast with particles of an attenuated strain of influenza and subsequently examined the tissue ultrastructurally and successfully to visualize the uptake of the particles into the syncytial cytoplasm (Keating and Ockleford, unpublished). Several organisms are of interest in this context. They include rubella, haemophilus, cytomegalovirus, treponema and toxoplasma.

4 Inborn errors of metabolism

Most potentially interesting is the final group of diseases. These are the inborn errors of metabolism known as the lysosomal storage diseases. Here obvious morphological pictures such as images of the Zebra bodies of Fabry's, Tay Sachs and Gaucher's disease are well recognized morphological markers for diagnostic ultrastructure. There are precedents for finding such markers in the trophoblasts of fetuses affected with gangliosidosis and mucolipidosis (Powell *et al.*, 1976; Lowden *et al.*, 1973) and there is one report of abnormally vacuolated placental tissue associated with hydrops fetalis as a result of Gaucher's disease (Ginsberg and Groll, 1973).

Several of these ultrastructural markers are better expressed in particular tissues and they all accumulate progressively with time. There is some evidence that accumulation of morphologically detectable inclusions typical of Gm1 Gangliosidosis is relatively fast in syncytiotrophoblast (Lowden *et al.*, 1973). Research is therefore needed on chorion sampling from a high-risk population of individuals to establish whether these structures can be demonstrated in the relevant setting as early as the eighth week of gestation. Similarly, research on metachromatic leukodystrophy, X-linked icthyosis, Pompes Type II glycogen storage disease, cystic fibrosis and Chediak–Higashi syndrome may yield potentially useful archetypal diagnostic images as a result of the possession of characteristic inclusions by affected cells.

Although these conditions are mostly rare, a population at relatively high risk may be identified via genetic counselling and further study is therefore indicated.

2.4 POTENTIAL ADVANTAGES OF DIAGNOSTIC ULTRASTRUCTURE OF CHORION SAMPLES

At a time where established and promising techniques of analysing chorion samples already include cell culture followed by cytogenetic analysis; cell culture followed by enzymology; direct analysis of chromosomes from whole villus squashes, and gene probing methods one is forced critically to analyse the potential usefulness of diagnostic ultrastructure in a competitive setting.

The potential advantages are as follows. First, it is expected to reduce the time required to obtain a result. The elapsed time may be as little as 24 hours to a result using modern rapid embedding methods. Secondly, biopsy size is important. The smaller the sample the less the risk to the normal development of an unaffected conceptus. Using Agar pre-embedding a single chorionic villus could be utilized. This sets the minimum useful sample size at approximately one-tenth of the 30–50 mg required for gene probing. Thirdly, the success rate is expected to be high. Methods which depend on cell culture are intrinsically more risky than those which do not because of the possibility of infection or poor growth of the culture.

Other considerations include the fact that although probably administered to establish or eliminate a specific diagnosis the ultrastructural analysis could reveal further unexpected risk. For example a sample taken to assess the likelihood of an inborn error of metabolism may incidentally reveal the presence of an infectious pathogen. Thus the results may not be inherently restricted to a single observation such as the presence or absence of a particular gene sequence.

2.5 CONCLUSION

The possible clinical advantage to be gained from diagnostic ultrastructural study of chorion villus sampling has been indicated. Further research is needed to examine the physiology and pathology of the tissue, particularly placental organelles to explore opportunities for additional diagnostic potential.

ACKNOWLEDGEMENTS

Part of this work was supported by the Medical Research Council. Thanks are due to Professor J. MacVicar and the obstetricians and gynaecologists of the Leicester Royal Infirmary for clinical co-ordination.

REFERENCES

Aherne, W. and Dunnill, M. S. (1966) Quantitative aspects of placental structure. *J. Path. Bact.*, **91**, 123–39.

Bailey, A. J., Robins, S. P. and Baltan, G. (1974) Biological significance of the intermolecular crosslinks of collagen. *Nature*, **251**, 105–9.

Byers, P. H., Holbrook, K. A., Hall, J. G., Bornstein, P. and Chandler, J. W. (1978) A new variety of spondyloepiphyseal dysplasia characterised by punctate corneal dystrophe and abnormal dermal collagen fibrils. *Hum. Gen.*, **40**, 157–69.

Booth, A. G. and Wilson, M. J. (1981) Human placental coated vesicles contain receptor bound transferrin. *Biochem. J.*, **196**, 355–62.

Boyd, J. D. and Hamilton, W. J. (1966) Electron microscopic observations on the cytotrophoblast contribution to the syncytium in the human placenta. *J. Anat.*, **100**, 535–48.

Chin-Tarng Lin (1980) Immunoelectron microscopic localisation of Immunoglobulin G in human placenta. *J. Histochem. Cytochem.*, **28**, 339–47.

Clint, J. M., Wakely, J. and Ockleford, C. D. (1979) Differentiated regions of human placental cell surface associated with attachment of chorionic villi, phagocytosis of maternal erythrocytes and syncytiotrophoblast repair. *Proceedings of the Royal Society* (B), **204**, 345–53.

Dearden, L. and Ockleford, C. D. (1982) Autoradiographic study of IgG transport in the human placenta. *J. Anat.*, **135**, 850.

Dearden, L. and Ockleford, C. D. (1983) Structure of human trophoblast, correlation with function. In *Biology of Trophoblast* (eds Y. W. Loke and A. Whyte), North Holland, Amsterdam. pp. 69–109.

Elston, C. W. (1983) Development and structure of trophoblastic neoplasms. In *Biology of Trophoblast* (eds Y. W. Loke and A. Whyte), North Holland, Amsterdam. pp. 188–232.

Enders, A. C. (1965) Amsterdam. A comparative study of the fine structure trophoblast in several haemochorial placentae. *Am. J. Anat.*, **116**, 29–67.

Fine, R. and Ockleford, C. D. (1984) The supramolecular cytology of coated vesicles. *Int. Rev. Cytol.*, **91**, 1–43.

Fox, H. (1978) Pathology of the Placenta. In *Major Problems in Pathology*, vol. VII (ed. J. L. Bennington), W. B. Saunders, London. pp. 1–491.

Fox, H. and Jones, C. J. P. (1983) Pathology of trophoblast. In *Biology of Trophoblast* (eds Y. W. Loke and A. Whyte), North Holland, Amsterdam. pp. 137–85.

Galton, M. (1962) DNA content of placental nuclei. *J. Cell Biol.*, **13**, 183–203.

Ginsberg, S. J. and Groll, M. (1973) Hydrops fetalis due to infantile Gaucher's disease. *J. Pediat.*, **82**, 1046–8.

Gitlin, J. D. and Gitlin, D. (1976) Protein binding by cell membranes and the selective transfer of proteins from mother to young across tissue barriers. In *Maternofetal Transmission of Immunoglobulins* (ed. W. A. Hemmings), Cambridge University Press, Cambridge. pp. 113–23.

Jones, C. J. P. and Ockleford, C. D. (1985) Nematosomes in the human placenta. *Placenta*, **6**, 355–61.

King, B. F. (1982) Absorption of Peroxidase-conjugated immunoglobulin G by Human Placenta: an *in vitro* study. *Placenta*, **3**, 395–406.

Levene, C. I., Ockleford, C. D. and Barber, C. L. (1977) Scurvy; a comparison between ultrastructural and biochemical changes observed in cultured fibroblasts and the collagen they synthesise. *Virchows Arch. B. Cell Path.*, **23**, 325–38.

Loke, Y. W. (1978) *Immunology and Immunopathology of the Human Foetal-*

maternal Interaction, Elsevier/North Holland, Amsterdam and London. pp. 1–328.

Lowden, J. A., Cruz, E., Conen, P. E., Rudd, N. and Doran, T. A. (1973) Prenatal diagnosis of Gm1-gangliosidosis. *New Eng. J. Med.*, **288**, 225–8.

Mayhew, T. M., Joy, C. F. and Haas, J. D. (1984) Structure function correlation in the human placenta: the morphometric diffusing capacity for oxygen at full term. *J. Anat.*, **139**, 691–708.

Martin, B. J. and Spicer, S. S. (1973) Ultrastructural features of cellular maturation and ageing in human trophoblast. *J. Ultrastr. Res.*, **43**, 133–49.

Matre, R. (1977) Similarities of Fc receptors on trophoblasts and placental endothelial cells. *Scand. J. Immunol.*, **6**, 953–8.

McNabb, T., Koh, T. Y., Dorrington, K. J. and Painter, R. H. (1976) Structure and function of immunoglobulin domains V. Binding of immunoglobulin G and fragments to placental membrane preparations. *J. Immunol.*, **117**, 882–8.

Niezgodka, M., Mikulska, J., Ugorski, M., Boratynski, J. and Lisowski, J. (1980) Human placental membrane receptor for IgG-1. Studies on the properties and solubilisation of the receptor. *Molec. Immunol.*, **18**, 163–72.

Olsen, B. R. (1980) Inherited disorders of collagen metabolism. In *The Biology of Collagen* (eds A. Viidik, J. Vuust), Academic Press, New York and London. pp. 153–73.

Ockleford, C. D. (1976) A three dimensional reconstruction of the polygonal pattern on placental coated vesicle membranes. *J. Cell Sci.*, **21**, 83–91.

Ockleford, C. D. and Clode, A. (1983) Microgibbosities in hydatidiform mole. *J. Pathol.*, **141**, 181–9.

Ockleford, C. D. and Wakely, J. (1982) The skeleton of the placenta. In *Progress in Anatomy*, vol. 2 (eds R. J. Harrison, V. Navaratnam), Cambridge University Press. pp. 19–47.

Ockleford, C. D. and Whyte, A. (1977) Differentiated regions of human placental cell surface associated with the exchange of materials between material and foetal blood. The structure, distribution, ultrastructural cytochemistry and biochemical composition of coated vesicles. *J. Cell Sci.*, **25**, 293–312.

Ockleford, C. D., Whyte, A. and Bowyer, D. E. (1977) Variation in the volume of coated vesicles isolated from human placenta. *Cell Biol. Int. Rep.* **1**, 2, 137–46.

Ockleford, C. D. and Clint, J. M. (1980) The uptake of IgG by human placental chorionic villi: a correlated autoradiographic and wide aperture counting study. *Placenta*, **1**, 91–111.

Ockleford, C. D., Wakely, J. and Badley, R. A. (1981) Morphogenesis of human placental chorionic villi: cytoskeletal, syncytioskeletal and extracellular matrix proteins. *Proceedings of the Royal Society* (Series B), **212**, 305–16.

Ockleford, C. D. (1982) Coated Vesicles in Electron microscopy of Proteins (ed. R. Harris), Academic Press, New York and London. pp. 255–99.

Powell, H. C., Benirschke, K., Favara, B. E. and Pflueger, O. H., Jr. (1976) Foamy changes of placental cells in fetal storage disorders. *Virchows Arch. A.*, **369**, 191–6.

Pearse, B. M. F. (1982) Coated vesicles from human placenta carry ferritin, transferrin and immunoglobulin G. *Proceedings of the National Academy of Sciences of USA*, 79, pp. 451–5.

Sideri, M., Fumagalli, G., De Virgiliis, G. and Remotti, G. (1980) The morphological basis of placental endocrine activity. In *The Human Placenta*, Serono Symposium 35 (eds A. Klopper, A. Genazzani and P. G. Crosignani), Academic Press, London. pp. 339–46.

Ungewickell, E. and Branton, D. (1981) Assembly units of clathrin coats. *Nature*, **289**, 420–2.
Williams, B. R., Cranley, R. E., Doty, S. B., Lichtenstein, J. R. and McKusick, V. A. (1974) Disorganization of collagen in individuals with procollagen peptidase deficiency (Ehlers-Danlos type VII). *Isr. J. Med. Sci.*, **10**, 1470.
Willingham, M. C. and Pastan, I. (1980) The receptosome an intermediate organelle of receptor-mediated endocytosis in cultured fibroblasts. *Cell*, **21**, 67–77.
Wislocki, G. B. and Dempsey, (1955) Electron microscopy of the human placenta. *Anat. Rec.*, **123**, 133–49.

3

The enzymology of chorionic villi and the first trimester diagnosis of metabolic disorders

A. H. Fensom

3.1 INTRODUCTION

The advantage of prenatal diagnosis of genetic metabolic disorders during the first 8–11 weeks of pregnancy using chorionic villi rather than at 18 weeks or later using cultured amniotic cells is so great that it is not surprising that many laboratories are now engaged in assessing the normal metabolic activities of chorionic villi. Indeed, in the short time since Kazy *et al.* (1982) first reported the presence of lysosomal enzymes in normal villi, diagnostic studies have been carried out in pregnancies at risk for several different diseases and some affected fetuses correctly detected. These diseases are almost all recessive conditions with a 25% risk of recurrence and comprise one of the highest risk groups for which second-trimester diagnosis is currently carried out. About 60 diseases have been diagnosed *in utero* in the second trimester and techniques exist for almost as many more (for review, see Benson and Fensom, 1985). It seems likely that most of these conditions will prove amenable to first trimester diagnosis although the specific techniques which are required for each disease and which have been developed for use with amniocytes need to be evaluated carefully before application to villi. The effect of gestational age on enzyme activities in normal villi over the whole diagnostic period must be studied and consideration must be given to the fact that the disease-specific enzyme assays developed for amniotic cells may lack this specificity when applied to villi, particularly when artificial substrates are employed. In the development of methods for second-trimester diagnosis, enzymatic properties of cultured fibroblasts from affected patients and their parents have been compared with those of normal amniotic cells, and this has been invaluable for optimizing the discrimination between affected, heterozygous and normal genotypes. Unfortunately, no exactly analogous postnatal equivalent to cultured fibroblasts from affected patients exists for comparison with normal villi, and the applicability of the assays for first trimester diagnosis will only be proven by carrying out test diagnoses in at-risk pregnancies. It is essential, therefore, that a confirmatory amniocentesis is carried out to verify a normal result while methods are being developed. Already some errors have occurred where affected fetuses were missed after analysis of villi and diagnosed at amniocentesis (Young and Patrick, 1983; Fensom *et al.*, 1984a; Simoni *et al.*, 1984; Fowler and Cooper, 1984), and while maternal contamination was probably responsible for some of these errors the possibility of non-optimal enzymology should also be considered. In addition to carrying out confirmatory amniocentesis the division of villus sample for direct assay, and assay after tissue culture, would appear to be prudent. In a pregnancy at risk for argininosuccinic aciduria, analysis of cultured villi allowed diagnosis of an affected fetus which was missed by direct assay of villi (Vimal *et al.*, 1984; see also below).

At the time of writing published data on the detailed properties of enzymes in chorionic villi or cultured villous cells are still scarce. The aim of the present chapter therefore is to give an indication of the enzymes which have been shown to be present in normal villi or cultured villi and to review the test diagnoses reported in the literature. Presentation is in terms of the related metabolic disorders rather than individual enzymes.

3.2 LYSOSOMAL STORAGE DISORDERS

The majority of prenatal diagnostic investigations for metabolic diseases are for lysosomal storage disorders, and the earliest studies of enzymes in chorionic villi were of lysosomal hydrolases. Kazy *et al.* (1982) assayed eight enzymes in villi and reported activity to be similar to that in amniotic cells. Later studies (Simoni *et al.*, 1983, 1984; Fensom *et al.*, 1984b; Poenaru *et al.*, 1984a) extended these findings and now most enzymes associated with lysosomal storage disorders have been found to be active in villi (Table 3.1).

3.2.1 Lipid disorders

The first indication that prenatal diagnosis of Tay–Sachs disease should be possible using chorionic villi was the report of Grebner *et al.* (1983). These workers found that hexosaminidase A (hex A) was deficient in homogenates of villi collected at sixteen weeks' gestation from a pregnancy where the fetus was found at amniocentesis to be affected with Tay–Sachs disease. More

Table 3.1 Lysosomal storage disorders where activity of the associated enzyme has been demonstrated in normal chorionic villi

Disorder	*Enzyme*	*References*
Lipid disorders		
GM_2-gangliosidosis type 1 (Tay-Sachs disease)*†	Hexosaminidase A	Pergament *et al.*, 1983 Grebner *et al.*, 1983† Simoni *et al.*, 1983 Fensom *et al.*, 1984b Grabowski *et al.*, 1984* Besançon *et al.*, 1984*
GM_2-gangliosidosis type 2 (Sandhoff's disease)†	Hexosaminidase A + B	Kazy *et al.*, 1982 Simoni *et al.*, 1983 Fensom *et al.*, 1984b Poenaru *et al.*, 1984a†
GM_1-gangliosidosis	β-galactosidase	Kazy *et al.*, 1982 Simoni *et al.*, 1983 Fensom *et al.*, 1984b Poenaru *et al.*, 1984a
Fabry's disease	α-galactosidase A	Fensom *et al.*, 1984b Poenaru *et al.*, 1984a
Farber's disease	Ceramidase	Fensom *et al.*, 1984b
Gaucher's disease	β-glucosidase	Kazy *et al.*, 1982 Fensom *et al.*, 1984b Poenaru *et al.*, 1984a
Niemann–Pick disease	Sphingomyelinase	Kazy *et al.*, 1982 Simoni *et al.*, 1983 Fensom *et al.*, 1984b
Krabbe's disease*	Galactocerebrosidase	Fensom *et al.*, 1984b Kleijer *et al.*, 1984a*
Metachromatic leucodystrophy†	Arylsulphatase A	Kazy *et al.*, 1982 Tsvetkova *et al.*, 1983 Simoni *et al.*, 1983 Fensom *et al.*, 1984a, b Poenaru *et al.*, 1984a
Wolman's disease	Acid esterase	Fensom *et al.*, 1984b
Mucopolysaccharidoses and related disorders		
Hurler's and Scheie's diseases	α-iduronidase	Simoni *et al.*, 1984 Fensom *et al.*, 1984b Poenaru *et al.*, 1984a
Hunter's disease*	Iduronate sulphatase	Lykkelund *et al.*, 1983 Kleijer *et al.*, 1984b* Upadhyaya *et al.*, 1984 Fensom *et al.*, 1984b

Table 3.1 continued

Disorder	*Enzyme*	*References*
Sanfilippo disease A	Heparan sulphamidase	Fensom *et al.*, 1984b Patrick *et al.*, 1984
Sanfilippo disease B	α-*N*-acetyl-glucosaminidase	Marsh & Fensom 1985
Sanfilippo disease C	Acetyl CoA: α-Glucosaminide *N*-acetyl transferase	Fensom *et al.*, 1984b
Morquio's disease	*N*-acetylgalacto-samine 6-sulphate sulphatase	Yuen & Fensom 1985
Maroteaux–Lamy disease	Arylsulphatase B	Fensom *et al.*, 1984b Poenaru *et al.*, 1984a
Sly's disease	β-glucuronidase	Kazy *et al.*, 1982 Simoni *et al.*, 1983 Fensom *et al.*, 1984b Poenaru *et al.*, 1984a
Mannosidosis	α-mannosidase	Fensom *et al.*, 1984b Poenaru *et al.*, 1984a
Fucosidosis	α-fucosidase	Kazy *et al.*, 1982 Fensom *et al.*, 1984b Poenaru *et al.*, 1984a Beyer & Wiederschain, 1984
Sialidosis	Neuraminidase	Simoni *et al.*, 1983
I-cell disease*	Multiple lysosomal enzymes (see text)	Poenaru *et al.*, 1984b*
Multiple sulphatase deficiency*	Multiple sulphatases	Patrick *et al.*, 1984*
Glycogen storage disorder		
Pompe's disease†	Acid α-glucosidase	Fensom *et al.*, 1984b Poenaru *et al.*, 1984a†

* Indicates an affected fetus had been diagnosed by assay of villi from an at-risk pregnancy.
† Indicates an enzyme deficiency has been demonstrated in villi obtained after termination of an affected fetus which was detected by amniocentesis.

recently, Grabowski *et al.* (1984) reported the actual diagnosis of two affected fetuses by analysis of chorionic villi taken from two at-risk mothers at 9 and 11 weeks' gestation, respectively. This was a very comprehensive study and the authors demonstrated deficient hex A activity in the supernatant fraction from disrupted villi by several methods: the heat-inactivation assay; DEAE-cellulose chromatography; cellulose acetate electrophoresis; and direct assay using two new substrates specific for hex A, 4-methylumbelliferyl-β-D-*N*-acetylglucosamine 6-sulphate and 4-methylumbelliferyl-β-D-*N*-acetylgalactosamine 6-sulphate. Both pregnancies were terminated by cervical dilatation and fetal extraction and the diagnoses confirmed by the finding of absent hex A activity in brain tissue and abnormal inclusions in neurones. The availability of Tay–Sachs villi enabled the authors to study the effects of time and temperature of incubation on the heat-inactivation assay and thus to optimize conditions for inactivation of hex A with minimal loss of hex B. They were also able to assess the amount of decidua or maternal blood which could lead to detectable hex A activity in affected villi. This study indicated that as little as 20–40 μg of decidua per mg of affected villi could cause appearance of hex A after cellulose acetate electrophoresis, possibly leading to misdiagnosis. The assay was less sensitive to contamination with plasma, requiring 50–100 μl per mg of villi for visualization of hex A.

Poenaru *et al.* (1984a) found low total hexosaminidase (3.8% of normal mean) in trophoblasts from a placenta obtained after abortion of a fetus affected with Sandhoff's disease, so it seems highly likely that first trimester diagnosis of this form of GM_2-gangliosidosis is also possible. We have monitored one pregnancy at risk for Sandhoff's disease by assaying total and heat-labile hexosaminidase in villi collected at ten weeks' gestation (Fensom *et al.*, 1984b). The total activity was within the normal range but the heat-labile component (84% of total) was high indicating a heterozygous fetus and this was confirmed at amniocentesis and in the new-born child.

The presence of α- and β-galactosidase in normal villi (Table 3.1) makes it likely that Fabry's disease and GM_1-gangliosidosis can be detected by direct assay, but Grabowski *et al.* (1984) have noted that β-galactosidase is particularly active in normal decidua indicating the possibility of misdiagnosis of GM_1-gangliosidosis if only a small degree of contamination of the villi occurs. Danesino (1983) tested β-galactosidase activity in villi at different gestational ages (6–12 weeks) but found no correlation between activity and increasing gestation.

β-glucosidase activity has been shown to be present in normal villi when assayed with an artificial substrate (Kazy *et al.*, 1982; Fensom *et al.*, 1984b; Poenaru *et al.*, 1984a) but it remains to be seen whether Gaucher's disease can be detected by this assay since artificial substrates are not suitable with some tissues for diagnosis of this condition. Unfortunately, techniques for carrying out this assay with a natural substrate are available in only a few laboratories. Enzymatic diagnosis of Farber's, Krabbe's and Niemann–Pick diseases is normally performed with labelled natural substrates and less diagnostic problems with villi might be expected for these disorders than for Gaucher's disease. Indeed, Kleijer *et al.* (1984a) have reported successful first trimester diagnosis of Krabbe's disease by direct assay of galactocerebrosidase in villi. A pregnancy at risk for Farber's disease was monitored by assay of ceramidase in cultured chorionic villi with prediction of an unaffected fetus (Dr H. W. Moser, personal communication).

At the time of writing the author is not aware of a detailed report on the diagnosis of metachromatic leucodystrophy by demonstration of deficient arylsulphatase A (ASA) activity in villi although Mikkelsen *et al.* (1984) indicate that an affected fetus has been detected. Poenaru *et al.* (1984a) found low activity in trophoblasts collected from placenta after abortion of an affected fetus and demonstrated absence of ASA by cellulose acetate electrophoresis. Tsvetkova *et al.* (1983) excluded the disease in two successive pregnancies in the same mother by demonstrating normal ASA activity in villi collected at eight weeks' gestation. An affected fetus was misdiagnosed as heterozygous in our laboratory after demonstration of low but not markedly deficient ASA activity in villi collected at twelve weeks' gestation (Fensom *et al.*, 1984a, b). Although it was not possible to exclude maternal contamination of the villi as the source of this error, further studies of the properties of ASA in normal villi (Sanguinetti *et al.*, 1986) have indicated that conventional assays for this enzyme using nitrocatechol sulphate as substrate may give rise to an overestimate of activity and subsequent misdiagnosis

3.2.2 Mucopolysaccharidoses and related disorders

Activity of α-iduronidase, the enzyme deficient in Hurler's disease, is low in normal villi but increases after tissue culture to levels comparable with those in amniotic cells (Fensom *et al.*, 1984a,b; Poenaru *et al.*, 1984a, 1985). Thus in our laboratory the normal range in fresh villi was 6.62 to 32.5, mean 14.6 nmol/h/mg protein (units), while after tissue culture the range was 59.5 to 354, with a mean of 154 units. The low activity in fresh tissue could perhaps lead to diagnostic uncertainties when monitoring pregnancies at risk for Hurler's disease, particularly in distinguishing an affected fetus from one that is heterozygous, and division of the sample for direct assay and tissue culture would certainly appear advisable for obtaining additional data.

Three errors in first trimester diagnosis of Hurler's disease have been documented (Young and Patrick, 1983; Simoni *et al.*, 1984; Fowler and Cooper, 1984). In each case the fetus was diagnosed as unaffected by direct assay of villi but was found to be affected at amniocentesis. The cause of the errors seems likely to have been maternal contamination in two instances (Young and Patrick, 1983; Fowler and Cooper, 1984) and an unidentified technical error in the third (Brambati *et al.*, 1985). Fowler and Cooper (1984) noted much higher α-iduronidase activity in contaminating material than in villi, again underlining the potential difficulties in first trimester diagnosis of this disease.

The feasibility of prenatal diagnosis of Hunter's disease using villi was demonstrated by Lykkelund *et al.* (1983) who found low iduronate sulphatase activity (5% of simultaneously-tested control) in extracts of villi obtained in the ninth week of pregnancy from an obligatory heterozygote for this X-linked mucopolysaccharidosis. The villi used in this study were separated from the aspirated material obtained after termination of pregnancy, which the patient had requested without prior diagnosis. Subsequent studies on cultured fibroblasts from the fetus confirmed that it was affected. Prenatal diagnosis was later reported by Kleijer *et al.* (1984b) on the basis of deficient iduronate sulphatase activity and 46XY karyotype in villi obtained at nine weeks' gestation from an obligatory heterozygote. The diagnosis was confirmed after termination of pregnancy by analysis of fetal organs, cultured fetal fibroblasts and cultured villous cells. It was of interest that the authors noted a low but significant iduronate sulphatase activity in the test villi and in villi obtained after abortion whereas the fetal tissues and both types of cultured cells showed virtually no activity. They speculated that this could indicate the presence of either a small amount of iduronate sulphatase of maternal origin in the villi or of a non-specific sulphatase which was absent in the other tissues.

A pregnancy at risk for Sanfilippo A disease was monitored in our laboratory by direct assay of heparan sulphamidase in villi with prediction of an unaffected, probably heterozygous, fetus (Marsh and Fensom, unpublished). Patrick *et al.* (1984) also found this enzyme to be present in normal villi but Gustavi *et al.* (1984) were unable to detect activity in chorionic tissue obtained from vacuum aspirated placentae.

Assays employing the 4-methylumbelliferyl substrate for α-*N*-acetylglucosaminidase are more sensitive than those employing colorimetric substrates and should have particular application in first trimester diagnosis of Sanfilippo B disease (Marsh and Fensom, 1985).

Activity of *N*-acetylgalactosamine 6-sulphate sulphatase, the enzyme deficient in classical Morquio's disease, is detectable in villi although the specific activity is lower than in amniotic cells (Yuen and Fensom, 1985). First trimester diagnosis is probably feasible by direct assay although division of the sample for culture is advisable for confirmatory studies in view of the higher specific activity of the enzyme in cultured cells.

In contrast to most lysosomal enzymes, the specific activity of α-fucosidase is lower in cultured villi than uncultured (Fensom *et al.*, 1984b; Poenaru *et al.*, 1984a, 1985). Beyer and Wiederschain (1984) have studied the isoenzymes of α-fucosidase in villi using isoelectric focusing and have found a similar pattern to those in fetal liver, kidney and lung.

I-cell disease (mucolipidosis II) is a disorder characterized by increased activity of many lysosomal enzymes in serum and decreased intracellular activity of some of them. The basic enzymatic deficiency is of *N*-acetylglucosamine phosphotransferase which leads to a lack of phosphomannosyl recognition markers on lysosomal enzymes. For first trimester prenatal studies the least equivocal diagnosis could probably be made by demonstrating phosphotransferase deficiency in villi, but this assay is available in very few laboratories. It is of particular interest therefore that Poenaru *et al.* (1984b) established correct diagnosis of two affected fetuses in different mothers at risk by demonstrating deficient lysosomal enzyme activities in villi, most notably a β-galactosidase deficiency. Nine enzymes were assayed in homogenates of villi sampled at nine and ten weeks' gestation, respectively. There was a marked deficiency of β-galactosidase (9% and 15% of normal mean) and partial deficiency of β-glucuronidase (18% and 26%), α-fucosidase (25% and 41%) and α-mannosidase (21% and 33%). β-glucosidase, β-glucosaminidase and arylsulphatases A and B activities were normal or high despite marked deficiency of the last three enzymes in fibroblasts from one of the index cases (values for fibroblasts from the other index case were not reported). The authors considered that both fetuses were affected in view of previously made observations that lysosomal enzyme deficiency in I-cell disease is limited to β-galactosidase deficiency in some other tissues, most notably liver (Leroy *et al.* 1972). Both pregnancies were terminated and the diagnoses confirmed by demonstration of β-galactosidase deficiency in fetal tissues and a typical pattern of multiple enzyme deficiency, including β-glucosaminidase and arylsulphatases A and B, in cultured fetal fibroblasts and cultured villous cells. It was concluded that although two correct diagnoses had been made by direct assay of villi some villi should also be cultured for this test in order to provide back-up studies, particularly in view of the more complete lysosomal enzyme deficiency expressed in cultured cells. Enzyme activity in fibroblasts from the index case should always be studied to exclude the possibility of an atypical case.

Multiple sulphatase deficiency is a disorder of unknown basic defect characterized by low activity of several sulphatases in tissues, leucocytes and cultured fibroblasts (for review see Benson and Fensom, 1985). First trimester diagnosis of an affected fetus was reported by Patrick *et al.* (1984) who demonstrated markedly deficient heparan sulphamidase and undetectable arylsulphatase A activity directly in villi. Since the expression of sulphatase deficiency in different patients with this disease is very variable, cultured cells from the index case should always be studied before attempting prenatal diagnosis in order to ascertain the most appropriate sulphatases to assay.

3.2.3 Lysosomal glycogen storage disease

The diagnosis of Pompe's disease using the sensitive 4-methylumbelliferyl substrate for assay of acid α-glucosidase is complicated by the presence of a neutral α-glucosidase in some tissues which obscures deficiency of the acid enzyme. We have studied the pH profile of α-glucosidase towards this substrate in villi and cultured villi (unpublished observations) and found both acid and neutral enzyme activity to be present. The acid enzyme showed optimal activity in the range pH 3–4 in villi and pH 4.0–4.5 in the cultured cells. It was strongly inhibited in the presence of turanose, an inhibitor of lysosomal α-glucosidase, whereas the neutral enzyme was not affected. These studies indicate that although a neutral enzyme is present in villous material its activity should not obscure that of the acid enzyme and that diagnosis of Pompe's disease should be possible using the simple fluorometric substrate. Poenaru *et al.* (1984a) have demonstrated acid α-glucosidase deficiency towards this substrate in villi obtained after abortion of an affected fetus which was detected following amniocentesis.

3.3 OTHER METABOLIC DISORDERS

A number of approaches to first trimester diagnosis of other metabolic disorders have been examined, in addition to enzymatic analysis of villi or cultured villi. These have included measurement of uptake of (^{35}S)-cystine by intact villi for detection of cystinosis, or of incorporation of label from (^{14}C)-citrulline into protein in villi for detection of citrullinaemia or argininosuccinic aciduria, and measurement of the long chain fatty acid content of villi for diagnosis of Zellweger syndrome. Disorders for which such diagnostic methods, or associated enzymology, have been reported are summarised in Table 3.2.

Table 3.2 Other metabolic disorders where activity of the associated enzyme or test parameter has been demonstrated in normal chorionic villi or cultured villi

Disorder	*Enzyme or test parameter*	*References*
Amino-acid and related disorders		
Homocystinuria	Cystathionine β-synthase (see text)	Benson *et al.*, 1983 Fensom *et al.*, 1984b Fowler & Cooper, 1984
Citrullinaemia*	[14C]-citrulline incorporation into protein	Kleijer *et al.*, 1983c*
Argininosuccinic aciduria†	[14C]-citrulline incorporation into protein	Vimal *et al.*, 1984†

Table 3.2 continued

Disorder	Enzyme or test parameter	References
Maple syrup urine disease	Branched-chain keto acid decarboxylase	Patrick *et al.*, 1984
Cystinosis*	[35S]-cystine uptake	Patrick *et al.*, 1984*
Hereditary tyrosinaemia	Fumarylacetoacetase	Holme *et al.*, 1985
Propionic acidaemia	[14C]-propionate incorporation into protein; propionyl-CoA carboxylase	Fensom *et al.*, 1984b
Methylmalonic acidaemia (B12 unresponsive)	[14C]-propionate incorporation into protein; methylmalonyl-CoA mutase	Fowler & Cooper, 1984 Kleijer *et al.*, 1984c
Carbohydrate disorders		
Galactosaemia	Galactose 1-phosphate uridyl transferase	Fensom *et al.*, 1984b
Glycogenosis IV	Brancher enzyme	Fensom *et al.*, 1984b
Purine disorders		
Lesch-Nyhan syndrome*	Hypoxanthine phosphoribosyl transferase	Gibbs *et al.*, 1984*
Adenosine deaminase deficiency	Adenosine deaminase	Simoni *et al.*, 1983
Miscellaneous disorders		
Menkes' disease*	Copper content	Tønnesen *et al.*, 1985*
X-linked ichthyosis	Steroid sulphatase	Benson *et al.*, 1983 Lam *et al.*, 1984
Adrenoleucodystrophy†	Very long chain fatty acid content; (also linkage analysis to a DNA probe)	Boué *et al.*, 1985†
Zellweger syndrome*	Acyl CoA: dihydroxy acetone phosphate acyltransferase; very long chain fatty acid content	Schutgens *et al.*, 1984b Hajra *et al.*, 1985*

* Indicates an affected fetus has been diagnosed by assay of villi from an at-risk pregnancy.
† Indicates an affected fetus has been diagnosed by assay of cultured villi from an at-risk pregnancy.

3.3.1 Amino-acid and related disorders

Activity of cystathionine β-synthase, the enzyme which is deficient in classical homocystinuria, is almost undetectable when assayed directly in villi, but increases after tissue culture to a value within the range found for amniotic cells (Benson *et al.*, 1983; Fensom *et al.*, 1984b). This excludes the possibility of direct assay for diagnosis of this disease, but nevertheless results from analysis of cultured villi should be available some 6–8 weeks earlier than those following amniocentesis. Attempts in our laboratory to stimulate cystathionine β-synthase activity by incubation of intact villi for periods up to five days in medium containing phytohaemagglutinin have been unsuccessful (Crees, Vimal and Fensom, unpublished observations).

First trimester diagnosis of citrullinaemia has been reported by Kleijer *et al.* (1984c). Intact villi were incubated in medium containing (^{14}C)-citrulline and (^{3}H)-leucine, and incorporation of label into trichloroacetic acid – precipitable protein was measured as the ratio (^{14}C) : (^{3}H). The values obtained (0.3, 0.9 and 16.0) in triplicate determinations for the patient were deficient when compared to three control villous specimens (128, 187 and 196), and the prediction of an affected fetus was confirmed by demonstration of a low incorporation ratio in fibroblasts cultured from the aborted fetus.

A pregnancy at risk for argininosuccinic aciduria was monitored in the author's laboratory (Vimal *et al.*, 1984) using a similar method except that single isotope labelling with (^{14}C)-citrulline was employed, and results were expressed as label incorporated per mg total protein. Further, one half of the specimen was used for tissue culture for confirmatory studies. In the direct assay a value within the normal range was obtained (189 patom per 6 h per mg protein (units); controls ($n = 15$) 15.5 to 304; mean 75.6), but after tissue culture a markedly deficient incorporation was noted (0.2 and 1.0 units on separate subcultures; three controls 373, 510 and 954), and an affected fetus was diagnosed. This was confirmed after termination of pregnancy by demonstration of an elevated argininosuccinic acid level in amniotic fluid and deficient (^{14}C)-citrulline incorporation in cultured fetal fibroblasts. Since villi collected at termination and assayed immediately gave an abnormal result (2.5 units), an unidentified technical error appears to have been the most likely cause of the high incorporation found in the test villi. Nevertheless, the precaution of use of half the sample for tissue culture avoided a late diagnosis and a prostaglandin termination following amniocentesis.

Patrick *et al.* (1984) monitored a pregnancy at risk for maple syrup urine disease by measuring branched-chain keto acid decarboxylase activity using 1-(^{14}C)-α-ketoisocaproic acid as substrate. The value obtained was within the range for control villi and the prediction of an unaffected fetus was confirmed at amniocentesis. In the same paper the authors reported successful first trimester diagnosis of cystinosis by direct analysis of villi. The biopsy was incubated overnight in 2 ml culture medium containing (^{35}S)-cystine, and then washed, lysed and tested for uptake of cystine by chromatography and autoradiography (Willcox and Patrick, 1974). The presence of a band in the region expected for cystine was diagnostic of the disease and the accuracy of the prediction was confirmed by analysis of fetal skin fibroblasts. Two further pregnancies were monitored by the same method, and in each case absence of a band in the cystine region was interpreted as indicating an unaffected fetus which was confirmed after amniocentesis.

Holme *et al.* (1985) have reported the presence of fumarylacetoacetase (FAA) activity in normal chorionic villi and suggested that first trimester prenatal diagnosis of hereditary tyrosinaemia should be possible. However, Pettit *et al.* (1985) have drawn attention to the fact that an allele exists which gives rise to a pseudo-deficiency of FAA in some individuals and that FAA activity measurements may lead to a false positive diagnosis if applied in families where carriers of the pseudo-deficiency gene occur.

Possible approaches to first trimester diagnosis of propionic acidaemia and methylmalonic aciduria are measurement of incorporation of label from (^{14}C)-propionate into protein in intact villi or direct assay of propionyl-CoA carboxylase or methylmalonyl-CoA mutase (for the mutase deficiency form of methylmalonic aciduria) in lysed villi. Kleijer *et al.* (1984c) employed both techniques in monitoring a pregnancy at risk for the latter disease, and from the normal values obtained predicted that the fetus was unaffected. This was confirmed at amniocentesis.

3.3.2 Carbohydrate disorders

At the time of writing there are few reported data on the enzymology of chorionic villi in relation to carbohydrate disorders. Galactose 1-phosphate uridyl transferase and glycogen brancher enzyme have been detected in a limited number of control specimens examined in the author's laboratory (Fensom *et al.*, 1984b), indicating the possibility of direct assay for diagnosis of galactosaemia and glycogen storage disease type IV. Glycogen storage disease type II is dealt with under lysosomal storage disorders above.

3.3.3 Purine disorders

First trimester diagnosis of three fetuses affected with Lesch–Nyhan syndrome in four pregnancies monitored has been reported by Gibbs *et al.* (1984). In the affected cases reduced hypoxanthine phosphoribosyl transferase (HPRT) activity was demonstrated directly in villi which were shown to be from male fetuses either by karyotyping or by using a Y-specific cDNA probe. In two cases HPRT activity was undetectable, and in the third case was about 10% of normal. This was thought to represent residual enzyme activity in an affected fetus. The two fetuses with undetectable activity were aborted three weeks after sampling and the diagnoses were confirmed by demonstration of absent HPRT activity in fibroblasts cultured from skin and umbilical cord. A confirmatory amniocentesis was arranged for further studies of the third fetus. However, this fetus aborted spontaneously at 14 weeks gestation, when again a low residual HPRT activity was found in villi obtained from the placenta. The fourth fetus was judged to be unaffected in view of normal villous HPRT activity and a female pattern after hybridization of villous DNA with the Y-specific probe.

3.3.4 Miscellaneous disorders

A fetus affected with Menkes' disease has been diagnosed by demonstration of increased copper content in chorionic villi collected at the tenth week of pregnancy (Tønnesen *et al.*, 1985). The villi, which had a male karyotype, contained a level of copper 16 times the highest control value, as determined by neutron activation analysis. The diagnosis was confirmed by demonstration of increased incorporation of ^{64}Cu into fibroblasts from the aborted fetus.

First trimester diagnosis of adrenoleucodystrophy has been reported by Boué *et al.* (1985). This X-linked disease is characterized by progressive cerebral demyelination and diminished adrenal function and is due to impaired capacity to degrade very long chain fatty acids (Singh *et al.*, 1984). In the pregnancy at risk the diagnosis was based initially on linkage analysis carried out directly on villi using the highly polymorphic probe St 14, which indicated that the fetus had a high probability ($> 90\%$) of being affected. The diagnosis was confirmed by demonstrating a high ratio (20 times control) of hexacosanoic acid (C26:0) to docosenoic acid (C22:0) in cultured chorionic villous cells. After termination a similar C26:0/C22:0 ratio was observed in cultured amniotic cells, and C26:0 was found to account for 28% of total fatty acids in post-mortem fetal adrenal cortex (controls 0.02%).

Zellweger (cerebro-hepato-renal) syndrome is a severe autosomal recessive disorder in which patients lack hepatic and renal peroxisomes (Goldfischer *et al.*, 1973). Biochemical markers for the disease have been delineated based on the peroxisomal deficiency, including elevated tissue levels of very long chain fatty acids (Brown *et al.*, 1982) and decreased activity of fibroblast acyl-CoA: dihydroxyacetone phosphate acyltransferase (Schutgens *et al.*, 1984a). Using both these parameters Hajra *et al.* (1985) have diagnosed an affected fetus by direct analysis of villi collected at eleven weeks' gestation. The hexacosanoic acid (C26:0) level in the sample was increased over control values, and the acyltransferase activity was reduced to 15% of control. Studies of fetal adrenal gland from the abortus showed inclusions characteristic of the disease, and C26:0 was found to account for 41% of total fatty acids in the cholesterol-ester fractions isolated from the fetal adrenal cortex (controls: less than 1%).

3.4 CONCLUSIONS AND FUTURE PROSPECTS

Considerable progress has already been made in assessing the enzymatic properties of chorionic villi and in applying methods to first trimester diagnosis of a variety of metabolic disorders. It does not seem over-confident to predict that methods will eventually be developed for all disorders for which second trimester diagnosis is currently available based on the study of amniotic cells. The direct assay of villi appears to be applicable to all disorders studied so far, with the exception of homocystinuria where the sample will have to be cultured for assay. However, even when direct assay is possible division of the sample for tissue culture for back-up studies is often advisable. Examples of disorders where this is particularly applicable are Hurler's and I-cell diseases.

There is still a scarcity of information on the basic properties of enzymes in villi, the applicability in some instances of artificial substrates, and the effect of gestation on activity. Laboratories engaged in prenatal diagnosis of metabolic disorders should attempt to make some study of these topics in order to increase the accuracy of the methods. Further studies are required on the enzymatic properties of normal decidua as indicated by Grabowski *et al.* (1984), to assess the degree of contamination likely to interfere with first trimester assays.

It remains to be seen whether any disorders which are not amenable to second trimester enzymatic diagnosis will prove to be so in the first trimester. It would perhaps be surprising to find activity of liver-specific enzymes such as phenylalanine 4-hydroxylase, and glucose 6-phosphatase in villi, but the tissue is still relatively unexploited, and should be tested for such enzymes, both directly and after stimulation with hormones or mitogenic agents.

Finally, even though the activity of such liver-specific enzymes may not be demonstrable in chorionic villi, it will be possible in some families to establish prenatal diagnosis of the associated diseases by demonstrating chorionic villi DNA polymorphisms. These techniques have been used for prenatal diagnosis of classical phenylketonuria using a cloned phenylalanine 4-hydroxylase gene probe to analyse cultured amniotic cell DNA (Lidsky *et al.*, 1985), and it seems highly likely that they will be applicable to DNA isolated from chorionic villi.

Since the completion of this review other enzymes have been shown to be active in chorionic villi. These include glycogen debranching enzyme (van Diggelen *et al.*, 1985), 3-methylcrotonyl-CoA carboxylase, pyruvate carboxylase, 4-aminobutyric acid aminotransferase, succinic semi-aldehyde dehydrogenase (Sweetman *et al.*, 1986), and several glycolytic enzymes, dehydrogenases and enzymes of glutathione and nucleotide metabolism (Dallapiccola *et al.*, 1985).

Grebner and Jackson (1985) have reported an extensive series of first trimester tests for Tay–Sachs disease, and correct prenatal diagnosis using chorionic villi has been reported for fetuses affected with Niemann–Pick disease type B (Vanier *et al.*, 1985), Sanfilippo disease type A (Kleijer *et al.*, 1986a), Pompe's disease (Besançon *et al.*, 1985) maple syrup urine disease (Kleijer *et al.*, 1985) and galactosaemia (Kleijer *et al.*, 1986b).

ACKNOWLEDGEMENTS

I thank my colleagues in the Paediatric Research Unit for their participation in many of the studies described in this review, and I am indebted to the obstetricians who have referred cases and provided control material. The critical comments of Dr Philip Benson were very much appreciated. Work was supported by Action Research, the National Fund for Research into Crippling Diseases and the Department of Health and Social Security.

REFERENCES

Benson, P. F. and Fensom, A. H. (1985) *Genetic Biochemical Disorders*, Oxford University Press.

Benson, P. F., Fensom, A. H., Crees, M. J., Lam, S. T. S., Coleman, D., Heaton, D. and Rodeck, C. (1983) Recent advances in prenatal diagnosis of inborn errors of metabolism. In *Progress in Perinatal Medicine* (ed. A. Albertini, P. G. Crosignani), Excepta Medica, Amsterdam. pp. 165–70.

Besançon, A. M., Belon, J. P., Castelnau, L., Dumez, Y. and Poenaru, L. (1984) Prenatal diagnosis of atypical Tay–Sachs disease by chorionic villi sampling. *Prenat. Diag.*, **4**, 365–70.

Besançon, A. M., Castelnau, L., Nicolesco, H., Dumez, Y. and Poenaru, L. (1985) Prenatal diagnosis of gylcogenosis type II (Pompe's disease) using chorionic villi biopsy. *Clin.Genet.*, **27**, 479–82.

Beyer, E. M. and Wiederschain, G. YA. (1984) Activity and multiple forms of α-L-fucosidase and hexosaminidase in chorion biopsy specimens and some fetal organs. *Prenat. Diag.*, **4**, 43–9.

Boué, J., Oberle, I., Heilig, R., Mandel, J. L., Moser, A., Moser, H., Larsen, J. W. Jr., Dumez, Y. and Boué, A. (1985) First trimester diagnosis of adrenoleucodystrophy by determination of very long chain fatty acid levels and by linkage analysis to a DNA probe. *Human Genet.*, **69**, 272–4.

Brambati, B., Simoni, G., Danesino, C., Oldrini, A., Ferrazzi, E., Romitti, L., Terzoli, G., Rossella, F., Ferrari, M. and Fraccaro, M. (1985) First trimester fetal diagnosis of genetic disorders: clinical evaluation of 250 cases. *J. Med. Genet.*, **22**, 92–9.

Brown, F. R. III, McAdams, A. J., Cummins, J. W., Konkol, R., Singh, I., Moser, A. B. and Moser, H. W. (1982) Cerebro-hepato-renal (Zellweger) syndrome and neonatal adrenoleukodystrophy: similarities in phenotype and accumulation of very long chain fatty acids. *Johns Hopkins Med. J.*, **151**, 344–51.

Dallapiccola, B., Novelli, G., Palloni, R., Catizone, F. and Magnani, M. (1985)

Activity of 30 nonlysosomal enzymes in chorionic villi. In *First Trimester Fetal Diagnosis* (eds M. Fraccaro, G. Simoni and B. Brambati), Springer-Verlag, Berlin, Heidelberg. pp. 242–5.

Danesino, C. (1983) Enzyme determinations on chorionic villi in the first trimester of pregnancy for prenatal diagnosis of metabolic disease. In *Progress in Perinatal Medicine* (ed. A. Albertini, P. G. Crosignani), Excepta Medica, Amsterdam. pp. 293–301.

Fensom, A. H., Jackson, M., Sanguinetti, N., Rodeck, C. H., Morsman, J. M., Coleman, D. V. and Heaton, D. (1984a) The use of chorionic villi for early prenatal diagnosis of metabolic disorders. *J. Med. Genet.* (abstract), **21**, 142.

Fensom, A. H., Chase, D., Crees, M., Jackson, M., McGuire, V. M., Marsh, J., Sanguinetti, N., Vimal, C. M. and Yuen, M. (1984b) Biochemical tests on chorion biopsy in *Early Prenatal Diagnosis: Present and Future* (ed. A. Paladini, D. Catalano, A. Di Lieto and F. Rullo). Proceedings of the International Symposium. Naples, Italy, 12–13 October, G.V.A. Press, Naples. pp. 63–77.

Fowler, B. and Cooper, A. (1984) Prenatal diagnosis of metabolic disease using chorionic villi – three cases. *Prenatal Diagnosis Group News Letter*, **8**(2) (ed. A. McDermott), Southmead Hospital, Bristol. pp. 32–3.

Gibbs, D. A., McFadyen, I. R., Crawfurd, M. d'A., De Muinck Keizer, E. E., Headhouse-Benson, C. M., Wilson, T. M. and Farrant, P. H. (1984) First trimester diagnosis of Lesch-Nyhan syndrome. *Lancet*, ii, 1180–3.

Goldfischer, S., Moore, C. L., Johnson, A. B., Spiro, A. J., Valsamis, M. P., Wisniewski, H. K., Ritch, R. H., Norton, W. T., Rapin, I. and Gartner, L. M. (1973) Peroxisomal and mitochondrial defects in the cerebro-hepato-renal syndrome. *Science*, **182**, 62–4.

Grabowski, G. A., Kruse, J. R., Goldberg, J. D., Chockkalingam, K., Gordon, R. E., Blakemore, K. J., Mahoney, M. J. and Desnick, R. J. (1984) First trimester prenatal diagnosis of Tay–Sachs disease. *Am. J. Hum. Genet.*, **36**, 1369–78.

Grebner, E. E., Wapner, R. J., Barr, M. A., and Jackson, L. G. (1983) Prenatal Tay–Sachs diagnosis by chorionic villi sampling. *Lancet*, ii, 286–7.

Grebner, E. E. and Jackson, L. G. (1985) Prenatal diagnosis for Tay–Sachs disease using chorionic villus sampling. *Prenat. Diag.*, **5**, 313–20.

Gustavi, B., Chester, M. A., Edvall, H., Iosif, S., Kristoffersson, U., Löfberg, L., Mineur, A. and Mitelman, F. (1984) First-trimester diagnosis on chorionic villi obtained by direct vision technique. *Hum. Genet.*, **65**, 373–6.

Hajra, A. K., Datta, N. S., Jackson, L. G., Moser, A. B., Moser, H. W., Larsen, J. W., Jr. and Powers, J. (1985) Prenatal diagnosis of Zellweger cerebrohepatorenal syndrome. *N. Engl. J. Med.*, **312**, 445–6.

Holme, E., Lindblad, B. and Lindstedt, S. (1985) Possibilities of treatment and for early prenatal diagnosis of hereditary tyrosinaemia. *Lancet*, i, 527.

Kazy, Z., Rozovsky, I. S. and Bakharev, V. A. (1982) Chorion biopsy in early pregnancy: a method of early prenatal diagnosis of inherited disorders. *Prenat. Diag.*, **2**, 39–45.

Kleijer, W. J., Mancini, G. M. S., Jahoda, M. G. J., Vosters, R. P. L., Sachs, E. S., Niermeijer, M. F. and Galjaard, H. (1984a) First trimester diagnosis of Krabbe's disease by direct enzyme analysis of chorionic villi. *New Engl. J. Med.*, **311**, 1257.

Kleijer, W. J., Van Diggelen, O. P., Janse, H. C., Galjaard, H., Dumez, Y. and Boué, J. (1984b) First trimester diagnosis of Hunter syndrome on chorionic villi. *Lancet*, ii, 472.

Kleijer, W. J., Thoomes, R., Galjaard, H., Wendel, U. and Fowler, B. (1984c) First trimester (chorion biopsy) diagnosis of citrullinaemia and methylmalonicaciduria. *Lancet*, ii, 1340.

Kleijer, W. J., Horsman, D., Mancini, G. M. S., Fois, A. and Boué, J. (1985) First-trimester diagnosis of maple syrup urine disease on intact chorionic villi. *New Engl. J. Med.*, **313**, 1608.

Kleijer, W. J., Janse, H. C., Vosters, R. P. L., Niermeijer, M., F. and van de Kamp, J. J. P. (1968a) First-trimester diagnosis of mucopolysaccharidosis IIIA (Sanfilippo A disease). *New Engl. J. Med.*, **314**, 185–6.

Kleijer, W. J., Janse, H. C., van Diggelen, O. P., Macek, M., Hajek, Z., Gillett, M. G. and Holton, J. B. (1986b) First-trimester diagnosis of galactosaemia. *Lancet*, i, 748.

Lam, S. T. S., Fensom, A. H., Coleman, D., Heaton, D., Morsman, J., Nicolaides, K. and Rodeck, C. H. (1984) Steroid sulphatase activity in trophoblast samples. *J. Obstet. Gynaecol.*, **5**, 24–6.

Leroy, J. C., Ho. M. W., MacBrinn, M. C., Zielke, K., Jacob, J. and O'Brien, J. S. (1972) I-Cell disease: biochemical studies. *Pediatr. Res.*, **6**, 752–7.

Lidsky, A. S., Güttler, F. and Woo, S. L. C. (1985) Prenatal diagnosis of classic phenylketonuria by DNA analysis. *Lancet*, i, 549–51.

Lykkelund, C., Søndergaard, F., Therkelsen, A. J., Tønnesen, T., Rasmussen, V., Mikkelsen, M., Guttler, F. and Nyland, M. H. (1983) Feasibility of first trimester prenatal diagnosis of Hunter syndrome. *Lancet*, ii, 1147.

Marsh, J. and Fensom, A. H. (1985) 4-methylumbelliferyl α-*N*-acetylglucosaminidase activity for diagnosis of Sanfilippo B disease. *Clin. Genet.*, **27**, 258–62.

Mikkelsen, M., Søndergaard, F., Tønnesen, T., Marsk, L. and Lindsten, J. (1984) First trimester biopsies of chorionic villi for prenatal diagnosis: experience of two laboratories. *Clin. Genet.* (abstract) **26**, 263–4.

Patrick, A. D., Young, E. and Mossman, J. (1984) The current experience of first trimester diagnosis for metabolic disorders. *Prenatal Diagnosis Group Newsletter,* **8** (2) (ed. A. McDermott), Southmead Hospital, Bristol. pp. 21–4.

Pergament, E., Ginsberg, N., Verlinsky, Y., Cadkin, A., Chu, L. and Trnka, L. (1983) Prenatal Tay–Sachs diagnosis by chorionic villi sampling. *Lancet*, ii, 286.

Pettit, B. R., Kvittingen, E. A. and Leonard, J. V. (1985) Early prenatal diagnosis of hereditary tyrosinaemia. *Lancet*, i, 1038.

Poenaru, L., Kaplan, L., Dumez, J. and Dreyfus, J. C. (1984a) Evaluation of possible first trimester prenatal diagnosis in lysosomal diseases by trophoblast biopsy. *Pediatr. Res.*, **18**, 1032–4.

Poenaru, L., Castelnau, L., Dumez, Y. and Thepot, F. (1984b) First trimester diagnosis of mucolipidosis II (I-cell disease) by chorionic biopsy. *Am. J. Hum. Genet.*, **36**, 1379–85.

Poenaru, L., Castelnau, L., Choiset, A., Rouquet, Y. and Thepot, F. (1985) Lysosomal hydrolase activity in chorionic villi and embryonic cells in culture. *Hum. Genet.*, **69**, 378–9.

Sanguinetti, N., Marsh, J., Jackson, M., Fensom, A. H., Warren, R. C. and Rodeck, C. H. (1986) The arylsulphatases of chorionic villi: Potential problems in the first trimester diagnosis of metachromatic leucodystrophy and Maroteaux-Lamy disease. *Clin. Genet.*, **30**, in press.

Schutgens, R. B. H., Romeyn, G. J., Wanders, R. J. A., van den Bosch, H., Schrakamp, G. and Heymans, H. S. A. (1984a) Deficiency of acyl-CoA: dihydroxyacetone phosphate acyl transferase in patients with Zellweger (cerebro-hepato-renal) syndrome. *Biochem. Biophys. Res. Commun.*, **120**, 179–84.

Schutgens, R. B. H., Heymans, H. S. A., Wanders, R. J. A., Bosch, H. V. D. and

Schrakamp, G. (1984b) Prenatal detection of Zellweger syndrome. *Lancet*, ii, 1339–40.

Simoni, G., Brambati, B., Danesino, C., Rossella, F., Terzoli, G. L., Ferrari, M. and Fraccaro, M. (1983) Efficient direct chromosome analysis and enzyme determinations from chorionic villi samples in the first trimester of pregnancy. *Hum. Genet.*, 63, 349–57.

Simoni, G., Brambati, B., Danesino, C., Terzoli, G. L., Romitti, L., Rossella, F. and Fraccaro, M. (1984) Diagnostic application of first trimester trophoblast sampling in 100 pregnancies. *Hum. Genet.*, **66**, 252–9.

Singh, I., Moser, A. B., Moser, H. W. and Kishimoto, Y. (1984) Adrenoleukodystrophy: impaired oxidation of very long chain fatty acids in white blood cells, cultured skin fibroblasts and amniocytes. *Pediatr. Res.*, **18**, 286–90.

Sweetman, F. R., Gibson, K. M., Sweetman, L., Nyhan, W. L., Chin, H., Swartz, W. and Jones O. W. (1986) Activity of biotin-dependent and GABA metabolizing enzymes in chorionic villus samples: potential for 1st trimester prenatal diagnosis. *Prenat. Diag.*, **6**, 187–94.

Tønnesen, T., Horn, N., Søndergaard, F., Boué, J., Damsgaard, E. and Heydorn, K. (1985) Measurement of copper in chorionic villi for first-trimester diagnosis of Menkes' disease. *Lancet*, i, 1038–9.

Tsvetkova, I. V., Zolotukhina, T. V., Bakharev, V. A., Rosenfeld, E. L. and Rosovsky, I. S. (1983) Prenatal exclusion of metachromatic leucodystrophy by estimation of arylsulphatase A activity in chorion and cultured amniotic fluid cells. *Prenatal Diagnosis*, **3**, 233–6.

Upadhyaya, M., Archer, I. M., Harper, P. S., Jasani, B., Roberts A., Shaw, D. J., Thomas, N. S. T. and Williams H. (1984) DNA and enzyme studies on chorionic villi for use in antenatal diagnosis. *Clin. Chim. Acta*, **140**, 39–46.

van Diggelen, O. P., Janse, H. C. and Smit, G. P. A. (1985) Debranching enzyme in fibroblasts, amniotic fluid cells and chorionic villi: pre- and postnatal diagnosis of glycogenosis type III. *Clin. Chim. Acta*, **149**, 129–34.

Vanier, M. T., Boué, J. and Dumez, Y. (1985) Niemann–Pick disease Type B: first-trimester prenatal diagnosis on chorionic villi and biochemical study of a foetus at 12 weeks of development. *Clin. Genet.*, **28**, 348–54.

Vimal, C. M., Fensom, A. H., Heaton, D., Ward, R. H. T., Garrod, P. and Penketh, R. J. A. (1984) Prenatal diagnosis of argininosuccinicaciduria by analysis of cultured chorionic villi. *Lancet*, ii, 521–2.

Willcox, P. and Patrick, A. D. (1974) Biochemical diagnosis of cystinosis using cultured cells. *Arch. Dis. Child.*, **49**, 209–12.

Young, E. and Patrick, A. D. (1983) First trimester diagnosis of metabolic diseases. *Prenatal Diagnosis Group Newsletter,* 7: no. 2 (ed. A. McDermott), Southmead Hospital, Bristol. pp. 4–5.

Yuen, M. and Fensom, A. H. (1985) Diagnosis of classical Morquio's disease: *N*-acetylgalactosamine 6-sulphate sulphatase activity in cultured fibroblasts, leucocytes, amniotic cells and chorionic villi. *J. Inher. Metab. Dis.*, **8**, 80–6.

4

Placental immunobiology in early pregnancy

—— Peter M. Johnson ——

4.1 INTRODUCTION

There has been a relentless ever-increasing interest in immunology as providing answers to many problems in medical science. Indeed, in recent years much exciting progress has been made in understanding the complex feto-maternal immunological interactions which occur normally in pregnancy and allow the genetically disparate fetus the privilege of evading transplant rejection reactions in the potentially hostile maternal environment (Faulk and McIntyre, 1983; Johnson, 1984; Clark, 1985; Johnson *et al.*, 1986). However, in the context of chorion-villus sampling, the most important role for immunology has been as a tool – that is, the provision of reagents to identify discrete cell populations by immunohistology and immunocytology. This can now best be done using monoclonal antibodies (mAbs) reactive with cell surface differentiation antigens, whereas previous reagents lacked the requisite degree of specificity and sensitivity. However, the situation is yet far from ideal, as will be illustrated.

4.2 HLA ANTIGENS

In the requirement to distinguish any maternal cells away from fetal cells, where there is doubt, the most obvious cell surface antigen markers that could be useful are the histocompatibility glycoproteins, HLA antigens. These are encoded from a large complex genetic region on chromosome 6 containing many separate loci, but the most relevant in this context are HLA-A and B antigens (so-called class I histocompatibility or transplantation antigens). All individuals inherit one haplotype from each parent, and hence the offspring must express a paternal haplotype. Since the HLA system is so incredibly polymorphic, the fetus in pregnancy will almost always express paternally inherited HLA antigens distinct from the maternal HLA type. Thus, if specific antibodies were available for each of these specificities, then it might be expected that there could be accurate distinction between maternal and fetal cells. However, there are two problems: first, that in many cases such antibodies do not yet exist with such single specificity as would be required; and secondly that fetal chorionic villous trophoblast does not express HLA! Undoubtedly, this failure of HLA expression by placental villous trophoblast is a major reason for the successful evasion by this tissue of a transplantation rejection reaction in pregnancy (Sunderland *et al.*, 1981a; Faulk and McIntyre, 1983; Johnson, 1984; Johnson *et al.*, 1986).

In contrast, some extravillous cytotrophoblast populations in the chorion laeve or placental bed are reactive with mAbs against common framework structures of class I HLA antigens, but these cells do *not* express polymorphic determinants (i.e. the characteristic tissue type) (Redman *et al.*, 1984). The nature of this apparent non-polymorphic class I HLA antigen expressed only by extravillous trophoblast is currently a matter of much speculation (Bulmer and Johnson, 1985a; Johnson *et al.*, 1986).

There has also been application of HLA-reactive antibodies for enriching fetal cells from samples of maternal blood early in pregnancy for prenatal diagnosis of chromosomal abnormalities and biochemical disorders (Herzenberg *et al.*, 1979; Parks and Herzenberg, 1982). This approach has been based on the sophisticated use of a fluorescence-activated cell sorter (FACS) machine to identify fetal cells specifically using fluorescein-tagged antibodies to cell surface antigens such as the paternally-inherited fetal HLA antigen tissue type. Initial studies indicated that this technique could separate at least some of the very trace amounts of fetal cells in maternal blood at any time of sampling. In the case of male fetuses, confirmation of fetal origin of separated cells was possible by quinacrine mustard staining of Y-chromatin in most but not all instances (Parks and Herzenberg, 1982). It was not feasible to make accurate estimations of the fraction of these fetal cells in maternal blood although, since all populations of trophoblast do not express HLA allotypic antigens, it must be assumed that these were non-trophoblastic fetal cells. Since most fetal cells which break away from the placental bed in early pregnancy and enter maternal circulation are thought to be trophoblastic, attention has recently focused more on the application of monoclonal antibodies reactive with characteristic cell surface differentiation antigens of trophoblast.

4.3 TROPHOBLAST SURFACE ANTIGENS

Several research groups have described the production of mAbs reactive with characteristic trophoblast surface antigens (Johnson *et al.*, 1981; Lipinski *et al.*, 1981; Sunderland *et al.*, 1981b; McLaughlin *et al.*, 1982; Rettig *et al.*, 1985). Of these, mAbs recognizing placental-type alkaline phosphatase (a major syncytiotrophoblast membrane protein) are of little value in the present application since this protein isoenzyme is only expressed in the placenta after the first trimester of pregnancy. However, other trophoblastic-reactive mAbs (such as H316 and NDOG1) have been shown to react with very early human pregnancy tissues (Bulmer *et al.*, 1984). Several trophoblast antigens defined by mAbs show restriction to certain anatomically-defined populations of fetal trophoblast (reviewed in Bulmer and Johnson, 1985a). For example, the NDOG1 antigen is expressed on placental syncytiotrophoblast and not by most populations of extravillous and villous cytotrophoblast. A similar situation is the case for the transferrin receptor (Bulmer and Johnson, 1985a), which is also expressed by proliferating leucocytes and hence is not an ideal marker for syncytiotrophoblast. Monoclonal antibodies reactive with every population of trophoblast seem largely restricted at present to those recognizing cytokeratins, cytoplasmic structures which are also present in endometrial gland epithelial cells within decidual tissues and other epithelia (Bulmer and Johnson, 1985a). There is clearly both scope and need for the development of further mAbs broadly specific for fetal trophoblast populations. Nevertheless the present mAbs, such as H315 which reacts in immunohistology with syncytiotrophoblast and several cytotrophoblast populations (Bulmer and Johnson, 1985a), represent reagents which can be used to identify a substantial amount of trophoblast in cell culture. Furthermore, these react with cell surface proteins and not soluble secreted products (e.g. human chorionic gonadotrophin, hCG) which may be picked up by other non-trophoblastic cells such as macrophages within primary cell cultures.

Similar mAbs have been used to characterize other (non-trophoblastic) cell populations within chorionic villus stroma and uterine decidual tissues. For example, many cells in chorionic villi and amniochorionic mesenchyme stain for the leucocyte common antigen (a marker of bone marrow-derived cells) and this highlights the number of fetal leucocytes within villous tissue in early pregnancy (Sutton *et al.*, 1983; Bulmer and Sunderland, 1984). These cells also stain with a mAb specific for tissue macrophages, leu-M3, and represent Hofbauer cells in placental villi (Loke *et al.*, 1982; Bulmer and Johnson, 1984); it is thought that these macrophages tend to dominate in prolonged cell cultures isolated from chorionic tissue. There are also many maternal leucocytes in uterine decidua, including both lymphocytes and macrophages (Bulmer and Sunderland, 1984; Bulmer and Johnson, 1984; Kabawat *et al.*, 1985). There is no immunological way (other than by HLA) to distinguish between maternal and fetal macrophages in cell culture.

Thus, there are numerous immunocompetent cells in fetal chorionic villi and also maternal decidual tissue in early human pregnancy. Indeed, these cells may be a central part of the cellular immunoregulation of deleterious cytotoxic response that could occur in pregnancy (Clark, 1985). One question that can be raised is whether chorion villus sampling techniques could cause iatrogenic disturbances to the immune balance between the maternal and fetal leucocytes which are closely apposite in these tissues. The answer to this is unknown, but probably not since there is evidence of some normal interplay of leucocytes across feto–maternal interfaces during pregnancy (Bulmer and Johnson, 1985b).

Finally, there is the notable phenomenon that substantial quantities of trophoblastic cellular elements break away from the placental bed throughout human pregnancy to reach maternal circulation and eventually lodge in maternal lung where they are mostly lysed (Douglas *et al.*, 1959; Attwood and Park, 1961). There have been interesting attempts to identify this material from maternal blood using antisera raised against human trophoblast (Goodfellow and Taylor, 1982). Preliminary studies using trophoblast-reactive mAbs and flow cytometry on a FACS machine have now shown it possible often to identify small numbers of such material in trophoblast-enriched leucocyte fractions from heparinized blood samples from 6 weeks of gestation (Covone *et al.*, 1984). Three types of cellular material were identified: (a) large polynucleated cells which presumably had a syncytiotrophoblastic origin, (b) diploid cells which presumably had a cytotrophoblastic origin, and (c) small anucleate material which presumably represented exfoliated syncytiotrophoblast microvilli. Chromosomal analysis may be difficult because it will be the diploid cell population alone that will be capable of cell division, and only very small numbers of fetal cells might be obtained. Clearly, further work needs to be pursued in this exciting area of a minimally invasive technique to obtain fetal cells for prenatal diagnosis – for example, the improved FACS separation of these cells and development of recombinant DNA analysis firstly to confirm fetal origin (such as with Y-specific probes) and subsequently to detect chromosomal abnormalities.

In conclusion, an immunological approach to the identification and possible separation of discrete cell populations from chorion villus samples or maternal blood is still in its infancy, but the information already obtained is promising.

REFERENCES

Attwood, H. O. and Park, W. W. (1961) Embolism to the lungs by trophoblast. *J. Obstet. Gynaecol. Brit. Cmwlth*, **68**, 611–17.

Bulmer, J. N., Billington, W. D. and Johnson, P. M. (1984) Immunohistologic identification of trophoblast populations in early human pregnancy with the use of monoclonal antibodies. *Amer. J. Obstet. Gynec.*, **148**, 19–26.

Bulmer, J. N. and Johnson, P. M. (1984) Macrophage populations in the human placenta and amniochorion. *Clin. Exp. Immunol.*, **57**, 393–403.

Bulmer, J. N. and Johnson, P. M. (1985a) Antigen expression by trophoblast populations in the human placenta and their possible immunobiological role. *Placenta*, **6**, 127–40.

Bulmer, J. N. and Johnson, P. M. (1985b) Identification of leucocytes within the human chorion laeve. *J. Reprod. Immunol.*, **7**, 89–92.

Bulmer, J. N. and Sunderland, C. A. (1984) Immunohistological characterization of lymphoid cell populations in the early human placental bed. *Immunology*, **52**, 349–57.

Clark, D. A. (1985) Materno-fetal relations. *Immunol. Letters*, **9**, 239–47.

Covone, A. E., Mutton, D., Johnson, P. M. and Adinolfi, M. (1984) Trophoblast cells in peripheral blood from pregnant women. *Lancet*, **ii**, 841–3.

Douglas, G. W., Thomas, L., Carr, M. C., Cullen, N. M. and Morris, R. (1959) Trophoblast in the circulating blood during pregnancy. *Amer. J. Obstet. Gynec.*, **78**, 960–9.

Faulk, W. P. and McIntyre, J. A. (1983) Immunological studies of human trophoblast: markers, subsets & functions. *Immunol. Rev.*, **75**, 139–75.

Goodfellow, C. G. and Taylor, P. V. (1982) The extraction and identification of trophoblast cells circulating in peripheral blood during pregnancy. *Brit. J. Obstet. Gynaecol.*, **69**, 65–8.

Herzenberg, L. A., Bianchi, D. W., Schroder, J., Cann, M. and Iveson, G. M. (1979) Fetal cells in the blood of pregnancy women: detection and enrichment by fluorescence-activated cell sorting. *Proc. Natl Acad. Sci. USA*, **76**, 1453–5.

Johnson, P. M. (1984) Immunobiology of human trophoblast. In *Immunological Aspects of Reproduction in Mammals* (ed. D. B. Crighton), Butterworths Press, London. pp. 109–31.

Johnson, P. M., Cheng, H. M., Molloy, C. M., Stern, C. M. M. and Slade, M. B. (1981) Human trophoblast-specific surface antigens identified using monoclonal antibodies. *Amer. J. Reprod. Immunol.*, **1**, 246–54.

Johnson, P. M., Risk, J. M., Bulmer, J. N., Niewola, Z. and Kimber, I. (1986) Antigen expression at human materno-fetal interfaces. In *Maternal Immunoregulation & Fetal Survival* (ed by T. G. Wegmann, T. J. Gill III), Oxford University Press.

Kabawat, S. E., Mostoufi-Zadeh, M., Driscoll, S. G. and Bhan, A. K. (1985) Implantation site in normal pregnancy. *Amer. J. Pathol.*, **118**, 76–84.

Lipinski, M., Parks, D. R., Rouse, R. V. and Herzenberg, L. A. (1981) Human trophoblast cell surface antigens defined by monoclonal antibodies. *Proc. Natl Acad. Sci., USA*, **78**, 5147–50.

Loke, Y. W., Eremin, O., Ashby, J. and Day, S. (1982) Characterisation of the phagocytic cells isolated from the human placenta. *J. Reticuloendothel. Soc.*, **31**, 317–28.

McLaughlin, P. J., Cheng, H. M., Slade, M. B. and Johnson, P. M. (1982) Expression on cultured human tumour cells of placental trophoblast membrane antigens and placental alkaline phosphatase defined by monoclonal antibodies. *Int. J. Cancer*, **30**, 21–6.

Parks, D. R. and Herzenberg, L. A. (1982). Fetal cells from maternal blood: their selection and prospects for use in prenatal diagnosis. *Meth. Cell. Biol.*, **26**, 277–95.

Redman, C. W. G., McMichael, A. J., Stirrat, G. M., Sunderland, C. A. and Ting, A. (1984) Class I major histocompatibility complex antigens on human extra-villous trophoblast. *Immunology*, **52**, 457–68.

Rettig, W. J., Cordon-Cardo, C., Koulos, J. P., Lewis, J. L., Oettgen, H. F. and Old, L. J. (1985) Cell surface antigens of human trophoblast and choriocarcinoma defined by monoclonal antibodies. *Int. J. Cancer*, **35**, 469–75.

Sunderland, C. A., Naiem, M., Mason, D. Y., Redman, C. W. G. and Stirrat, G. M. (1981a) The expression of MHC antigens by human chorionic villi. *J. Reprod. Immunol.*, **1**, 323–31.

Sunderland, C. A., Redman, C. W. G. and Stirrat, G. M. (1981b) Monoclonal antibodies to human syncytiotrophoblast. *Immunology*, **43**, 541–6.

Sutton, L., Mason, D. Y. and Redman, C. W. G. (1983) HLA-DR positive cells in the human placenta. *Immunology*, **49**, 103–12.

Section II

TRANSCERVICAL CHORION — VILLUS SAMPLING —

PART ONE

Devices

5

The method of chorion villus sampling under real-time ultrasound guidance using the 'Portex' cannula

—— *Humphry Ward and Bernadette Modell* ——

5.1 INTRODUCTION

Until recently, the established method available for fetal diagnosis of the haemoglobinopathies was by globin chain analysis using samples of fetal blood obtained either by placentacentesis or fetoscopy during the second trimester (Fairweather *et al.*, 1980).

In 1978 Kan and Dozy showed that sickle cell disease could be diagnosed by the new methods of gene mapping using DNA, and Dozy *et al.* (1979) applied these methods to fetal DNA extracted from amniotic fluid for the intra-uterine diagnosis of α-thalassaemia hydrops fetalis in the second trimester. In the meantime we were becoming increasingly aware that while our own patients at risk for haemoglobinopathies welcomed the availability of a fetal diagnostic test, they were extremely distressed by the associated 25% risk of a late therapeutic abortion in each pregnancy (Modell *et al.*, 1980). It was therefore proposed that perhaps the most valuable immediate clinical use that could be made of the new advances in DNA technology would be to use direct gene analysis of chorionic villi to diagnose some of the haemoglobinopathies in the first trimester of pregnancy (Williamson *et al.*, 1981).

We first considered, but then dismissed, the possibility of using a trans-abdominal approach similar to placentacentesis, as high quality ultrasound with an appropriate needle guide was not then available. Moreover, at least where the haemoglobinopathies are concerned, it seemed desirable to develop a simple approach that would also be suitable for use in the developing countries where these diseases are so common. A transcervical approach had already been used for fetal sexing in the mid-1970s, apparently without significant complications, by a Chinese group (Anshan, 1975). Villi were aspirated at 8–12 weeks' gestation 'blind', i.e. without ultrasound guidance, through a specially designed metal cannula. Fetal sexing was done directly by examination for Barr bodies, without the need for tissue culture, which was not then available. The subjects involved were young women. There were strict criteria for exclusion which may have eliminated a number of non-viable or potentially unsuccessful pregnancies, and a low rate of fetal loss (4 out of 70 continuing pregnancies = 6%) following the procedure.

The small number of fetal losses is surprising in view of the generally accepted figure of about 10% spontaneous abortion in the first trimester of pregnancy, even among young women (Gustavii, 1985; Gilmore and McNay, 1985). However, the approach was discontinued in China for a time because of the high demand for therapeutic abortion of fetuses of the 'wrong' sex, but it has recently been revived for genetic diagnosis.

The Chinese work was valuable because it showed that chorionic villi could be obtained without necessarily entraining undesirable consequences, and it seemed reasonable to use it as a model for further development. We began the attempt to obtain chorionic villi under ultrasound guidance immediately prior to suction termination performed under general anaesthesia, with Ethical Committee permission and informed patient consent.

We started using a 16-gauge Medicut cannula, as the first suitably sized instrument available, but as it had an open end it often became blocked with cervical epithelium as it was introduced through the cervix, and this then made it impossible to aspirate villi. We therefore abandoned it and started work with Dr J. Sutherland and Portex Ltd to develop a more suitable instrument. The first model was longer, with a blind tip and side holes. Although this permitted us to reach the placental site, we frequently had difficulty in negotiating the cervical canal, and the side holes turned out not to be ideal for aspirating villi. Sampling was done under real-time ultrasound guidance, but there were several technical problems. For instance, the 9 cm linear array probe on the available machine (Toshiba SAL-20A) was unsuitable for scanning deep in the pelvis, and there was often poor resolution because of fasciculation of the anterior abdominal wall musculature related to the type of anaesthetic used, while the urinary bladder had invariably been emptied. We were therefore not unduly discouraged to achieve a success rate in obtaining villi of only 31% (a result similar to that later obtained by Loeffler without ultrasound guidance (Horwell *et al.*, 1983)).

In the next stage the anaesthetic technique was modified and the patients were asked not to empty their bladders pre-operatively. Ultrasound resolution was greatly improved, so that we were able to follow the passage of the cannula into the uterus and direct its tip towards the appropriate area. The cannula was also modified to have an end hole only, and a specially created stainless steel obturator which could be curved within the cannula immediately before introduction. We also introduced a low-power dissecting microscope into the operating theatre so that samples could be checked immediately to see if villi were present. If not, another sample could be taken. With these changes the success rate for obtaining villi rose to 90%. This performance was maintained in the next stage when we routinely gave the samples of villi to colleagues for fetal karyotyping (Dr D. Coleman) or for DNA extraction (Dr J. Old), to confirm the quantity and its suitability for diagnostic purposes.

In mid-1982 we were approached by a patient at risk of bearing an infant with sickle cell disease who wished to have a first trimester test (Old *et al.*, 1982). In order to obtain experience in the non-anaesthetized patient and a short-term follow up, we asked three patients for permission to take samples in out-patients within a week of their planned admission for suction termination: samples were successfully obtained with no immediate ill effect for the pregnancy. Subsequently we found that surgeons could obtain a 67% success rate having observed the technique once in the anaesthetized patient. This gave us confidence that the method utilizing the 'Portex' cannula under guidance of real time ultrasound was easy to learn and yielded material suitable for biochemical analysis and chromosomal study without the need for tissue culture (Ward *et al.*, 1983).

5.2 THE 'PORTEX' CANNULA TECHNIQUE

Ideally a geneticist should counsel couples at risk either before pregnancy or as early in pregnancy as possible. Unfortunately it is traditional that pregnant patients tend not to be referred to antenatal clinics until after the second missed period, so that many women who might prefer a first trimester approach are not able to take advantage of it. For mothers at genetic risk it will be necessary to build up a system for immediate referral and early access to ultrasound, and this calls for an organized effort to inform general practitioners, community nurses and health visitors about the possibility of first trimester diagnosis. However, since we deal with a specific limited group of patients at risk for thalassaemic offspring, it has proved possible to contact most of the families and warn them to present themselves early in any further pregnancies. Patients that do present early enough have been told that experience of the technique is limited and that neither the short- nor long-term complications are yet known. At the counselling session a detailed ultrasound examination is performed to confirm pregnancy and fetal viability, and the date for the procedure is selected. Ideally it is planned for 9 weeks (range 8–10½ weeks).

At the time of chorion villus sampling (CVS) another detailed scan is performed. Both longitudinal and transverse scans are performed with the patient's bladder partially filled, so that the limits of the chorion frondosum and the umbilical cord insertion are located. At this stage of pregnancy it is not uncommon to find a major lateral component to the placenta. Ideally the obstetrician requires an assistant with a microscope and an ultrasonographer, although the same person may double for both these tasks.

The patient is not premedicated and no anaesthetic is used. With the patient in the lithotomy position a vulval and vaginal toilet is performed with aqueous cetrimide. Despite having done a preliminary ultrasound examination it is prudent to do a gentle bimanual examination to confirm the size and position of the uterus. Either a Sims' or Cusco's speculum is used to visualize the cervix, which is cleaned with aqueous betadine. An instrument may be needed to steady the cervix, and rather than use a tenaculum, which can readily make the cervix bleed, we now use 9 in Babcock forceps. The passage of a uterine sound is not essential in every case but does allow the team to appreciate the direction of the cervical canal and the site of the internal os. It also allows the operator to estimate the distance between the intended sampling site and internal os, and to know to what degree the assembled cannula needs to be curved.

The 'Portex' cannula now used is 1.5 mm in external diameter with an overall length of 21 cm (see Fig. 5.1). The removable stainless steel obturator protrudes sufficiently to obliterate the open end, which has smoothed edges. The complete instrument is bent to allow satisfactory intra-uterine placement. The technique differs according to the placental site. The anteriorly placed placenta in an anteverted uterus is readily reached with the cannula bent with an anterior concavity. On the other hand, for a posterior placenta in an anteverted uterus, the cannula can be rotated through 180° when the internal os is reached, and gently advanced. The cannula tip is continuously visualized on ultrasound and placed well within the placental substance, equidistant between the gestational sac and decidua. Time should be taken at

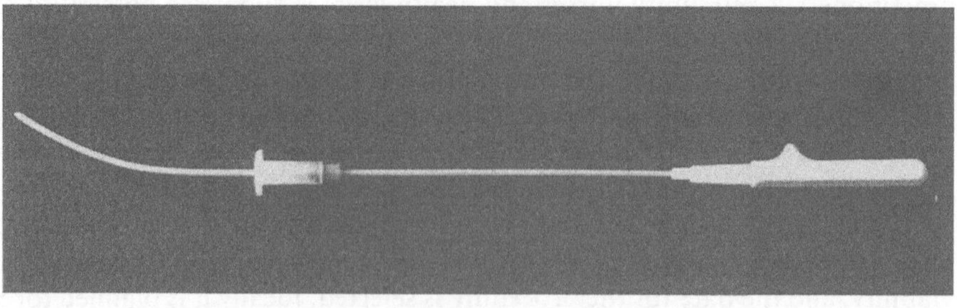

Figure 5.1 The assembled 'Portex' cannula, the adjustable 'stop' is optional.

this point to confirm the exact position of the cannula tip with both longitudinal and transverse scans before proceeding. The site of the cord insertion is best avoided because of the increased vascularity. Once the catheter is optimally situated, the obturator is removed while holding the cannula firmly and is replaced by a 20 ml syringe containing 3–4 ml of heparinized culture medium. Provided the tip has been placed well within the chorion frondosum there is little danger of it being dislodged by these actions. While applying intermittent suction (5–10 ml) the catheter tip is moved very gently to and fro; a manoeuvre we have called 'hoovering'. This is an essential part of the technique, as seems necessary for avulsing the chorionic villi so that they can be aspirated into the cannula. The hollow cannula shows ultrasonically as two parallel lines and the 'plucking' of the villi and their movement by the cannula can be readily visualized as they are aspirated. Suction is maintained to the level of the internal os as the cannula is removed. With this technique the quantity of villi obtained at one aspiration attempt is usually between 10 and 40 mg.

Although villi are often readily recognized using the naked eye, it is essential that the specimen be immediately transferred to a Petri dish and examined under sterile conditions, using a strong magnifying glass or a dissecting microscope. If villi have not been obtained a second attempt is made, but we recommend limiting aspiration attempts to two on any one occasion (a new cannula should be used each time). In our first diagnostic cases we set no limit to the number of attempts made, but there was a high incidence of complications and five losses in the first 11 singleton pregnancies, in which 51 separate attempts at sampling were made. We concluded that repeated unsuccessful attempts, particularly when only decidua are obtained, are likely to injure the uterus and cause bleeding, and can be a major factor in subsequent fetal loss. When the operator is not confident about the siting of the cannula, we believe it is safer to remove the cannula and repeat the passage rather than to attempt sampling 'blind'. Furthermore, third and fourth attempts cannot be justified, as improvements in the success rate are only marginal (Simoni *et al.*, 1983). It is preferable and safer to reschedule the CVS attempt for a few days later.

If the patient is unduly anxious, and uterine contractions are present and form a contributory factor to the failure of the initial procedure, premedication should be considered. While the presence of decidua in the aspirate is of concern as regards subsequent fetal loss, blood staining is not necessarily an adverse prognostic sign. Many patients report slight spotting for up to 48 hours without any subsequent complications.

We have allowed patients home after 6 hours and invited them for another ultrasound at the time the fetal diagnosis is known (usually 10–14 days later). Rhesus negative patients should all receive anti-D immunoglobulin as the maternal serum AFP level rises significantly in 74% of patients after CVS

(Ward *et al.*, 1985a). There is no evidence that maternal serum AFP screening for neural tube defects is subsequently complicated by CVS.

What are the contra-indications to CVS? Many surgeons have deliberately avoided CVS where there is doubt about the pregnancy continuing and when there has been vaginal bleeding. When time allows, a delay and repeat scan will invariably resolve whether a pregnancy is continuing but when the indication for CVS is one with a low genetic risk, it may still be advisable to avoid first trimester sampling. A history of recurrent early abortions should not be considered an absolute contra-indication; the parents should be karyotyped beforehand because one could be a translocation carrier, which would in fact be an extra indication for the procedure.

There is inevitably concern about introducing infection (Garden *et al.*, 1985), particularly when a cervicitis is present. Ideally at the initial counselling session, a preliminary bacteriological screen would allow for treatment but the stage of pregnancy limits the scope for adequate therapy, although Chlamydia trachomatis would respond to a course of erythromycin. We have evidence that some of our earlier fetal losses that occurred after a considerable delay may have been secondary to chorio-amnionitis (Ward *et al.*, 1985b). More recently, a patient who had an intra-uterine contraceptive device (IUCD) *in situ* subsequently aborted eleven weeks after a straightforward CVS, and the same organism (*Staphylococcus aureus*) was cultured from the coil as had previously been found in the cervical canal. However, this does not constitute evidence that infection was introduced by the catheter.

We have not experienced any problem negotiating the cervix in nulliparous patients or following cone biopsy, and successful sampling using this technique can be expected in all but 1–2% of patients. Failure is more likely if CVS is attempted after eleven weeks, partly because the chorion frondosum may be relatively less accessible and also because greater suction is required to avulse the villi.

Our policy of deliberately restricting the technique to those couples with a high genetic risk, especially the haemoglobinopathies (see Table 5.1) has limited the size of our diagnostic series. The fetal losses and failures of

Table 5.1 Indications for CVS (all cases)

	1982–83	*1984*	*1985**	*Total*
Haemoglobinopathies	19	37	21	77
Metabolic disease	1	2	1	4
Fetal sexing	–	4	–	4
Fetal Karyotyping	–	4	9	13
Total	20	47	31	98

* To 11 June 1985.

sampling have been largely confined to the early days when we were breaking new ground and had no one else's experience to draw upon. However, we were able to identify what the problems were (principally inadequate ultrasound facilities) and have since noted a dramatic improvement, with no failure and only one loss (the patient with an IUCD – *vide supra*) in the last 61 singleton pregnancies (see Table 5.2). Thus to an extent the benefit of our early experience has been available to others who subsequently set up a diagnostic CVS service.

Table 5.2 Results of CVS in singleton pregnancies

	1982–83		*1984–85*		
Patients sampled	18	20	19	20	17
Failures	3	1	0	0	0
Affected fetuses and termination of pregnancy	5	7*	5	4	3
Fetal losses	4	2	0	1†	0
Continuing pregnancies	9	11	14	15	14
Delivered	8	11‡	14§	–	–

* Two late therapeutic abortions of viable pregnancies.
† Patient had IUCD *in situ*.
‡ Stillbirth: misdiagnosis of α-thalassaemia.
§ Neo-natal death at 28 weeks.

Nevertheless the technique is now well established with several individual series of over 500 patients. A total of over 2000 diagnostic cases has been reached by combining the series from Milan (Brambati), Rotterdam (Jahoda), Philadelphia (Wapner) and Chicago (Ginsburg) (Jackson, 1985). Their low failure and fetal loss rates confirm our initial hopes that the technique would prove to be safe, reliable and readily learnt, as well as acceptable to our patients.

ACKNOWLEDGEMENTS

Many colleagues have been involved in this work. It is a pleasure for us to acknowledge the contribution of Dr J. Hooker, Dr F. Karagozlu, Dr E. Douratsos, Dr R. Penketh, Dr S. Kanokpongsukdi, Miss M. Petrou and Professor D. V. I. Faithweather. We are grateful for the co-operation of Dr W. Watson of Portex Ltd and and the invaluable suggestions of Dr I. Sutherland.

REFERENCES

Anshan Department of Obstetrics and Gynaecology. (1975) Fetal sex prediction by sex chromatin of chorionic villi cells during early pregnancy. *Chin. Med. J.*, **1**, 117.

Dozy, A. M., Forman, E. N., Abuelo, D. N., Barsel-Bowers, G., Mahoney, M. J., Forget, B. G. and Kan, Y. W. (1979) Prenatal diagnosis of homozygous α-thalassaemia. *J. Am. Med. Assoc.*, **241**, 1610–12.

Fairweather, D. V. I., Ward, R. H. T. and Modell, B. (1980) Obstetric aspects of midtrimester fetal blood sampling by needling or fetoscopy. *Brit. J. Obstet. Gynaecol.*, **87**, 87.

Garden, A. S., Reid G. and Benzie R. J. (1985) Chorionic villus sampling. *Lancet*, i, 1270.

Gilmore, D. H. and McNay, M. D. (1985) Spontaneous fetal loss rate in early pregnancy. *Lancet*, i, 107.

Gustavii, B. (1985) Chorionic biopsy and miscarriage in first trimester. *Lancet*, i, 562.

Horwell, D. H., Loeffler, F. E. and Coleman, D. V. (1983) Assessment of a transcervical aspiration technique for chorionic villus biopsy in the first timester of pregnancy. *Brit. J. Obstet. Gynaecol.*, **90**, 196.

Jackson, L. G. (1985) Chorionic villi sampling. *Newsletter*, 17 April (1985).

Kan, Y. W. and Dozy, A. M. (1978) Antenatal diagnosis of sickle cell anaemia by DNA analysis of amniotic fluid cells. *Lancet*, ii, 910.

Modell, B., Ward, R. H. T. and Fairweather, D. V. I. (1980) Effect of introducing antenatal diagnosis on reproductive behaviour of families at risk for thalassaemia major. *Brit. Med. J.*, **162**, 1347.

Old, J. M., Ward, R. H. T., Karagozlu, F., Petrou, M. and Modell, B. (1982) First trimester fetal diagnosis for haemoglobinopathies: three cases. *Lancet*, ii, 1413.

Simoni, G., Brambati, B., Danesino, C., Rossella, F., Terzoli, G. L., Ferrari, M. and Fraccaro, M. (1983) Efficient direct chromosome analysis and enzyme determinations from chorionic villi samples in the first trimester of pregnancy. *Hum. Genet.*, **63**, 349.

Ward, H., Grudzinskas, G., Bolton, A. G., Model, B., Kanakpongsukdi, S. and Petrou, M. (1985a) Chorionic villus sampling in a high risk population using the Portex catheter. In *First Trimester Fetal Diagnosis* (eds M. Fraccaro, G. Simoni and B. Brambati), Springer-Verlag, Berlin, pp. 19–24.

Ward, R. H. T., Modell, B., Petrou, M., Kanakpongsukdi, D. and Penketh R. (1985b) Fetoplacental products as a prognostic guide following chorionic villus sampling. In *First Trimester Fetal Diagnosis* (eds M. Fraccaro, G. Simoni and B. Brambati), Springer-Verlag, Berlin, pp. 19–24.

Ward, R. H. T., Modell, B., Petrou, M., Karagozlu, F. and Douratsos, E. (1983) Method of sampling chorionic villi in first trimester of pregnancy under guidance of real time ultrasound. *Brit. Med. J.*, **286**, 1542.

Williamson, R., Eskdale, J., Coleman, D. V., Niazi, N., Loeffler, F. E. and Modell, B. (1981) Direct gene analysis of chorionic villi a possible technique for first trimester antenatal diagnosis of haemoglobinopathies. *Lancet*, ii, 1125.

6

Transcervical chorion villus aspiration by a single operator technique

Richard C. Warren, Christina F. McKenzie, Lyndal Kearney and Charles H. Rodeck

6.1 INTRODUCTION

Of the estimated 8% of all pregnancies sufficiently at risk to warrant prenatal diagnosis (PND) in England and Wales (Brock, 1982) only 2–3% are investigated by mid-trimester amniocentesis (Turnbull and Mackenzie, 1983). It is likely that the demand for chorion villus sampling (CVS) will be even greater than the resulting 17 000 amniocenteses performed per annum in the United Kingdom, as a number of patients who would not consider second trimester PND because of the possibility of late therapeutic abortion may accept CVS which allows earlier, easier and safer therapeutic abortion at a time when a private decision can be taken and before fetal movements are perceived.

If first trimester prenatal diagnosis by CVS is to become widely available the technique must be a simple, quick and painless outpatient procedure. The single-operator method of CVS using a malleable silver cannula (Down's PLC) for ultrasound guided transcervical biopsy (Rodeck *et al.*, 1983) has, after the evaluation of several methods, been our preferred method of CVS and has been used for prenatal diagnosis in over 200 cases.

The Down's cannula is made of 16-gauge silver tubing and measures 23 cm in length (see Fig. 6.1). A suction control valve is positioned on the finger plate which incorporates a tubing mount with internal luer connector. A stilette passes through the lumen; its smooth rounded end protrudes 1–2 mm to allow atraumatic transcervical introduction, to prevent decidual 'coring' and to maintain the lumen during shaping. After withdrawal of the stilette, a

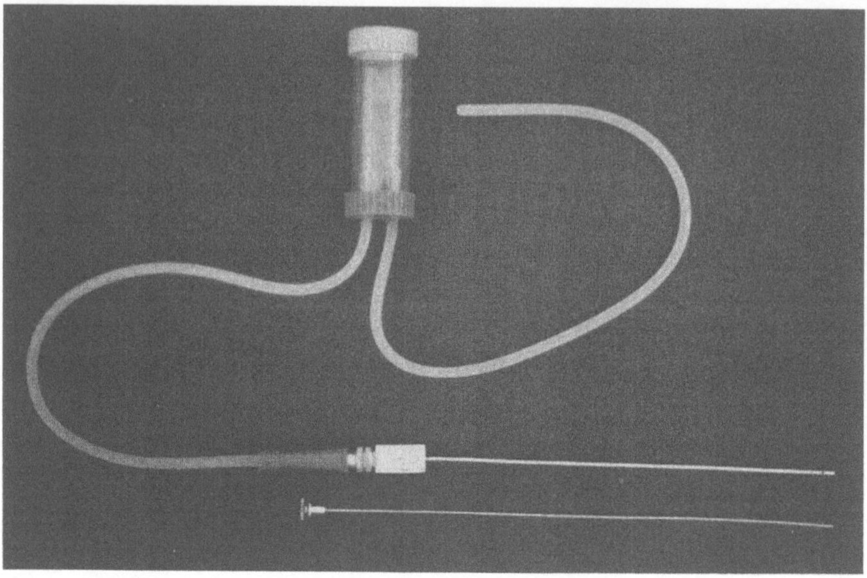

Figure 6.1 The 23 cm 16-gauge malleable silver cannula showing finger plate for suction control, and with stilette removed, is connected via a neonatal mucus aspirator to a standard vacuum pump.

disposable neonatal mucus aspirator and trap is connected to the cannula which in turn leads to a standard theatre vacuum pump.

6.2 TECHNIQUE

All patients referred for chorion villus sampling are counselled, preferably before the day of sampling. The nature of the procedure is explained in depth and the implications and risks discussed and quantified from our experience as well as from collated world experience (Jackson, 1985).

We prefer to scan all our patients one to two weeks prior to sampling to confirm gestation and subsequent adequate and expected growth of gestation sac volume and crown rump length.

The sample is performed on an out-patient basis. It is a painless procedure requiring no sedation, analgesia or anaesthesia. Ultrasound scanning confirms a single or multiple gestation, allows measurement of gestation sac volume and crown rump length and identifies the shape and position of the uterus and cervical canal. The position of the implantation site, umbilical cord insertion and yolk sac are recorded and uterine fibroids, placental lakes and evidence of haemorrhage are noted. The presence of a uterine contraction will often distort the uterine cavity as well as the apparent site and thickness of the implantation; if seen, sampling should be delayed until the contraction regresses.

Sampling takes place with the patient comfortably positioned on a colposcopy couch. To avoid unnecessary embarrassment, we restrict those in attendance to an absolute minimum, viz. one assistant and one 'visitor' under instruction. Because of the intimacy of the examination it is also preferable if the operator has previously met and counselled the patient.

Careful and thorough cleansing of the vulva, inner thigh and vagina is essential and is performed using chlorhexidine solution; the vagina is then irrigated with normal saline and dried thoroughly.

The silver cannula with stilette *in situ* is bent to shape according to the uterine position and implantation site within. Once inserted into the cervical canal the passage of the highly echogenic cannula is monitored closely by ultrasound from the external cervical os onwards. The operator guides the cannula with the forefinger and thumb of one hand while holding the ultrasound transducer through the sterile drapes in the other. This technique avoids the necessity of having additional skilled personnel with ultrasound experience in attendance and allows easy and accurate guidance of the catheter tip as it is passed around the gestation sac into the implantation site. Rarely, an assistant may be useful to maintain cervical traction or adjust a speculum but the majority of samplings can be performed quite simply by a single operator.

Once in position within the implantation site the stilette is carefully removed. Sampling is achieved by attaching a neonatal mucus aspirator connected to a standard theatre vacuum pump. Suction is commenced and may be controlled by finger tip occlusion of the hole in the finger plate. The cannula, being metal, maintains its shape on withdrawal of the stilette, and fine accurate control of the cannula tip is possible. Aspiration (400–500 mmHg) continues for approximately 30 seconds with a limited 'hoovering' action over a few millimetres along the path of insertion – side to side and up and down movement is avoided to reduce the risk of damage to the placenta. Suction is discontinued as the cannula is withdrawn from the implantation. The cannula is then removed carefully while still under ultrasound guidance.

The sampled villi are flushed from within the lumen of the cannula into the mucus trap by gentle aspiration of tissue culture medium. Naked eye inspection can confirm the presence of chorionic villi but microscopic examination is essential to confirm quantity and quality of the specimen as well as to enable removal of decidual contamination.

6.3 RESULTS/DISCUSSION

Of 226 referrals, 15 had spontaneous pregnancy losses before consultation, eight had losses diagnosed on ultrasound at preliminary consultation and three were unsuitable for sampling because of threatened abortion with heavy vaginal bleeding at the planned time of sampling. Two hundred patients proceeded to CVS (Table 6.5).

Table 6.1 shows the indications for sampling which are further detailed in Tables 6.2, 6.3 and 6.4.

Initial restriction of CVS to those at high risk of congenital disease has subsequently been modified as improved safety has been achieved; pregnancy

Table 6.1 Indications for diagnostic chorion villus sampling (CVS)

Karyotyping	96
DNA analysis	79
Inborn errors of metabolism	25
Total	200

Table 6.2 Diagnostic chorion villus sampling (CVS)

Karyotyping	
Maternal age	35
Previous affected child	40
Abnormal parental chromosomes	11
Fetal sexing	10
Total	96

Table 6.3 Diagnostic chorion villus sampling (CVS) DNA analysis

Fetal sexing	
Duchenne muscular dystrophy	30
Haemophilia A	4
Ornithine carbamyl transferase deficiency	3
X-linked mental retardation	9
Centronuclear myopathy	1
Incontinentia pigmentii	1
Norrie disease	1
X-linked micropenis	1
Haemoglobinopathies	
Sickle cell disease	16
β-thalassaemia	8
Haemophilias	
Haemophilia A	4
Others	
Alpha-1 antitrypsin deficiency	1
Total	79

Table 6.4 Diagnostic chorion villus sampling (CVS) metabolic disorders

Gaucher's disease	2
Niemann–Pick disease	1
Tay–Sachs disease	3
Metachromatic leukodystrophy	2
Sandhoff disease	2
Hurler's disease	4
Sanfilippo 'A' disease	1
Multiple sulphatase deficiency	2
Pompe's disease	1
Maple Syrup Urine disease	1
Citrullinaemia	1
Congenital hypophosphatasia	1
Hunter's disease	1
Glutaric aciduria type I	1
GMI Gangliosidosis	1
β-glucuronidase deficiency	1
Total	25

Table 6.5 Outcome of diagnostic chorion villus sampling (CVS)

Total number of patients	200	
Successful sampling	197	(98.5%)
Repeat sampling	7	(3.5%)
Outcome		
Abortion/intra-uterine death	11	(7.1† – 5.5%*)
Therapeutic abortion	44	(22%)
Continuing pregnancies	145	(72.5%)
undelivered	79	
delivered	66	

* As % of procedures.
† As % of continuing.

losses have fallen from 16.7% of continuing pregnancies in the first 50 cases to 4.2% in the subsequent 150 samples (Table 6.6). Such improvement comes from research experience and improvements in technique and operator skill. Indeed the recent low level of pregnancy losses after sampling is similar to the calculated 3.3% background risk of spontaneous abortion prior to 16 weeks (Christiaens and Stowtenbeek, 1984). The combined world experience (Jackson, 1985) reports similar results, with those centres with the greatest experience reporting the lowest losses. Such figures, however, are cumulative and include the heavier losses experienced in those centres which pioneered the research and development of CVS.

The demand for CVS has recently increased considerably. The majority of referrals are now for those at lower risk, viz. advanced maternal age.

Although we perform a direct chromosome preparation after a 48-hour culture we have not been as successful as Simoni *et al.* (1983) in obtaining good quantity and quality chromosomes and therefore rely on cultured cells for a definitive result (Heaton *et al.*, 1984). The use of 'Y' specific probes for fetal sexing (Table 6.3) (Gosden *et al.*, 1982) has been superseded by cheaper and quicker 'direct' karyotyping.

At King's we have on-site facilities for karyotyping and for the use of 'Y' specific probes. A diverse PND service, however, requires the collaboration of a number of specialized centres. Dr J. Old (The John Radcliffe Hospital, Oxford) has performed the DNA diagnosis of haemoglobinopathies (Table 6.3) and Professor A. D. Patrick (Institute of Child Health, London) and Dr A. Fensom (Guy's Hospital, London) have carried out biochemical analysis of a variety of inborn errors of metabolism (Table 6.4). The number of inborn errors of metabolism amenable to first trimester diagnosis is extensive. In this field alone we maintain a policy of confirmatory amniocentesis in all continuing pregnancies to complement the analysis of direct and of cultured chorionic villi.

Most centres agree that the optimum time for sampling lies between 8 and 12 weeks. Before eight weeks the implantation site is poorly localized and thin, active embryogenesis is occurring and any damage to the implantation at biopsy represents a relatively larger area. The reason for an upper gestation limit is less clear; in our early experience after the first 35 samplings, we suffered six pregnancy losses. Of these, two of the four performed at less than eight weeks gestation and two of four at greater than 12 weeks resulted in pregnancy loss. Nevertheless, when referral has been late, we have subsequently performed sampling without complication on a number of occasions after 12 weeks gestation. Apart from difficulty in reaching a fundal implantation in the larger uterus, it has become apparent that even when sampling within the implantation site, which is easily distinguishable in the more advanced pregnancy, a successful biopsy cannot be guaranteed; possibly the villi themselves become more organized and with mesenchymal differentiation, stronger and more resistant to aspiration. We are at present assessing a longer and slightly larger bore cannula as well as sampling forceps for use in such cases.

We have found a very full bladder to be a disadvantage; it pushes the uterus upwards, makes it less mobile and causes anterior vaginal wall ballooning making cervical visualization more difficult. Some urine in the bladder is, however, usually required to act as an ultrasound 'window' for clear visualization.

Manipulation of the uterus by bladder filling, cervical traction or by digital examination may be indicated where there is acute ante- or retroflexion. Such manoeuvres may make the passage of the cannula easier by straightening the required path. The effect of these measures is usually minimal on the steeply retroverted uterus which is best left for one to two weeks before attempt at sampling, by which time uterine growth has invariably straightened the necessary pathway.

After sampling 60% of our patients had some revealed vaginal bleeding. Usually this was only spotting and in those who have been examined the source of bleeding has nearly always been from the site of application of the cervical tenaculum. Nevertheless, our recent study (Warren *et al.*, 1985) has shown that, following sampling, 49% of patients had a significant rise in maternal serum alpha fetoprotein (MSAFP). Although Kleihauer–Betke tests were always negative, such a rise in MSAFP must be taken to represent a small fetomaternal haemorrhage and therefore we recommend that all rhesus negative women having CVS receive anti-D immunoglobulin prophylaxis.

It seems likely that repeated passages of the cannula in an attempt to obtain sufficient villi for diagnosis is associated with increased risk of pregnancy loss. We now limit the number of passages to two (rarely three). As laboratory experience in handling CVS specimens has increased so we have noticed a fall in the size of sample required for analysis. In conjunction with this, improvements in CVS technique and operator experience has significantly reduced the number of attempts necessary to obtain a suitable sized sample.

In the last 150 cases (Table 6.6) we failed to achieve an adequate specimen on three occasions and six patients had to re-attend before sampling was successful. Of the three failures, two patients were over 12 weeks and only two passages were carried out in each. The third patient was extremely obese and the procedure was technically so difficult that it was curtailed after a single unsuccessful attempt. Those patients required to re-attend, owing to difficulties related to uterine position and implantation site, returned for sampling one to two weeks later; in all cases sampling was then successful at the first attempt.

Table 6.6 Diagnostic chorion villus sampling (CVS) outcome

	First 50 cases		*Subsequent 150*	
	n	*(%)*	*n*	*(%)*
Success within three attempts	45	90	147	98
Repeat procedures	1	2	6	4
Failed sample	0	0	3	2
Therapeutic abortion	14	28	30	20
Spontaneous abortion/IUD	6	12	5	3.3
Continuing pregnancies	30	60	115	77
Loss as % of procedures		12%		3.3%
Loss as % of continuing		16.7%		4.2%

Although the transcervical route has been criticized because of the potential risk of introducing infection (Garden *et al.*, 1985), we, like many centres, have had no cases of septic abortion or infected culture. Our pre-sampling cleaning regime is meticulous, including drying the vagina; the cannula must then be introduced into the cervical canal without touching the vaginal walls.

Recognition of the difficult sample is not always possible. Careful ultrasound assessment immediately prior to sampling is nevertheless essential. We have often been surprised how even small changes in the patient's position and posture can effectively change the required path of the cannula. The careful guidance of the cannula from its insertion through the cervical canal to the implantation site is of critical importance; unnecessary or incorrect manipulation must be avoided during introduction and withdrawal.

The 'single operator technique' is simple and easy to learn and practise. Such advantages are extremely important if the anticipated workload of CVS is to be achieved. Further multi-centre evaluation (*Lancet*, 1985) is awaited to see whether the early success and safety of CVS will be confirmed. Comparison of the short-term and possible long-term effects of CVS with those of amniocentesis by a randomized study is planned and is a vital part of this evaluation.

ACKNOWLEDGEMENTS

Richard Warren and Christina McKenzie are supported by Medical Research Council grant No. 8209273 CA.

REFERENCES

Brock, D. J. H. (1982) In *Early Diagnosis of Fetal Defects. Current Reviews in Obstetrics and Gynaecology*, vol. 2. Churchill Livingstone, London.

Christiaens, G. C. M. L. and Stowtenbeek, Ph. (1984) *Lancet*, ii, 571–2.

Garden, A. S., Reid G. and Benzie R. J. (1985) *Lancet*, i, 1270.

Gosden, J. R., Mitchell A. R., Gosden C. M., Rodeck C. H. and Morsman J. M. (1982) *Lancet*, ii, 1416–19.

Heaton, D. E., Czepulkowski B. H., Horwell D. H. and Coleman D. V. (1984) *Prenat. Diagn.*, 4, 279–87.

Jackson, L. (1985) Chorionic Villus Sampling Newsletter. Personal communication.

Lancet leading article (1985) *Lancet*, i, 735–6.

Rodeck, C. H., Morsman J. M., Nicolaides K. H., McKenzie F. C., Gosden C. M. and Gosden J. R. (1983) *Lancet*, ii, 1340–1.

Simoni, G., Brambati B., Danesino C., Rossella F., Terzoli G. L., Ferrari M. and Fraccaro M. (1983) *Hum. Genet.*, 63, 349–57.

Turnbull, A. C. and MacKenzie I. Z. (1983) *Br. Med. Bull.*, 39(4), 315–21.

Warren R. C., Butler J., McKenzie F. C., Morsman J. M. and Rodeck C. H. (1985). *Lancet*, i, 691.

7

Tipped metal cannulae

—— W. E. MacKenzie and J. R. Newton ——

7.1 INTRODUCTION

Transcervical chorion villus sampling is the most popular technique in diagnostic antenatal practice. In a report of a survey of 56 centres offering chorion villus sampling (CVS), it was found that 55 were using a transcervical method as the preferred technique (Jackson, 1985). The most favoured procedure is aspiration of chorionic villi through a cannula, which is passed into the placental site using real-time ultrasound visualization.

The instrument first described – Portex Trophocan – consisted of a plastic outer sheath with an inner aluminium obturator which added malleability as well as enhancing the instrument's image on the ultrasound screen (Ward, 1983).

As experience with this device was gained in clinical practice, certain problems were encountered. First, the plastic cannula lost its malleability and shape after the aluminium obturator was withdrawn. Accurate identification of the tip of the device on the ultrasound image was lost after the obturator was withdrawn, and the tip of the plastic cannula moved as the curved aluminium obturator was withdrawn. This shift in the tip cannot be seen on ultrasound and therefore the original position can be lost.

In an attempt to remedy the problems, we designed two cannulae and subsequently compared them in a randomized cannula study with the Portex cannula (MacKenzie *et al.*, 1986).

7.2 CHARACTERISTICS OF THE METAL CANNULAE

Both cannulae were designed with certain objects in mind, namely:

1. Malleability, i.e. the ability to retain shape when bent to the curve of the utero-cervical canal.
2. Good ultrasound visualization especially the tip of the cannula.

Chorion Villus Sampling. Edited by D. T. Y. Liu, E. M. Symonds and M. S. Golbus. Published in 1987 by Chapman and Hall Ltd, 11 New Fetter Lane, London EC4P 4EE.
© 1987 Chapman and Hall.

3. Small diameter, such that minimal stretching of the cervical canal would be necessary.
4. Easily sterilized.
5. Ease of use by a single operator using one hand to insert the cannula and the other to operate the ultrasound transducer.

Two cannulae were subsequently designed. In one, made of malleable stainless steel, the tip was olive shaped to enhance its ultrasonic visualization. In the other, made of aluminium, the tip was rounded. Both cannulae had opposing 'eyes' through which villi could be sucked (Fig. 7.1 and Table 7.1). These cannulae were tested to determine the vacuum developed along them when 10 cc of suction was applied. Each cannula was tested five times using a Sensym LX0503A pressure transducer linked by a three-way tap. The results of this test can be seen in Table 7.2.

The Portex and malleable stainless steel cannulae were found to have a higher negative pressure than the aluminium cannulae. This could lead to fragmentation and destruction of villi more often than with the aluminium cannulae.

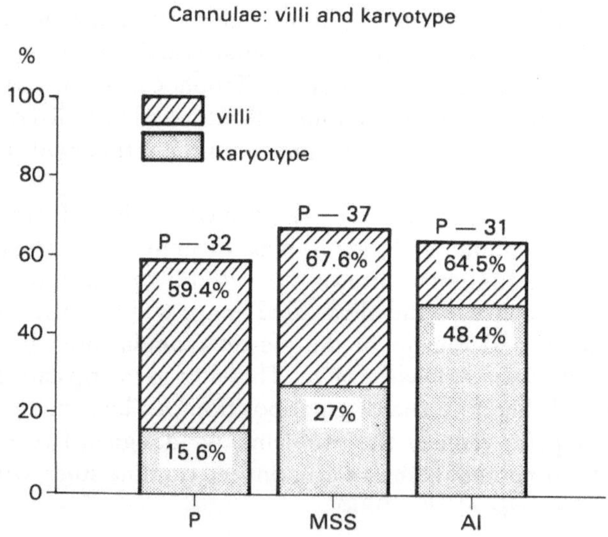

P — procedures
1 procedure = 2 Sampling attempts

	Chi squared	p
Villus recovery	0.5	$p > 0.05$
Karyotype success	8.3	$0.05 > p > 0.01$

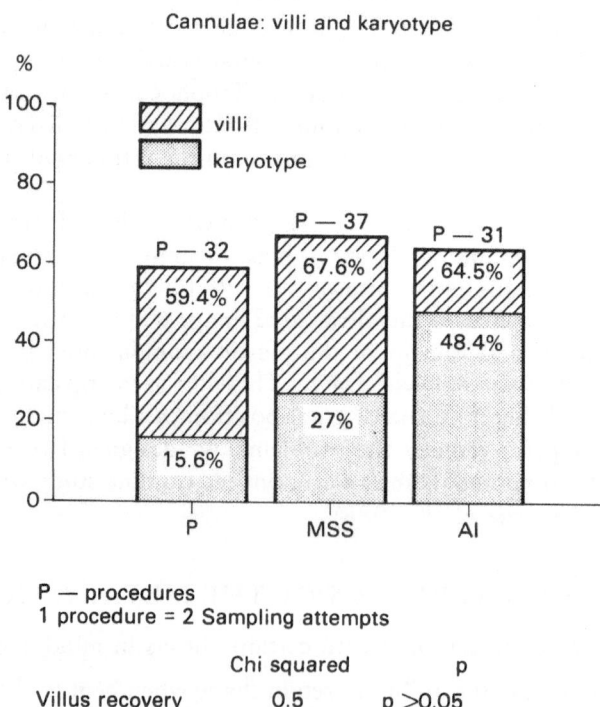

Figure 7.1 Cannulae: villi and karyotype.

Table 7.1 Characteristics of cannulae

	Length (mm)	*Internal diameter (mm)*	*Outer diameter (mm)*
Tipped cannula (MSS)†	210	1.80*	2.70
Aluminium cannula (AL)†	210	1.30	2.30

* At olive tip.
† Manufactured by Rocket of London.

Table 7.2 Suction pressures of cannulae

Cannula	*Pressure (mmHg) 10 ml syringe*		
	Mean	*Standard error*	*Dead space volume (ml)*
Portex	−671.40	0.25	0.6
MSS	−671.40	0.25	0.7
AL	−659.40	0.25	0.8

7.3 RANDOMIZED CANNULAE STUDY

In a randomized cannulae study, involving 200 chorionic villus samples taken without analgesia or anaesthesia between 8–11 weeks gestation, reported elsewhere, it was found that there was a variation in the ability of each of these cannulae to recover villi (MacKenzie, 1986). This is further reflected in the subsequent karyotype success which was recorded for each cannula (Fig. 7.1 and Table 7.3).

Previous reports have indicated that 10 mg or greater of villus material is required for reliable karyotyping (Simoni, 1983) and in Table 7.3 from our randomized cannulae study we found that the metal cannulae consistently recovered > 10 mg of villi two to three times better than the Portex cannula. A further study was carried out to assess the variation in villus recovery depending on the placental site, as assessed on ultrasound. From our

Table 7.3 Villus recovery by weight

	% of samples where villi obtained			
Weight of villi (mg)	*<5*	*5–10*	*>10*	*Total no. samples*
Portex	31.5	15.6	12.5	64
MSS	32.4	8.1	27.0	74
AL	12.9	16.1	35.5	62
Total	26.0	13.0	25.0	200

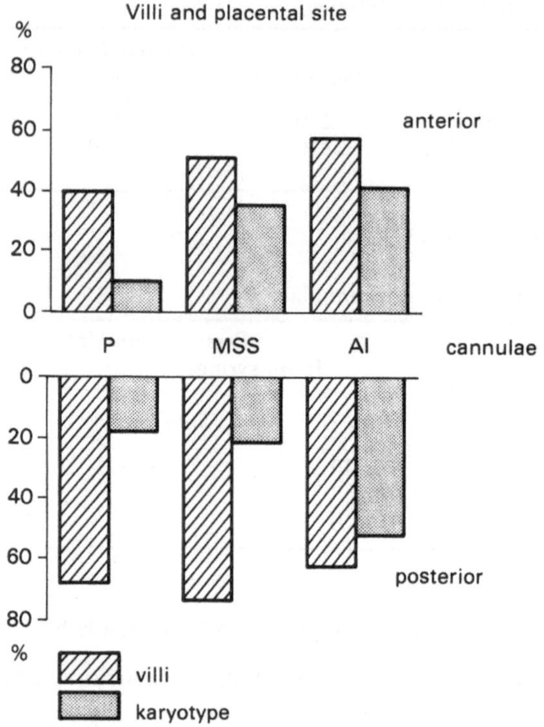

	F	P
Villi obtained	6.2	>0.05
Karyotype success	0.7	>0.05

Figure 7.2 Villi and placental site.

randomized study the effect of an anteriorly or posteriorly sited placenta can be seen in Fig. 7.2. Although there was little difference in the ability of any of the cannulae to obtain villi from a posteriorly sited placenta, there is a marked difference in the ability of the Portex cannula to obtain villi in an anteriorly sited placenta.

7.4 CONCLUSIONS

We have found in a randomized cannula study that in terms of overall villus recovery and subsequent karyotyping success, a malleable metal cannula produces consistently better results than a Portex flexible plastic cannula. This is especially so when the placental site is anteriorly placed. Subsequent work has shown that it may be preferable to apply a transabdominal technique to anteriorly or fundally placed placentae rather than a transcervical technique, which we feel is more suited for sampling villi from posteriorly sited placentae.

REFERENCES

Jackson, L. (1985) *Chorionic Villus Sampling Newsletter*, 17 April.

MacKenzie, W. E., Holmes, D. S., Webb, T., Whitehouse, C. and Newton, J. R. (1986) A randomised study of three cannulae for transcervical chorionic villus sampling. *Am. J. Obstet. Gynecol.*, **154**, 34–9.

Simoni, G., Brambati, B. *et al.* (1983) Efficient direct chromosome analyses and enzyme determinations from chorionic villi samples in the first trimester of pregnancy. *Hum. Genet.*, **63**, 349–57.

Ward, R. H. T., Modell, B., Petrou, M. *et al.* (1983) Method of sampling chorionic villi in first trimester of pregnancy under guidance of real time ultrasound. *Br. Med. J.*, **283**, 1542–4.

8

The Nottingham brush for chorion villus sampling

— David T. Y. Liu and E. Malcolm Symonds —

In the first trimester the embryo is enveloped in a dense coat of chorionic villi. This villus coat is maintained until after the 12th week when enlargement of the gestation sac and its approximation to the uterine wall results in attenuation of most of this material, apart from the chorion frondosum which develops to form the definitive placenta. Chorionic villi are filamentous in nature and access to it is readily available via the transcervical route. It is, therefore, conceivable that a small brush can be introduced through the cervix to entwine and subsequently retrieve chorionic villi for prenatal diagnosis. We describe our experience in advancing this concept to fashion an implement suitable for clinical application.

8.1 THE IMPLEMENT

The Nottingham chorion villus sampling brush is designed in conjunction with Rockets of London Ltd. The implement consists of a brush, and an introducer with its obturator (Fig. 8.1). Nylon bristles are pleated into place by two entwined strands of malleable wire (diameter 0.38 mm) to produce the 1–1.2 cm brush with a width of 3.0 mm (Fig. 8.2). The brush is 22 cm in total length and allows easy access to the fundus of a 12-week gestation uterus without the operator's hand having to encroach into the vagina. A plastic knob mounted on the caudal end facilitates rotation of the brush for collection of villi (Fig 8.1). The brush is delivered to the chosen sampling site by a 13-gauge hollow steel introducer (length 20 cm; diameter 2.4 mm). An imprinted curve towards the tip of the introducer assists introduction through the cervix and direction to the sampling site in both the anteverted and retroverted uterus. An obturator is used during introduction to minimize

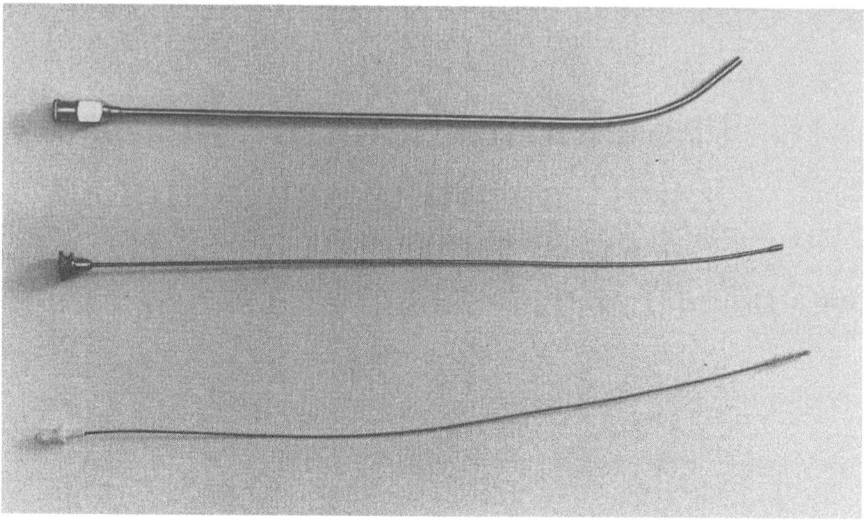

Figure 8.1 Brush, introducer and obturator.

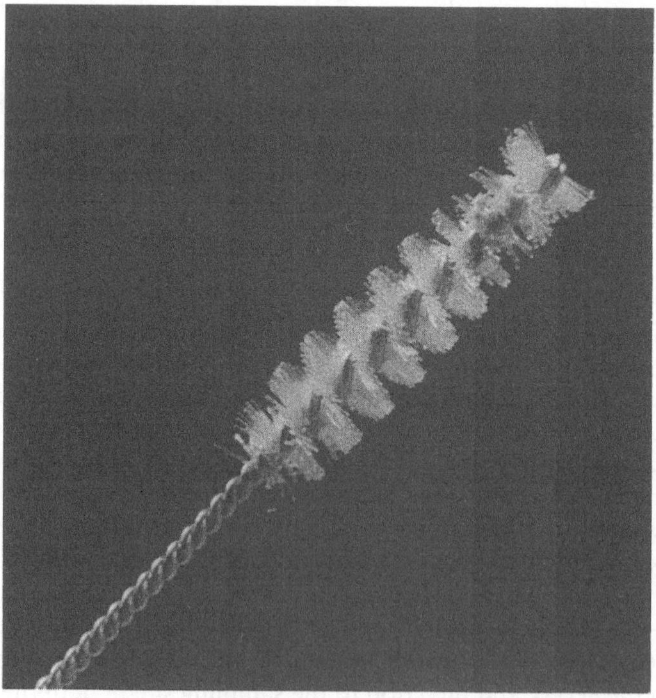

Figure 8.2 The brush.

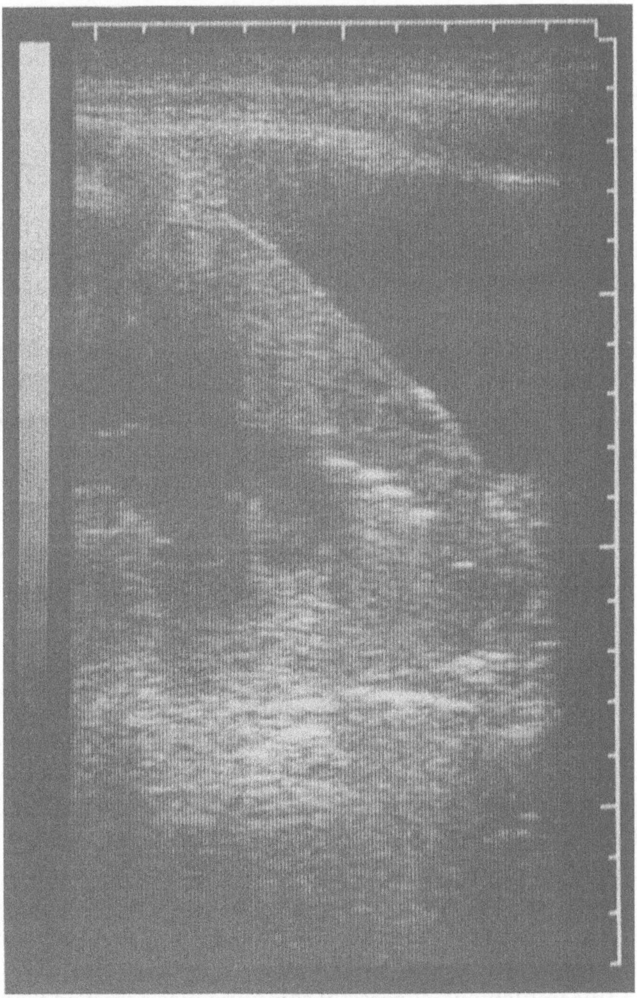

Figure 8.3 Localization of brush by ultrasound.

trauma to both cervical canal and intra-uterine structures. The highly echogenic metal introducer and air trapped among the bristles of the brush ensure easy localization of this implement by ultrasound (Figure 8.3).

8.2 TECHNIQUE

Before sampling an ultrasound examination is performed to determine gestational age and an appropriate sampling site, and to ensure normality. A full bladder is found to be most helpful and patients are thus advised accordingly. Sampling is conducted with the patient in the lithotomy position. Detailed explanation of the procedure is offered. No premedication or anaesthetic is used. Ultrasound scanning (Hitashi, EUB-25) with a 3.5 megaHertz probe is maintained to direct the brush to the area where chorionic villi is most abundant. Neither a vosellum nor dilatation of the cervix was found necessary for introduction of the brush. The obturator is withdrawn once the introducer is correctly sited. The brush is designed to protrude beyond the introducer. This fact must be taken into account to avoid unnecessary damage or inadvertent perforation of the gestation sac. When the brush is in position gentle rotation of the plastic knob clockwise and anti-clockwise through 180° helps gather the villus tissue. The brush is withdrawn into the introducer before removal through the cervix. This precaution avoids lost of sample material and reduces contamination by maternal cells. Collected material is teased from the brush into a Petri dish containing normal saline for examination under a phase contrast microscope. One sample attempt is usually all that is required to obtain sufficient villi for diagnostic purposes. Electron microscopic examination suggests this method of collection does not damage the chorionic villi.

8.3 RESULTS

In our study with 83 informed and consenting patients requesting first trimester termination of pregnancy, passage of the implement through the cervix, localization by ultrasound and guidance to the sampling site were all found to be relatively easy (Liu *et al.*, 1985). The procedure was found to be well accepted by patients when performed in an out-patient setting. A gentle curve at the tip of the non-malleable introducer assists ready direction to the sampling site. Easy localization contributed to the fact that no gestation sac was perforated. Like other techniques, collection of villus material was most successful from gestations between 9 and 11 weeks. In the initial phase of our experience with this implement, successful sampling was achieved from 65% of patients (Table 8.1). As with other techniques further practice resulted in collection rates in excess of 80%. Since techniques which can successfully retrieve villus material more than 80% of the time are considered suitable for diagnostic usage (Ward *et al.*, 1983; Simoni *et al.*, 1983) it is anticipated that the brush will find clinical application.

Some bleeding associated with 89% of sampling attempts was the major complication of concern. Although most of the bleeding was of a minor degree and merely produced a faint discoloration of the normal saline in the receiving Petri dish, the incidence is more than 58% observed when blind aspiration was used for collection of villi (Liu *et al.*, 1983). Bleeding following 3.6% of samples was considered excessive (Table 8.1).

Table 8.1 Chorionic villus collection and associated bleeding at various gestations using a brush technique

Chorionic villi				*Bleeding*		
Gestation in weeks	*Patients studied*	*No*	*Yes*	*Nil or minimal*	*Moderate*	*Heavy*
7 or less	8	3	5	8	–	–
8	17	4	13	14	3	–
9	6	2	4	4	1	1
10	26	10	16	21	4	1
11	16	4	12	10	5	1
12 or more	10	6	4	6	4	–
Total	83	29	54	63	17	3
Percentage		35	65	76	20	4

8.4 CONCLUSION

Many implements and techniques have been suggested for chorion villus sampling (Rodeck and Morsman, 1983). The question of a safe level of negative pressure and the potential for added trauma and infection following multiple sampling attempts is inherent in the aspiration technique (Ward *et al.*, 1983; Simoni *et al.*, 1983; Liu *et al.*, 1983; Liu *et al.*, 1984). Our experience has shown that the brush can be adapted for villus sampling and since acceptable collection rate following a single sampling attempt is achieved, this alternative approach has clinical potential and deserves consideration for early prenatal diagnosis.

REFERENCES

Liu, D. T. Y., Mitchell, J., Johnson, J. and Wass, D. M. (1983) Trophoblast sampling by blind transcervical aspiration. *Br. J. Obstet. Gynaecol.*, **90**, 1119–23.

Liu, D. T. Y., Slater, E. and Norman, S. (1984) Aspiration as a technique for biopsy of chorionic villi. *J. Obstet. and Gynaecol.*, **5**, 75–7.

Liu, D. T. Y., Symonds, E. M., Jeavons, B. and Norman, S. (1985) Transcervical chorion villus biopsy with a brush. *Prenat. Diag.*, **5**, 349–55.

Rodeck, C. H. and Morsman, J. M. (1983) First trimester chorion biopsy. *Br. Med. Bull.*, **39**, 338–42.

Simoni, G., Brambati, B., Danesino, C., Rosella, F., Terzoli, G. L., Ferrari, M. and Fraccaro, M. (1983) Efficient direct chromosome analysis and enzyme determination from chorionic villi samples in the first trimester of pregnancy. *Hum. Genet.*, **63**, 349–57.

Ward, R. H. T., Modell, B., Petrou, M., Karagozlu, F. and Douratsos, E. (1983) Method of sampling chorionic villi in first trimester of pregnancy under guidance of real-time ultrasound. *Br. Med. J.*, **286**, 1542–4.

9

Chorion villus sampling using rigid forceps

M. Dommergues and Y. Dumez

9.1 INTRODUCTION

The original method of chorion villus sampling developed in our centre consists of a transcervical sampling using rigid forceps under ultrasound guidance. This technique is simple and efficient. Although the number of cases is still limited, the decreasing trend of the fetal loss rate seems to confirm the safety of the procedure.

9.2 MATERIAL AND METHODS

Our diagnostic experience started in December 1982, and, by June 1985, 200 procedures had been performed. Informed consent was obtained from all couples. Apart from the gestational age which was required to be less than 12 weeks of amenorrhoea, no obstetrical criterion led to the exclusion of any patient.

9.2.1 Material

The sampling forceps manufactured by Stortz (ref. 8. 591 A, paediatric device), is 25 cm long and 2 mm in diameter. It is resistant, easy to clean and sterilize, and can be operated by a single hand. It is highly echogenic, and can be easily and accurately located on the ultrasound scan, throughout the whole procedure.

The tip of the closed forceps is smooth and rounded, so it can be atraumatically introduced through the cervix, to the sampling site. The jaws open wide enough to be seen on the ultrasound scan and will grasp an adequate amount of chorionic tissue. The scanner used is a Toshiba SAL 22, real-time linear electronic scanning, with a 3.5 MHz probe.

The remaining testing material comes in a standardized sterile pack and includes an autostatic speculum (single posterior valve), a Pozzi tenaculum and containers for antiseptic solution and sampling medium.

9.2.2 Method

This method is suitable only as an outpatient procedure. No anaesthesia or premedication is needed and cervical dilatation is not necessary. A single operator, assisted by a trained nurse, can perform the whole procedure in a relatively short time. A vaginal and cervical bacteriological swab is taken a few days before sampling. This may lead to the need for preoperative treatment. An ultrasound scan is made immediately before the sampling to assess gestation, fetal viability, the number of embryos, placental location, uterine position and any ovular or uterine anomalies. The patient is placed in the lithotomy position, and the external genitalia, vagina and cervix are cleansed with an antiseptic solution. The autostatic speculum is gently inserted, and each stage of the procedure is explained to the patient to encourage relaxation.

The cervix is grasped with a Pozzi tenaculum to allow modification of the

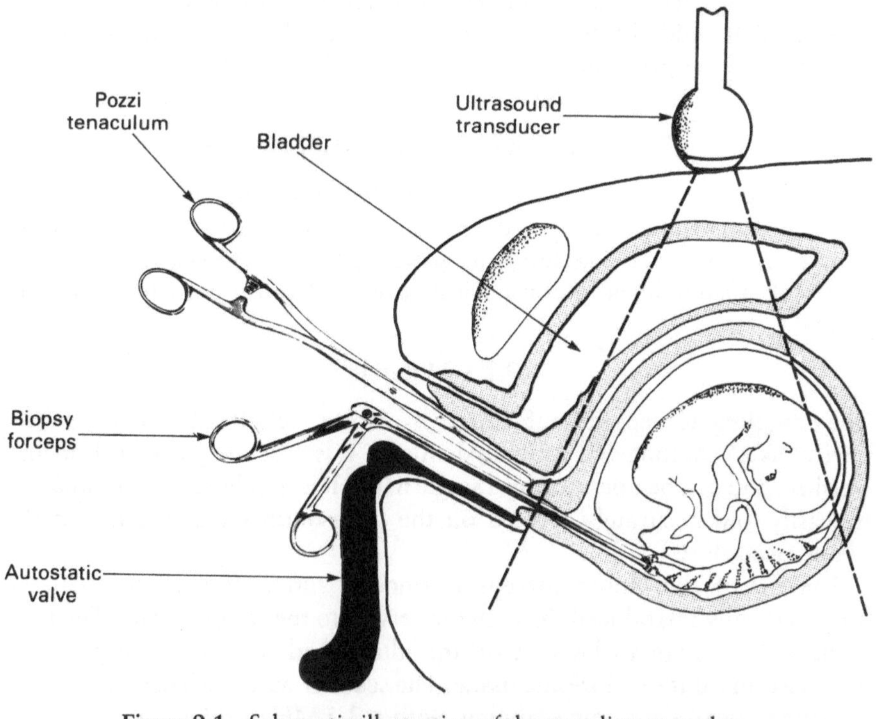

Figure 9.1 Schematic illustration of the sampling procedure.

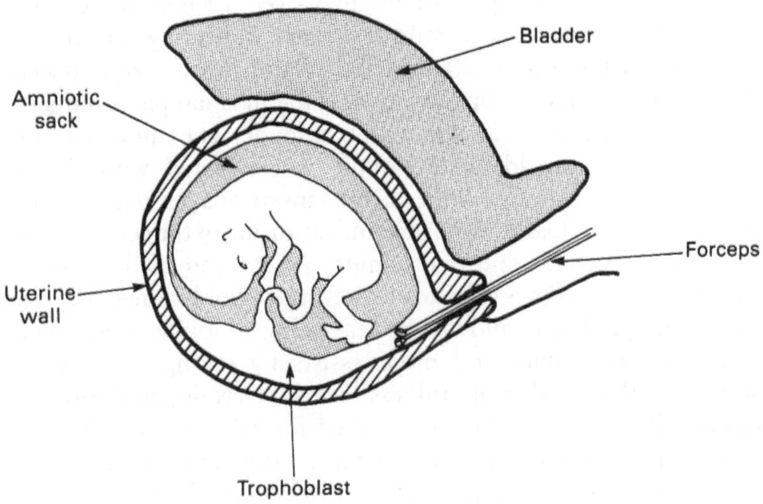

Figure 9.2 Opened forceps.

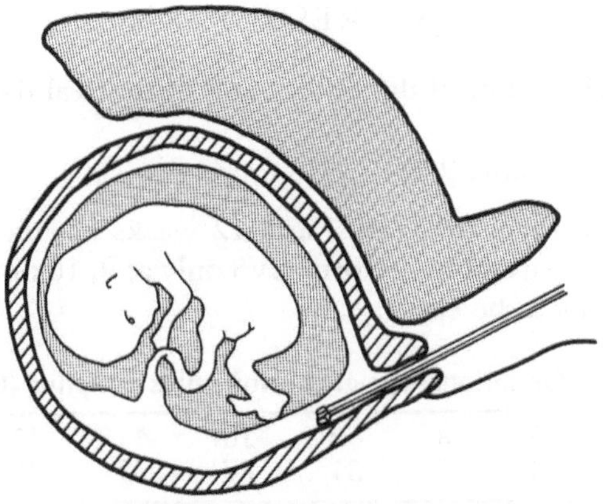

Figure 9.3 Closed forceps.

orientation of the uterus. This is the only slightly painful step of the procedure. The ultrasound transducer is then aligned to produce an image of the internal os and the thickest part of the trophoblast. The fullness of the bladder is not important. The closed forceps are pushed very slowly through the cervix. Progression of the forceps tip from the internal os towards the thickest part of the trophoblast is easily followed on the ultrasound screen. When the most echogenic zone, nearly in contact with the chorionic plate is reached, the forceps are opened, whilst being moved slowly forward. The jaws are then closed, grasping the base of the villi. The forceps detach from the villi when they are carefully withdrawn.

With experience, the operator learns to see a small depression on the chorionic plate, and to feel a mild resistance indicating the success of the sampling. The villus is immediately checked and, if necessary, dissected from the decidua under microscopic control. If the first sample is not sufficient a second and sometimes a third insertion is made. The number of insertions needed to obtain an adequate sample is correlated with the technical difficulty of the sampling. A limit of three insertions per patient is imposed.

The sampling itself, after exposure and cleansing of the cervix usually takes between thirty seconds and one minute. At the end of the procedure the ultrasound examination is repeated to detect trophoblast hematoma and fetal viability. The patient is allowed to leave the sampling room immediately following the procedure and often assists by taking the sample to the laboratory. Although their usefulness seems uncertain, antibiotics and anti-spasmodic drugs are routinely prescribed for 10 days. If indicated, anti-D antibodies are administered to prevent fetomaternal rhesus isoimmunization. An ultrasound scan is repeated two to three weeks later.

9.3 RESULTS

9.3.1 Technical difficulties and obstetrical data

Gestational age (see Table 9.1)

Sampling was performed between 7 and 12 weeks of amenorrhoea. With experience, it became usual to perform CVS only at 9, 10 or 11 weeks, when the procedure seems to be easier.

Table 9.1 Gestational age at chorion villus sampling (CVS)

Weeks	7	8	9	10	11	12
n	1	5	31	87	49	27

Placental location and uterine position (see Tables 9.2 and 9.3)

No correlation could be demonstrated between these data and the number of forceps insertions. Nevertheless, the only sampling failure in this series occurred in a patient with lateral placental implantation, which we subjectively consider as the least convenient placental location.

Other obstetrical data

Eight women were older than 38 years. In ten cases bleeding of uterine origin was noticed before sampling. Nine myomas were discovered at the

Table 9.2 Placental location and number of attempts

	Location				
Insertions	*Post.*	*Ant.*	*Fund.*	*Lat.*	
1	58	58	26	13	NS
2	7	5	3	1	
3	13	7	7	2+1*	

* Failure.

Table 9.3 Uterus position and number of attempts

	Position			
Insertions	*Ant.*	*Retro.*	*Indiff.*	
1	99	22	33	NS
2	8	5	3	
3	15	8	7	

ultrasound examination. None of these conditions seemed to be correlated with technical difficulties or with a higher risk of fetal loss, but the number of cases studied is limited. Two pairs of twins underwent chorion villus sampling. The sampling was taken near the cord insertion of each fetus.

9.3.2 Quality of samples (see Table 9.4)

Weight of samples

The weight of the samples was evaluated as described by Simoni and Brambati (visual comparison with photographs of samples of known weight). 94% of the samples weighed over 10 mg, and all were sufficient to achieve the required biological assays.

Table 9.4 Quality of samples (n=200)

Quality		*n*
Pure		183 (91.5%)
Mixed		15
<10% decidua	8	
10% – 50% decidua	4	
>50% decidua	3	
Bloody		1
Failure		1

Decidual contamination (see Table 9.4)

91.5% of the samples were not contaminated by decidua. The contaminated fragments were easily separated under the dissecting microscope.

Sampling failure

In one case with lateral placentation at ten weeks of amenorrhoea it was impossible to obtain any villus after three forceps insertions.

9.3.3 Obstetrical follow up (see Table 9.5)

Fetal loss rate

There were nine fetal losses. Six fetal deaths were discovered at the planned ultrasound scan two to three weeks after sampling. In three patients, clinical features of miscarriage occurred between one and three weeks after sampling. In one case, a pseudomolar aspect of the chorion was suggestive of a triploidy.

Infection was obvious in three cases. No clear explanation was detected in the other patients. In one of these three cases, the mother had shown symptoms of influenza when the sampling was performed, and in two patients, the sampling was considered technically difficult.

Therapeutic abortion

The high rate of therapeutic abortion is explained by the high genetic risk in our patient population. 55 pregnancies (27.5% of cases) were interrupted by vacuum suction or prostaglandin administration.

Continuing pregnancies

79 pregnancies continued without complication and 57 women have now been delivered.

Table 9.5 Obstetrical follow up

Spontaneous abortion	9
Therapeutic abortion	55
Continuing pregnancy	79
Delivered	57
Bleeding >2 days	5
Hematoma	4
Amniotic fluid leakage	0
Abruptio placenta	0
Premature labor	3
Small for date	2

Some minor complications were observed. Five patients showed vaginal bleeding for more than two days after the sampling, but without any consequence for their babies. Four echographic hematomas were diagnosed, again without clinical consequence. Premature labour occurred in three patients between 32 and 36 weeks. One of the patients was known to have severe cervical incompetence. All infants delivered after sampling are now doing well.

Two babies were small for dates, with birth weights between the 3rd and 9th percentiles. One of these mothers had induced hypertension. No amniotic fluid leakage was noticed.

9.3.4 Indications (see Tables 9.6 to 9.9)

At the beginning of our experience we were uncertain of the risk of the method and chose to limit our indications to high risk genetic problems.

DNA analysis (see Table 9.6)

52 pregnancies at risk for sickle cell anaemia have been screened by Goossens *et al.* (1983). All diagnoses were confirmed at birth or after abortion. One case of adrenoleucodystrophy has been evaluated simultaneously by DNA and enzyme assay (Mandel *et al.*).

In one case of thalassemia, the family history was not informative and although the sampling was successful, the diagnosis had to be made by fetal blood sampling. 12 patients have been screened for Duchenne muscular dystrophy (DMD), ornithine transcarbamylase (OTC) deficit and congenital adrenal hyperplasia. As far as DMD diagnosis is concerned, suitable genetic information was available only in two cases. The decision for therapeutic abortion was based on sexing for the other patients. For congenital adrenal hyperplasia, a genetic diagnosis was possible on only one occasion.

Table 9.6 DNA analysis (n=66)

Sickle-cell anaemia	52
β-thalassaemia	1
Adrenoleukodystrophy	1
Duchenne muscular dystrophy	6
Ornithine transcarbamylase (OTC) deficit	1
Congenital adrenal hyperplasia	5

Metabolic diseases (see Table 9.7)

46 patients at risk for various metabolic diseases underwent sampling. Except for the Hurler and the Fanconi cases, the assay was performed on uncultured

Table 9.7 Metabolic diseases (n–46)

Disease	*No. of cases*	*In collaboration with*
Metachromatic leucodystrophy	4††††	Poenaru
Mucolopidosis II	3**†	,,
Glycogenosis II	5**†††	,,
Mannosidosis	1†	,,
Tay–Sachs disease	3*††	,,
Sandhoff's disease	3†††	,,
Landing's disease	1†	,,
Fabry's disease	1†	,,
Hurler's syndrome	2††	,,
Gaucher's disease	2††	,,
Niemann–Pick's disease	1*	Vanier
Menkes' syndrome	2*†	Horn and Tonnesen
Cystinosis	2††	Patrick
Maple syrup urine disease (MSUD)	1*	Kleijer
Hunter's syndrome	3*††	Kleijer
Fanconi's anemia	4*†††	Auerbach
Lesch–Nyhan syndrome	2*†	Kleijer
Citrullinemia	1†	Kamoun
Methylmalonic aciduria	1†	Saudubray
Argininosuccinic aciduria	1†	Kleijer
Neuraminidase deficiency	1†	Poenaru
Adrenoleukodystrophy	1*	Mandel and Moser
Refsum syndrome	1†	Schutgnens

* Affected; † normal.

villi, and therefore the diagnosis was available within a very short time after sampling. They were all confirmed on aborted or born children. Amniocentesis was performed only at the beginning of our experience.

Sexing (see Table 9.8)

86 diagnoses of fetal sex were performed using the direct method together with karyotyping on villus cultures. All the fetuses were at risk for X-linked

Table 9.8 Sexing (n=86)

Duchenne muscular dystrophy	68	(6*)
Fragile X syndrome	2	
Wiskott–Aldrich syndrome	3	
OTC deficit	3	(1*)
Congenital adrenal hyperplasia	5	(5*)
X-linked immune deficiency	2	
Incontinentia pigmenti	1	
X-linked microcephalus	1	
Lesch–Nyhan	1	

* Sexing + DNA.

diseases. Male fetuses aborted, except when a non-ambiguous diagnosis was made possible by DNA analysis, or when the finding of a male fetus led to fetoscopy for fetal blood sampling (X-linked immune deficiencies) or for fetal liver sampling (OTC deficit). All diagnoses were confirmed after abortion or birth.

Chromosomal anomalies (see Table 9.9)

Before commencing mass cytogenetic screening for low-risk patients, we undertook a precise evaluation of the forceps sampling risk. We considered CVS was indicated in women over 38 for whom late therapeutic abortion could be hazardous (e.g. patients who had previously undergone cesarean section). In two cases of high risk of fetal chromosomal aberration (parental translocation) CVS was performed and chromosomal aberration was found in one patient. She was carrying twins. One fetus showed an abnormal cytogenetic pattern (45,XO) and this misaborted during the first trimester while the other fetus continued to do well.

Table 9.9 Karyotype (n=9)

Maternal age		7
Translocation	14/21	1
Translocation	16/21	1

9.4 DISCUSSION

9.4.1 Potential inconvenience due to the rigidity of the forceps

It had been thought by some that rigid and straight forceps would fail to reach a posterior placenta in a retroverted uterus, an anterior placenta in an anteverted uterus, or a mainly fundal trophoblast. In fact, with traction on the cervix caused by using the Pozzi tenaculum or sometimes by modifying the bladder fullness, sampling was nearly always possible. Despite one failure, the success rate remains high (99.5%), although no obstetrical or anatomical criteria led to any patient exclusion.

9.4.2 Fetal loss rate (Fig. 9.4)

The fetal loss rate needs further evaluation because of our high rate of the therapeutic abortion (27.5%). This status is accounted for by our choice to restrict the indication of CVS to patients with high genetic risk. The drawback of this position is the small number of continuing pregnancies, thus accurate assessment of fetal risk is impaired.

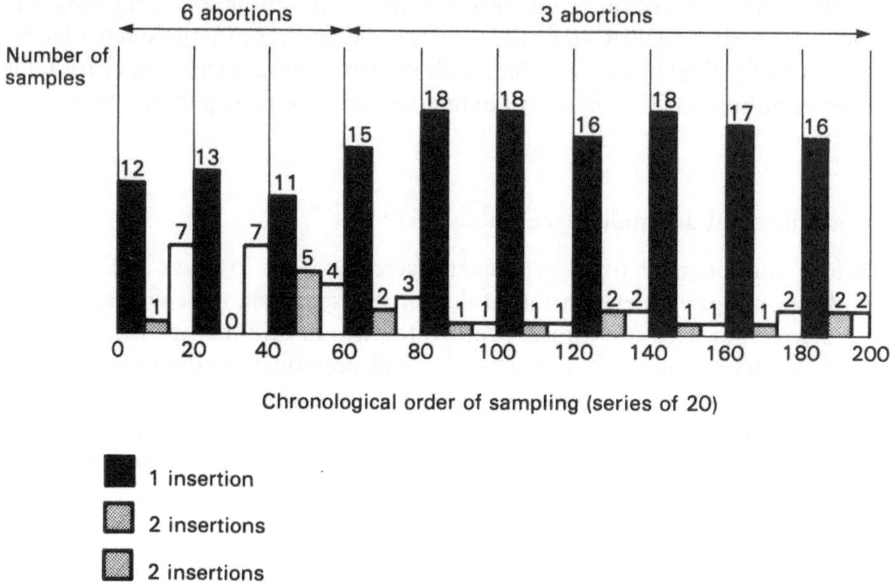

Figure 9.4 Fetal loss rate

All terminated pregnancies showed normal growth at ultrasound examination before therapeutic abortion 10 to 15 days after sampling. The frequency of fetal loss decreased with the increasing experience of the operator; 6 out of 9 fetal deaths occurred within the first 60 attempts.

9.5 CONCLUSION

The rigid sampling forceps method has four major advantages:

1. It is efficient. The rate of successful sampling was 99.5% for unselected patients. Of the samples 91.5% were uncontaminated and 94% weighed over 10 mg – sufficient for repeat assays or for other analyses to verify the diagnosis.
2. It is convenient and quick. The sampling itself usually takes from thirty seconds to one minute. It does not cause discomfort and can be performed by a single operator.
3. It can be reproduced. Other teams have adopted the technique with similar results without a long training period (Pachi, Roma; G. Monni, Cagliari; Y. Rouquet, Paris).
4. It is relatively cheap. The forceps costs less than US $100 and can be used for hundreds of samplings. An ultrasound scanner used in routine obstetrical practice is sufficient to monitor the sampling.

These data advocate the widespread use of this technique, providing the low fetal loss rate is confirmed and is comparable with that of other methods.

ACKNOWLEDGEMENTS

We would like to thank Dr M. Goossens, Dr J. L. Mandel, Dr A. Moser, Dr J. Boué, Dr L. Poenaru, Dr S. Girard and Dr F. Thepot for their help with conducting and confirming the diagnoses.

REFERENCES

Y. Dumez, M. Goossens, J. Boué, L. Poenaru, M. Dommergues and R. Henrion (1985) Chorionic sampling using rigid forceps under ultrasound control. In *First Trimester Fetal Diagnosis* (ed. F. Fracaro *et al.*), Springer-Verlag, Berlin Heidelberg.

Y. Dumez, M. Goossens, L. Poenaru and R. Henrion (1984) La biopsie de villosités choriales à la pince sous contrôle ultrasonore: technique et résultats. *J. Genet. Hum.*, **32**, 335–44.

M. Goossens and Y. Dumez (1982) First trimester fetal diagnosis of haemoglobin disorders. In *Fetal Diagnosis During the First Trimester* (eds. B. Brambati, G. Simoni and M. Fabio) Marcel Dekker, New York.

M. Goossens, Y. Dumez, L. Kaplan, M. Lupker, C. Chabret and R. Henrion (1983) Prenatal diagnosis of sickle-cell anemia in the first trimester of pregnancy. *N. Eng. J. Med.*, **309**, 831–3.

W. J. Kleijer, O. P. Van Diggelen, H. C. Janse, H. Galjaard, Y. Dumez and J. Boué (1984) First trimester diagnosis of Hunter syndrome on chorionic villi. *Lancet*, **11**, 472.

L. Poenaru, L. Kaplan, Y. Dumez and J. C. Dreyfus (1984) Evaluation of possible first trimester prenatal diagnosis in lysosomal diseases by trophoblast biopsy. *Pediat. Res.*, **18**, 1032–4.

PART TWO

Techniques

10

Blind chorion villus aspiration

—— *David H. Horwell* ——

10.1 INTRODUCTION

There is an obvious attraction to any technique for obtaining tissue of fetal origin for prenatal diagnosis, in which the amniotic sac is not transgressed and which uses simple, cheap and readily available equipment. 'Blind' chorion villus aspiration – the transcervical aspiration of chorionic villi without visual or ultrasonic localization of their position – achieves these aims but has failed to become established as a clinical technique. The origins of blind aspiration and the reasons for its failure will be examined in this chapter.

10.2 EARLY REPORTS OF CHORION VILLUS SAMPLING

The earliest investigation of the use of chorionic villi for antenatal diagnosis was by Hahnemann and Mohr (1968). Their use of hysteroscopy to visualize the villi predated similar attempts by other workers such as Kullander and Sandahl (1973), but their success in obtaining villi was low and initially there were considerable difficulties in culturing the cells for karyotyping. In an expanded study, Hahnemann (1974) described his experience with a total of 95 hysteroscopies for chorion villus sampling in patients about to undergo termination of pregnancy. In twenty of these cases, visibility via the hysteroscope was so poor that samples had to be taken completely blindly. Chorionic villi or chorion were present in four such samples (20%), the remaining samples consisting of decidua (75%) or amnion (one case). This was therefore the first report of 'blind' chorion villus sampling.

The earliest report of blind chorion villus aspiration for antenatal diagnosis came from China (Department of Obstetrics and Gynaecology, Tietung

Hospital, 1975). The work was stimulated by the need to obtain reliable samples of fetal cells for sex prediction 'in order to help women desiring family planning'. A 3 mm diameter metal cannula with a fine inner suction tube was introduced through the cervix to a point of 'sensation of soft resistance', which was presumed to be the gestation sac. The inner tube was then pushed forward by 0.5–1.0 cm and suction applied using a 5 ml syringe. The contents of the tube and cannula were expelled to make smears on slides and after Papanicolaou staining the nuclei were examined for sex chromatin. A series of one hundred successful aspirations was described. In 94 cases the fetal sex, assessed at abortion or birth, was diagnosed correctly. There were four spontaneous abortions following the procedure. Unfortunately, no mention at all was made of the number of cases in which aspiration was attempted but which did not yield villi. It was therefore impossible to assess whether the method would be universally applicable to antenatal diagnosis, as a high rate of success in obtaining suitable material is an essential requirement for any such technique to be acceptable.

A different approach to sampling trophoblast was taken by Rhine *et al.* (1975) who sought and found exfoliated trophoblast cells above the cervical mucous plug in the region of the internal cervical os. These cells were considered suitable for fetal sexing by Y-chromosome fluorescence. Rhine *et al.* (1977) later devised the Antenatal Cell Extractor (ACE), a 3.5 mm diameter plastic tube with a moveable bulbous tip which occluded the lumen during its passage through the cervical mucus into the lower, extraovular part of the uterine cavity. A small quantity of saline solution was injected and then aspirated and examined for trophoblast cells. Fetal chromosomes were identified in 26% of the samples. In a further series, Rhine and Milunsky (1979) applied this technique to 53 patients in the first trimester of pregnancy. Trophoblast cells could be identified in 37 cases (70%) and fetal chromosomes were identified after subsequent tissue culture in 26 (49%). The authors concluded that the technique held promise for early antenatal diagnosis of chromosome disorders, but that the small quantities of tissue obtained and the poor quantity and quality of the chromosome preparations were serious disadvantages.

The latter conclusion was supported by Goldberg *et al.* (1980) who also used the Antenatal Cell Extractor. They were unable to show that the cells obtained were of fetal origin. In twelve patients with male fetuses, cells from nine ACE specimens were cultured successfully and the karyotypes in all nine cases were female. It is of interest that previous workers (e.g. Bobrow and Lewis, 1971) had similar disappointing experiences with cells obtained from the cervical mucus itself.

It appeared that the best source of actively dividing cells of fetal origin in the first trimester would therefore be the chorionic villi themselves. Niazi *et al.* (1981) from St. Mary's Hospital, London, overcame the problem of poor growth of villous cells in tissue culture by a process of trypsinization and filtering to expose the mesenchyme cores of the villi. Specimens of the villi were initially obtained from pregnancies terminated by suction curettage, but in three patients specimens were obtained by blind transcervical aspiration using a 20-gauge Medicut intravenous cannula attached to a 20 ml syringe. All three samples were successfully cultured and karyotyped and the origin of the cells confirmed by examination of fetal tissue. This was the first report of chorion villus sampling by aspiration in the Western literature and it was followed closely by the classical report of Williamson *et al.* (1981), also from St. Mary's Hospital, of direct gene analysis from chorionic villi obtained by the same technique. These two reports established chorion villus sampling as a potentially valuable method for first trimester antenatal diagnosis.

10.3 ASSESSMENTS OF THE SUCCESS OF BLIND CHORION VILLUS SAMPLING

Having demonstrated that chorionic villi could be used for reliable antenatal diagnoses, it was necessary to establish the value of the blind sampling method. The first report of an objective assessment of the technique was by the present author and colleagues at St Mary's Hospital (Horwell *et al.*, 1983). In this first series of blind aspirations, a 16-gauge (1.6 mm outer diameter, 1.3 mm bore) Medicut polyethylene intravenous cannula attached to a 20 ml syringe was passed through the cervical canal into the uterine cavity immediately before dilatation of the cervix for termination of pregnancy at 7–13 weeks gestation. Two samples were taken from each of 82 women and were examined histologically for the presence of chorionic villi. These were identified in samples from 33 of the 82 women (40%). In an attempt to assess the feasibility of the technique for out-patient sampling, it was found that the cannula had been introduced easily, without strong traction on the cervix and without the prior passage of a uterine sound in 44 of the women; villi were present in the first aspirate in 21 cases (48%) but these represented only 26% of the original 82 patients. The presence of the villi was unrelated to gestation, parity or the length of the cervical canal, but only in parous women was it possible to introduce the cannula in every case. The amniotic sac was punctured in three cases (two at 13 weeks) and bleeding was recorded as moderate or heavy in eleven.

The low success rate in obtaining villi was disappointing and was thought to be related to three principal factors. The first was the difficulty encountered in the introduction of the Medicut cannula due to its thin sharp flexible tip being caught in folds of cervical mucosa or at the internal os. Secondly, its length (6.8 cm) may have been insufficient to reach the gestation sac in many cases. Finally, its straight configuration necessitated excessive traction to straighten the cervical canal.

For these reasons a new cannula was devised and was used for our second blind aspiration study between November 1982 and September 1983 (Horwell, 1984). This cannula was longer than the Medicut (15 cm), was constructed from 16-gauge stainless steel and incorporated a gentle curve and a bulbous tip of 2.5 mm diameter, reproducing the shape of a standard uterine sound. Using this cannula, villi were found in one or both aspirates in 104 of 212 pregnancies sampled, a success rate of 49%. This was an improvement, but still not a high enough proportion for blind aspiration to be offered as a viable diagnostic procedure. However, the new instrument had the considerable advantage over the Medicut cannula of easy introduction in all but three cases, irrespective of parity.

These studies of blind aspiration were valuable in that they established success rates with precision and because they yielded villi obtained under clinical conditions, rather than villi from pregnancy termination material, for the development of laboratory methods. During the first series, the work of Elles *et al.* (1983) using restriction fragment length polymorphisms showed that chorionic villi were a source of fetal DNA for analysis which was free from contamination by maternal DNA. Villi from the second series were used by Heaton *et al.* (1984) to develop a new and considerably simpler technique for tissue culture and karyotyping from chorionic villi. Samples were also provided to other laboratories working on the diagnosis of haemoglobinopathies and on microbiochemical assays for inborn errors of metabolism.

Only three other studies dealing with blind chorion villus aspiration have been reported. In a detailed paper, Liu *et al.* (1983) showed that trophoblast was present in single aspirates from 45 out of 137 patients about to undergo first-trimester termination of pregnancy. The cannula used was a 14-gauge Longdwell Teflon intravenous cannula, attached to a 2 ml syringe. This success rate of 33% was not dissimilar to that using intravenous cannulae in the first St. Mary's series. Interestingly, the one amniotic sac puncture in this series was in a pregnancy at 13 weeks gestation, identical to that of two out of three punctures in the first St. Mary's series. No fetal cells were detected in maternal blood using the Kleihauer technique, but five of the patients had significant increases in serum alpha-fetoprotein (AFP) levels.

Rodeck *et al.* (1983) reported on six different approaches to chorion villus sampling. Among these, blind aspiration was carried out on 15 patients using four different cannulae or tubes varying between 1.7 mm and 4 mm outer diameter. No chorionic villi were obtained from any of these patients. The series was small and the operators clearly could not have developed sufficient experience with blind sampling before proceeding to more sophisticated methods. The third report gave very different results. MacKenzie *et al.* (1983) referred to a series of 60 patients scheduled for first trimester termination of pregnancy, in which a 10F soft plastic aspiration catheter with a 20 ml syringe was used. Suction was applied while it was rotated and withdrawn. Chorionic villi said to be suitable for diagnostic purposes were obtained in 78% of cases. An additional case at 11 weeks gestation in which the diagnosis of an unbalanced chromosome translocation was made was also reported; the patient aborted spontaneously five days after sampling. The reasons for the difference in results between this series and those of the other series reviewed above remain unclear.

10.4 REASONS FOR POOR SUCCESS RATES

The reasons for the generally poor success of blind chorionic villus aspiration are not difficult to determine. The first is that the gestation sac may not have been reached by the cannula at all, or that even if reached, the decidua capsularis may not have been punctured in order to gain access to the villi themselves. The former may well have been the case when Medicut cannulae were used. Some evidence for this may be deduced from Ward's initial series of chorionic villus aspirations under ultrasound guidance (Ward *et al.*, 1983), when Medicut cannulae and early side-holed Portex cannulae were used. In the first 26 patients, villi were obtained from only eight (31%). No mention was made of their success in placing the tips of the cannulae in the implantation sites, but the success rate of 89% in the next 19 patients when the prototype of the much longer Trophocan cannula (Portex) was used implied that part of the problem might well have been that of cannula length. However, the cannula used in the second St. Mary's series should have overcome this.

The second and more fundamental reason for the failure of blind aspiration to obtain chorionic villi in every case lies in their distribution around the gestation sac. Blind aspiration relies on the presence of villi in all areas, not only at the implantation site (Fig. 10.1). While this may often be the case at six to eight weeks gestation, the relentless expansion of the gestation sac and the degeneration of the chorionic villi other than at the implantation site mean that increasingly large areas of the chorion are left bare (Fig. 10.2). These areas, the chorion laeve, generally appear after 10 weeks gestation, but in some cases the process may occur considerably earlier (Boyd and Hamilton, 1970). Clearly, unless the tip of the sampling device is actually in the chorion frondosum at the implantation site, it is merely a matter of chance that it will be in contact with chorionic villi. Blind aspiration cannot achieve such precision of location.

10.5 DOES BLIND CHORION VILLUS ASPIRATION HAVE A PLACE IN ANTENTAL DIAGNOSIS?

This review has shown that chorionic villi can indeed be obtained by blind aspiration, but that when assessed objectively the success rate is too low for it

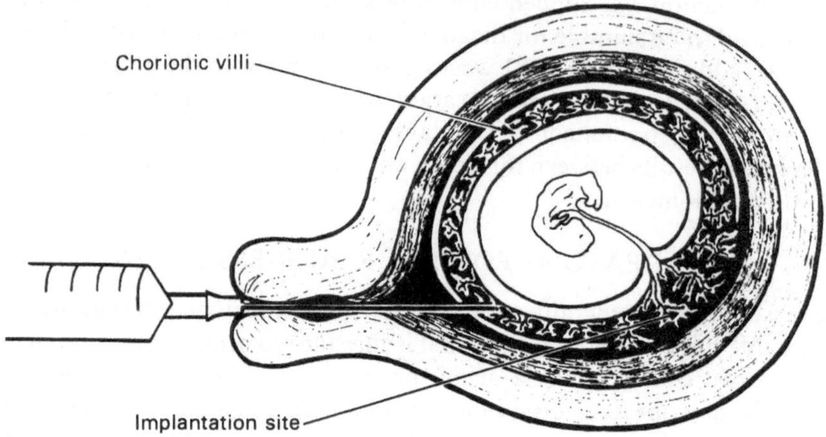

Figure 10.1 Theoretical model for blind chorionic villus aspiration. The villi surround the gestation sac and should be accessible at any point reached by the cannula. (Department of Medical Illustration, St Mary's Hospital Medical School.)

to be a viable diagnostic procedure. Other disadvantages include the risk of amniotic sac puncture, which appears to be negligible with sampling under ultrasound control, and the inability of the operator to assess fetal viability at the time of sampling. The advantages of the avoidance of the use of expensive equipment and the need for only a modicum of skill are undoubtedly outweighed by the disadvantages already mentioned.

Heaton (personal communication), with her extensive experience of culturing and karyotyping of cells from villi obtained by both methods, is of the opinion that villi from ultrasound-directed sampling provide better material for laboratory analysis, presumably because viable villi from the implantation site are sampled on every occasion. In blind aspiration, a proportion of the samples will inevitably be taken from degenerating or even degenerate villi of the prospective chorion laeve.

The only indication for blind sampling now recognized by the author is the occasional need to obtain genuinely aspirated chorionic villi for laboratory research, when pregnancies about to be terminated will yield villi in 40–50% of cases without significant prolongation of anaesthesia and without the requirement for sophisticated equipment (and the personnel to operate it) to be present in the operating theatre. Such sampling was continued at St. Mary's Hospital using the stainless steel curved bulbous-tipped cannula despite the commencement of regular sampling under ultrasound guidance in September 1983.

Blind chorion villus aspiration flourished in the form of research studies in 1982 and 1983. The large studies reviewed in this chapter rapidly and objectively established the need for precision in localization of the implantation

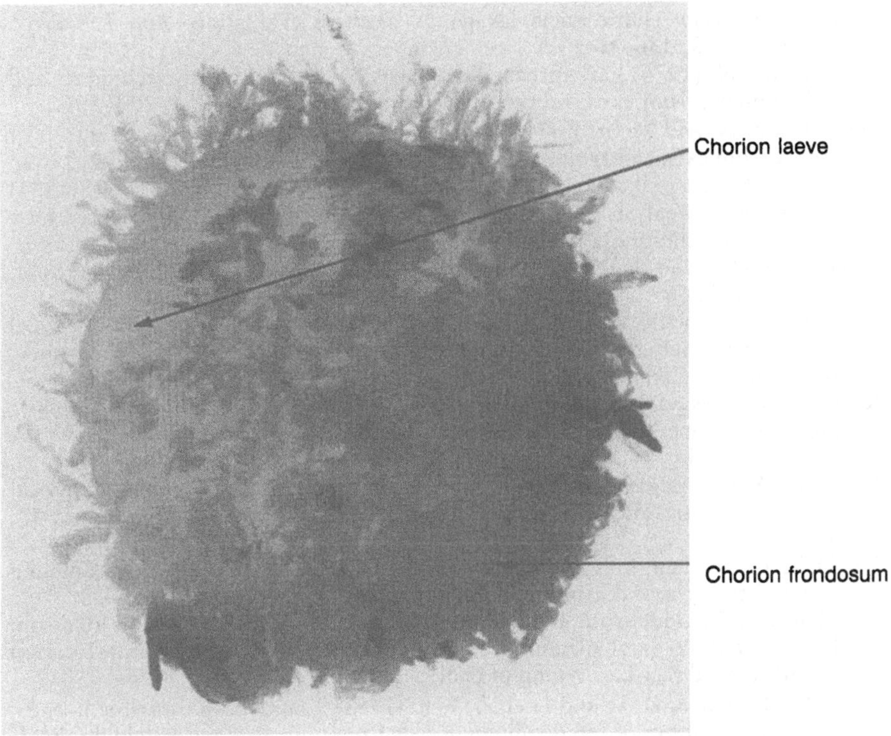

Figure 10.2 Gestation sac from a spontaneous complete abortion at 9 weeks gestation. Significant areas of the chorion already lack chorionic villi. The villi remaining on the chorion laeve are long and thin, while at the implantation site the villi of the chorion frondosum are thick and densely clustered.

site and it was the advent of the use of real-time ultrasound (Kazy *et al.*, 1982; Old *et al.*, 1982) that led to the safety and success of chorion villus sampling as practised today.

REFERENCES

Bobrow, M. and Lewis, B. V. (1971) Unreliability of fetal sexing using cervical material. *Lancet*, ii, 486.

Boyd, J. D. and Hamilton, W. J. (1970) *The Human Placenta*. Heffer, Cambridge.

Department of Obstetrics and Gynaecology, Tietung Hospital of Anshan Iron and Steel Company (1975) Fetal sex prediction by sex chromatin of chorionic villi cells during early pregnancy. *Chin. Med. J.*, 1, 117–26.

Elles, R. G., Williamson, R., Niazi, M., Coleman, D. V. and Horwell, D. H. (1983) Absence of maternal contamination of chorionic villi used for fetal-gene analysis. *New Engl. J. Med.*, **308**, 1433–5.

Goldberg, M. F., Chan, A. T. L., Ahn, Y. W. and Reidy, J. A. (1980) First trimester diagnosis using endocervical lavage: A negative evaluation. *Am. J. Obstet. Gynecol.*, **138**, 436–40.

Hahnemann, N. (1974) Early prenatal diagnosis; A study of biopsy techniques and cell culturing from extraembryonic membranes. *Clin. Genet.*, **6**, 294–306.

Hahnemann, N. and Mohr, J. (1968) Genetic diagnosis in the embryo by means of biopsy from extraembryonic membranes. *Bull. Eur. Soc. Hum. Genet.*, **2**, 23–9.

Heaton, D. E., Czepulkowski, B. H., Horwell, D. H. and Coleman, D. V. (1984) Chromosome analysis of first trimester chorionic villus biopsies prepared by a maceration technique. *Prenat. Diag.*, **2**, 39–45.

Horwell, D. H. (1984) Further experience with chorionic villus aspiration. *J. Obstet. Gynaecol.*, 5, 66.

Horwell D. H., Loeffler F. E., Coleman D. V. (1983) Assessment of a transcervical aspiration technique for chorionic villus biopsy in the first trimester of pregnancy. *Br. J. Obstet. Gynaecol.*, **90**, 196–8.

Kazy, Z., Rozovsky, I. S. and Bakharev, V. A. (1982) Chorion biopsy in early pregnancy: a method of early prenatal diagnosis of inherited disorders. *Prenat. Diag.*, **2**, 39–45.

Kullander, S. and Sandahl, B. (1973) Fetal chromosome analysis after transcervical placental biopsies during early pregnancy. *Acta Obstet. Gynaecol. Scand.*, **52**, 355–9.

Liu, D. T. Y., Mitchell, J., Johnson, J. and Wass, D. M. (1983) Trophoblast sampling by blind transcervical aspiration. *Br. J. Obstet. Gynaecol.*, **90**, 1119–23.

MacKenzie, I. Z., Lindebaum, R. H., Patel, C., Clarke, G., Crocker, M. and Jonasson, J. A. (1983) Prenatal diagnosis of an unbalanced chromosome translocation identified by direct karotyping of chorionic biopsy. *Lancet*, **ii**, 1426–7.

Niazi, M., Coleman, D. V. and Loeffler, F. E. (1981) Trophoblast sampling in early pregnancy. Culture of rapidly dividing cells from immature placental villi. *Br. J. Obstet. Gynaecol.*, **88**, 1081–5.

Old, J. M. Ward, R. H. T., Karagozlu, F. Petrou, M., Modell, B. and Weatherall, D. J. (1982) First trimester fetal diagnosis for haemoglobinopathies: three cases. *Lancet*, ii, 1413–16.

Rhine, S. A., Cain, J. L., Cleary, R. E., Palmer, C. G. and Thompson, J. F. (1975) Prenatal sex detection with endocervical smears: successful results using Y body fluorescence. *Am. J. Obstet. Gynecol.*, **122**, 155–60.

Rhine, S. A. and Milunsky, A. (1979) Utilization of trophoblast for early prenatal diagnosis. In *Genetic Disorders and the Fetus* (ed. A. Milunsky), Plenum Press, New York. pp. 536–7.

Rhine, S. A., Palmer, G. C. and Thompson, J. F. (1977) A simple first trimester alternative to amniocentesis for prenatal diagnosis. *Birth Defects Original Article Series XII*, 3D, pp. 231–47.

Rodeck, C. H., Morsman, J. M., Gosden, C. M. and Gosden, J. R. (1983) Development of an improved technique for first-trimester microsampling of chorion. *Br. J. Obstet. Gynaecol.*, **90**, 1113–18.

Ward, R. H. T., Modell, B., Petrou, M., Karagozlu, F. and Douratsos, E. (1983) Method of sampling chorionic villi in first trimester of pregnancy under guidance of real time ultrasound. *Br. Med. J.*, **286**, 1542–4.

Williamson, R., Eskdale, J., Coleman, D. V., Niazi, M., Loeffler, F. E. and Modell, B. M. (1981) Direct gene analysis of chorionic villi: a possible technique for first-trimester antenatal diagnosis of haemoglobinopathies. *Lancet*, **ii**, 1125–7.

11

Ultrasound for transcervical chorion villus sampling

—— *R. E. Richardson and D. T. Y. Liu* ——

The use of ultrasound for guiding sampling needles is now well established. Amniocentesis is invariably successful when performed under ultrasound control and the risk to the fetus minimized. Sophisticated intra-uterine techniques such as blood transfusion and catheterization of the fetal bladder are now possible with the help of ultrasound. The use of ultrasound in chorion villus sampling is an obvious extension of the role of ultrasound during pregnancy.

11.1 WHICH TYPE OF ULTRASOUND MACHINE?

Real-time ultrasound machines come in various different forms and price range. In general, machines can be divided into:

1. Linear arrays.
2. Phased arrays (electronically steered).
3. Sector scanners (mechanically steered).
4. Hybrid – curvilinear arrays.

The actual type of machine used does not matter. What is required is that an adequate view of the uterus and contents, maternal bladder, vagina and cervix is obtained.

Different scanners have different advantages and disadvantages and these will be discussed in detail. Points that apply to all scanners are:

1. It must be of a reasonable quality, which means a reasonable price. The cheapest scanners give poorer resolution than the more expensive ones. However, it should be emphasized that there is no necessity to buy the very top of the range: mid-range equipment is perfectly adequate.

2. For accurate localization of the cannula it is desirable to have a scanner with a narrow slice width, that is a narrow beam dimension in the plane perpendicular to the scan plane. It is advisable to have this measured before purchase.
3. Sampling is performed with the patient in the lithotomy position. Probe design, particularly the position of the insertion of the cable into the probe, may limit the accessibility of the probe.

It is advisable to test equipment before purchase to ensure that the operators are happy with all aspects of the machine design and performance.

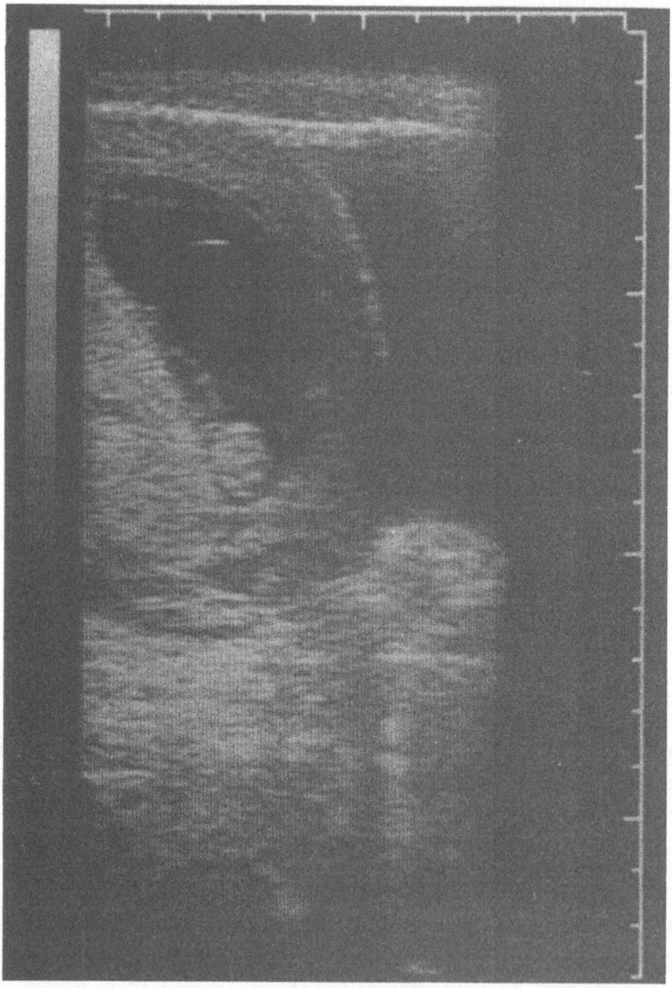

Figure 11.1 Linear array image showing the uterus, cervix and maternal bladder.

11.1.1 Linear arrays

A linear array probe consists of an array of small transducers, typically 10–15 cm long. The real-time image is produced by sequentially firing off groups of transducers so the image consists of parallel lines of ultrasound information. Electronic smoothing is frequently employed so that the individual lines are not apparent. A typical illustration of this is shown in Fig. 11.1.

The advantages of this type of machine are that a good viewing window is obtained even if the uterus is near the probe and scan plane orientation is very easy. The long probe length does lead to some disadvantages including loss of contact if the anatomy is very uneven. The image may be obscured by bowel gas and the design of the linear array probe does not lend itself to manipulation to overcome this problem.

11.1.2 Phased arrays

A phased array probe is also made up of an array of small transducers, but a sector image is produced by electronically steering the beam. This steering is achieved by phasing the firing of the cystals so the image consists of radial lines of ultrasound information. The probe is very light, small and easy to manoeuvre. This means that there are no contact problems and the sector image means that it is possible to view under bowel gas and so obtain a better image of the uterus. A typical phased array image is shown in Fig. 11.2.

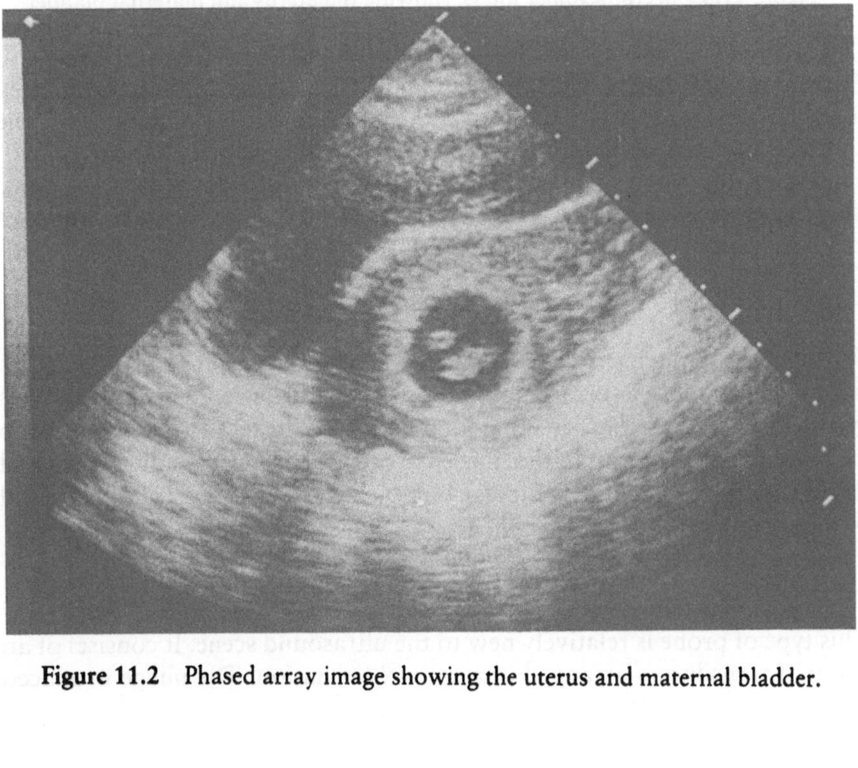

Figure 11.2 Phased array image showing the uterus and maternal bladder.

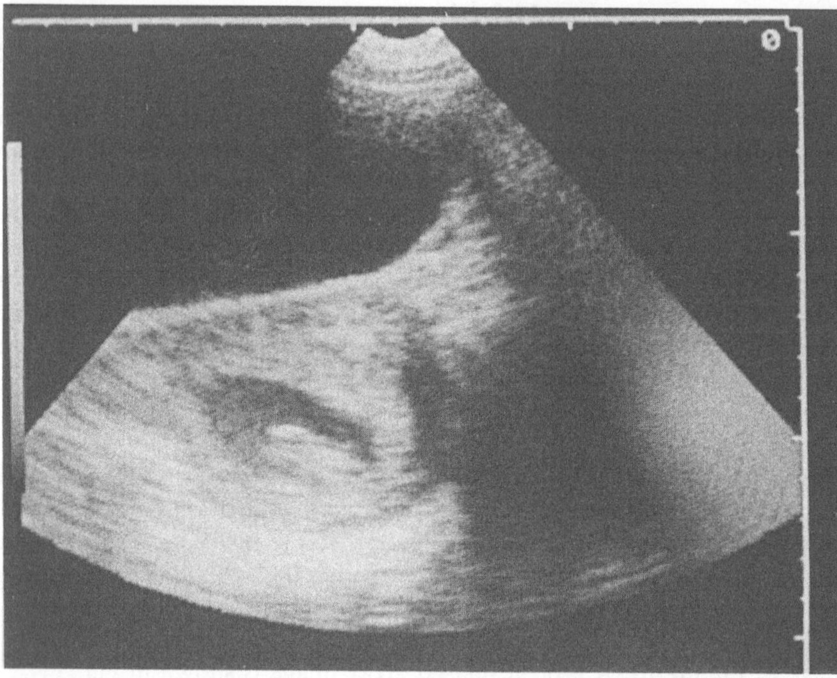

Figure 11.3 Sector scanner image showing the uterus and maternal bladder

A major disadvantage of this type of probe is that it is much harder to determine the orientation of the scan plane (see section 11.3 on technique). This can cause problems when attempting to insert the cannula into the uterus along the scan plane. The scan field is invariably limited to 90° maximum due to the problems of steering the beam at oblique angles and this could cause problems if the uterus is near the skin surface. The uniformity of the scan tends to be poor at the edges of the image.

11.1.3 Sector scanners

A single oscillating transducer or a rotating ring of three or four transducers are used to produce a sector image. These probes are steered mechanically as opposed to the electronic steering used in phased arrays. The probes tend to be marginally heavier than the phased array probes but the advantages and disadvantages are similar. An image obtained with a single oscillating crystal is shown in Fig. 11.3.

11.1.4 Curvilinear arrays

This type of probe is relatively new to the ultrasound scene. It consists of an array of transducers arranged in a convex formation. The image produced

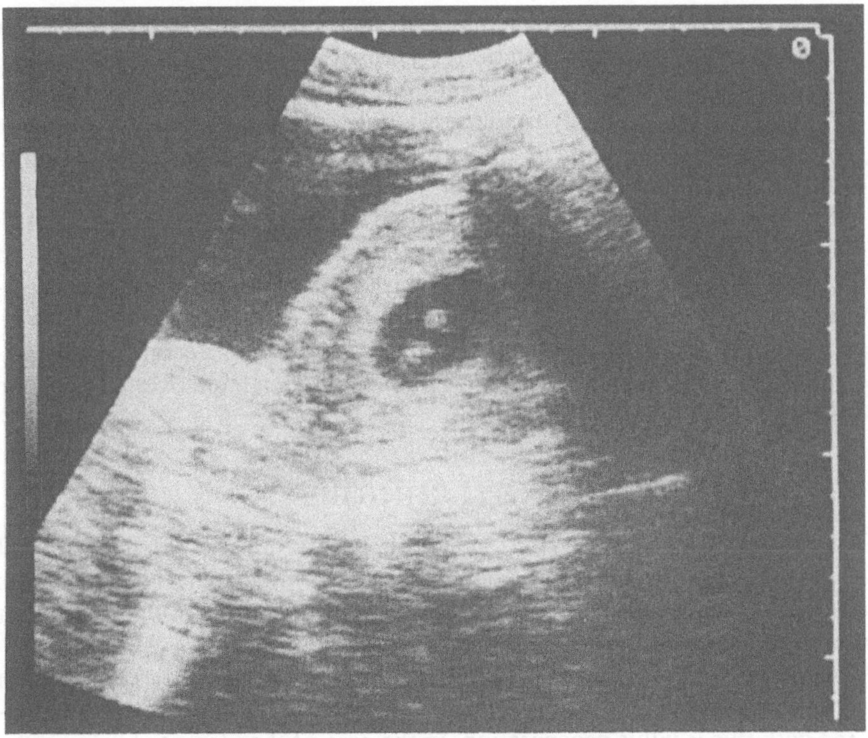

Figure 11.4 Curvilinear array image showing the uterus, cervix and maternal bladder.

has both the advantages of the linear array (wide field of view, particularly in the near field, and ease of orientation) and the advantages of sector scanners (fewer contact problems and the ability to 'see' under bowel gas). The type of image obtained with this type of probe is shown in Fig. 11.4.

Multi-element probes, such as linear arrays, phased arrays and curvilinear arrays, have the advantage that they can be focused electronically in the plane of the scan, which means that a narrow beam can be produced. Sector scanners cannot be focused electronically so the beam width at depth tends to be quite wide.

11.2 WHO SHOULD SCAN?

The person operating the ultrasound machine must be knowledgeable about the normal and abnormal anatomy of pregnancy, have a good understanding of the interaction of ultrasound with tissue and its very different interaction with the cannula materials and be able to identify artefactual images. A feel for three-dimensional geometry is also an advantage.

Radiographers who have experience in ultrasound or midwives are the best people to scan in these situations. The radiographers may need some additional information about the anatomy and physiology of early pregnancy and midwives will certainly need to be taught in depth about ultrasound.

Scanning and sampling can be performed simultaneously if the sampling cannula is attached to some sort of suction device (Warren and Rodeck, 1985). If such a system is not available then it is necessary to have one person who scans and another person to perform the sampling. The advantages of the single-handed approach is that lining up the scan plane and the orientation of the cannula is easier. If two people are involved there needs to be good co-ordination between them. A working compromise is for the obstetrician to scan while manipulating the cannula and then hand over to someone else while the sample is being taken.

11.3 TECHNIQUE

The intention in chorion villus sampling is to remove a small sample of healthy chorionic tissue without endangering the pregnancy. To achieve this it is necessary to know the best sampling site, where the cannula is and that there is no risk of rupturing the membranes.

As described in previous chapters, chorionic villi surround the conceptus in early pregnancy. The placental site gradually becomes apparent and associated with this is villus degeneration, in the area of the placenta however the villi proliferate. The best place to take a sample is from the thickest part of the placenta. The placenta can be implanted anteriorly, posteriorly or fundally and to the right, left or centre of the uterine cavity. The cannula will need to be manipulated to reach these different sites. For example, to sample from an anterior placenta requires that the cannula is manipulated upwards as soon as it is passed through the cervical canal.

In very early pregnancy the placenta appears on scanning to surround the fetus and it is not easy to determine where the implantation site will be. At this stage it may not be necessary to define this site should patients present this early.

As the pregnancy progresses, the site of implantation appears on the scan as a defined thickening of part of the sac. Most of the villi will be degenerating except at the implantation site so it is very important to identify this area. Serial longitudinal sections across the uterus should be taken at a separation of a probe thickness. Once the placental thickening has been identified the probe should be manipulated until the placental thickening, the cervix and the vagina can all be viewed together. The doctor performing the sampling can see from the angle of the probe the direction he or she must place the cannula to reach the optimal sampling site. After the cannula is inserted it must only be moved minimally. If the direction of insertion lies along the plane of the scan the cannula should be instantly identifiable on the screen. In cases where this does not happen the cannula should be kept stationary and the probe should be slowly rocked so that the ultrasound plane sweeps across the uterus. Once the cannula is identified the angulation of the probe is noted to redirect the cannula. In practice, suitable sampling sites are presented over a reasonable area of the uterine wall so it may be possible to sample without moving the cannula.

If the cannula is inserted at an angle to the plane of scan then it can be more difficult to locate. Once located, if the cannula is not viewed along its length it is difficult to identify the tip. When this happens the probe should be rotated until the cannula and the scan plane coincide. The angle between the original and new scan planes determines how the cannula can be repositioned correctly. It is vitally important to spend time during this part of the procedure – patience is invariably rewarded!

Once the cannula is correctly positioned sampling can begin. In some cases, depending on the cannula used, it should be possible to see the tissue moving along the cannula as it is removed.

11.4 SAMPLING CANNULAE

Many different sampling cannulae have been used by different centres. Discussion of the advantages and disadvantages of each type is given in other chapters. In this chapter we will confine ourselves to the ultrasound images of different cannulae materials. Current sampling procedures either suck the villi into a syringe or entwine them onto a brush. Suction cannulae can be made of either metal or plastic and each device produces a very different ultrasound image.

11.4.1 Brush

A sampling brush is illustrated in Fig. 11.5 along with the ultrasound image. The head consists of many angled bristles which all scatter the ultrasound. The image of the head, therefore, shows up as a fairly bright area with a small degree of shadowing behind it. The handle of the brush is not always seen as its cross-sectional dimension is small. Careful scanning, however, will demonstrate it.

11.4.2 Suction cannulae

(a) Plastic

The difference in acoustic impedance between the plastic and the surrounding tissue is not large. The acoustic impedance for polythene is 1.84×10^5 compared to 1.70×10^5 for muscle (units are g/cm^{2}s). This means that the

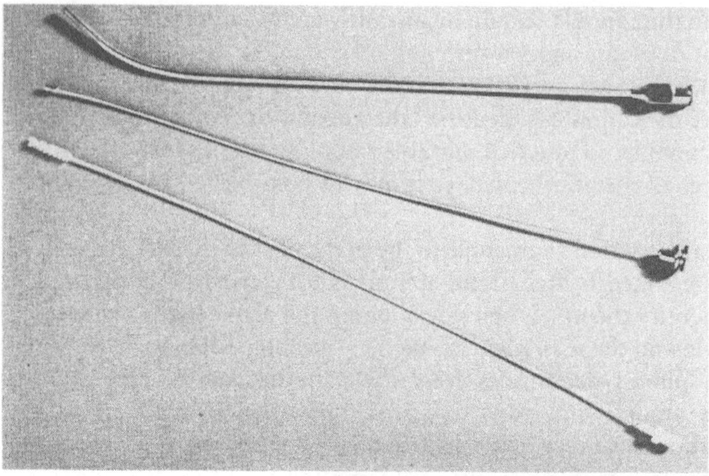

Figure 11.5 Brush and ultrasound image.

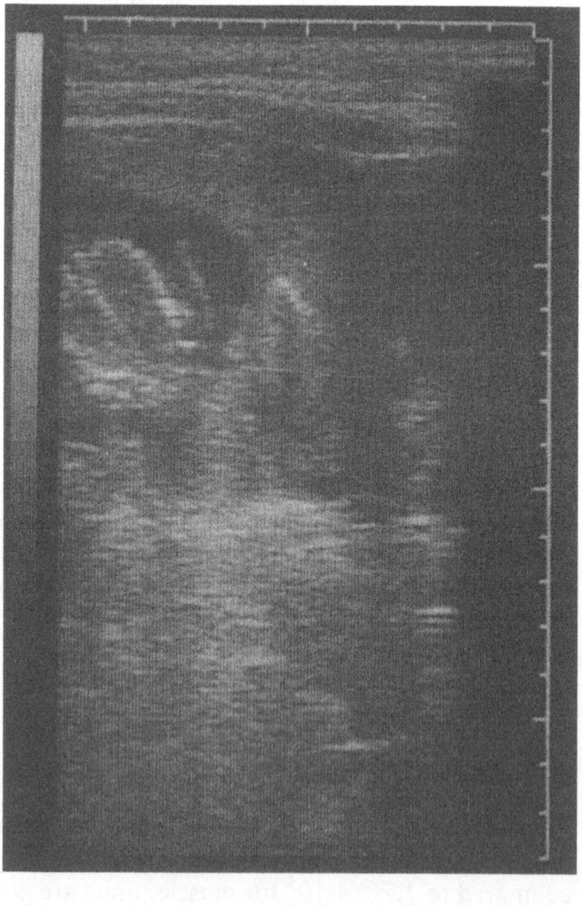

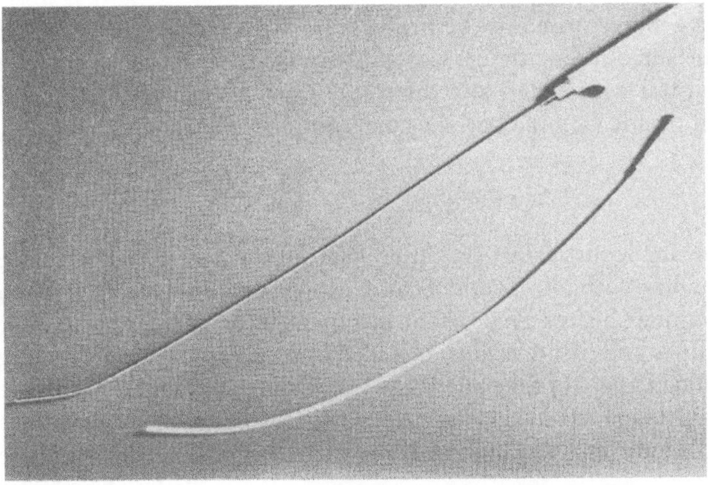

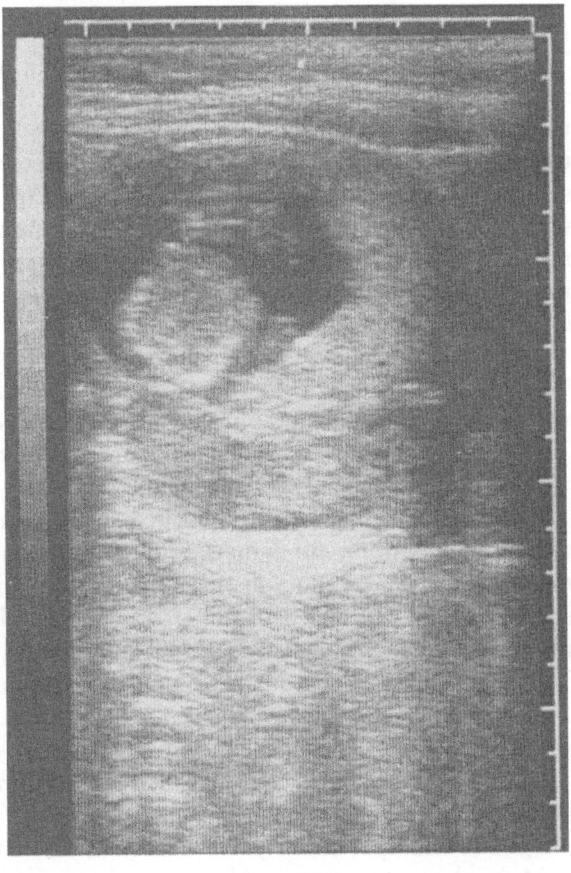

Figure 11.6 Plastic cannula and ultrasound image.

strength of the echo returned to the probe is not vastly different from the echoes from the surrounding tissue. Careful scanning is essential to detect a plastic cannula, but with experience there should be no problem. Fig. 11.6 shows a typical plastic cannula and the corresponding ultrasound image.

(b) Metal

Metal cannulae are acoustically very different from soft tissue and therefore are easy to visualize with ultrasound. Strong echoes are returned even when the cannula is at quite a steep angle to the beam. It should be possible to view both walls of the cannula and in some instances see the sample moving along the bore. A metal cannula of the sort we use is illustrated in Fig. 11.7 with the corresponding ultrasound image. The large difference in acoustic impedance between the cannula and the surrounding soft tissue does lead to some artefacts.

(i) Slice-width artefact

The ultrasound beam is not infinitely small but has dimensions both in the scan plane and perpendicular to the scan plane. Slice width is used to describe the dimension of the beam perpendicular to the scan plane. For single transducer systems (mechanically steered sectors) the beam has circular symmetry so the slice width equals the lateral resolution in the plane of the scan. All array systems have non-circular symmetry so the slice width is unlikely to equal the lateral resolution. It is important that the slice width is investigated before purchasing a scanner so that the slice width artefact can be minimized.

The artefact occurs because the slice width is much greater for strong reflectors such as metal than it is for soft tissue. Images can be produced where the metal cannula appears to be positioned right in the sac (see Fig. 11.8). In actual fact the cannula is passing to one side of the sac but the slice-width problem results in an artefactual image.

This artefact must be distinguished from tenting the membranes where there is the possibility of damage to the sac. When the membranes are tented movement of the cannula disturbs the amniotic fluid and fetus. This is not seen when the cannula is to one side of the sac. In most cases we find that tenting the membranes also produces an artefact such as shown in Fig. 11.9. This is a beam width or diffraction grating artefact.

(ii) Beam width: diffraction grating artefact

As stated in the previous section, the beam has dimensions in the plane of the scan. For a single element transducer this shows up as point sources being imaged as lines, particularly in the far field where the beam width is greater.

Multi-element transducers have an exaggerated form of this artefact. The

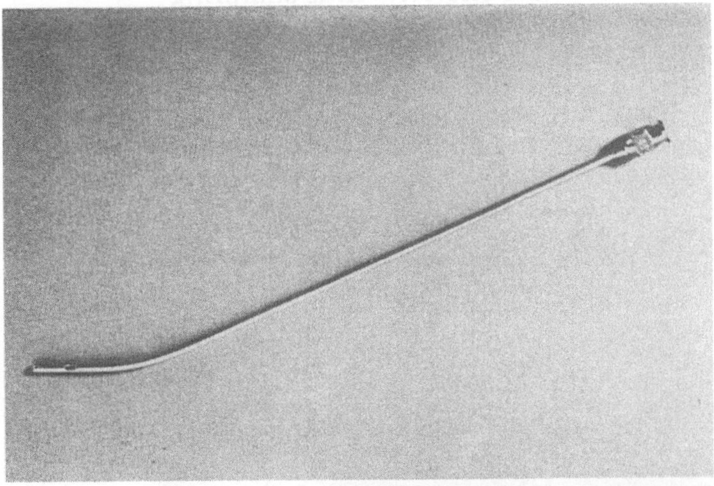

Figure 11.7 Metal cannula and ultrasound image.

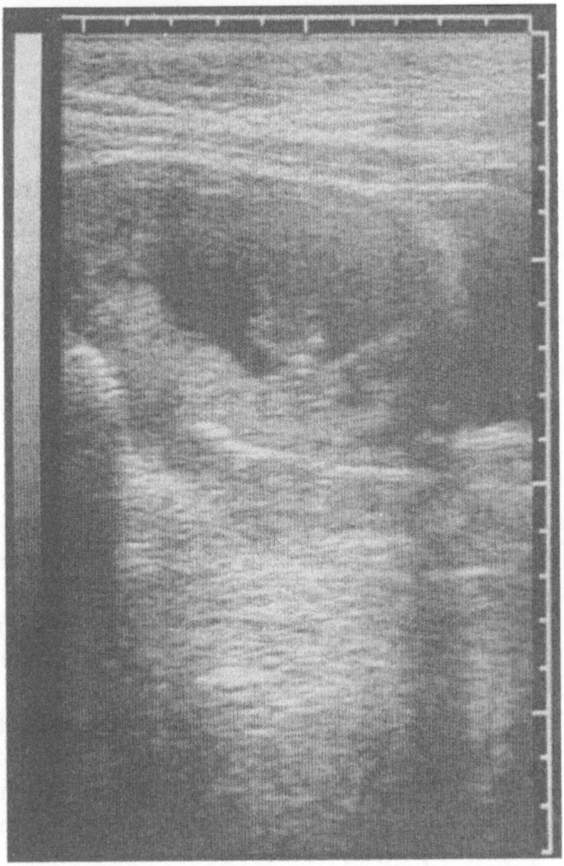

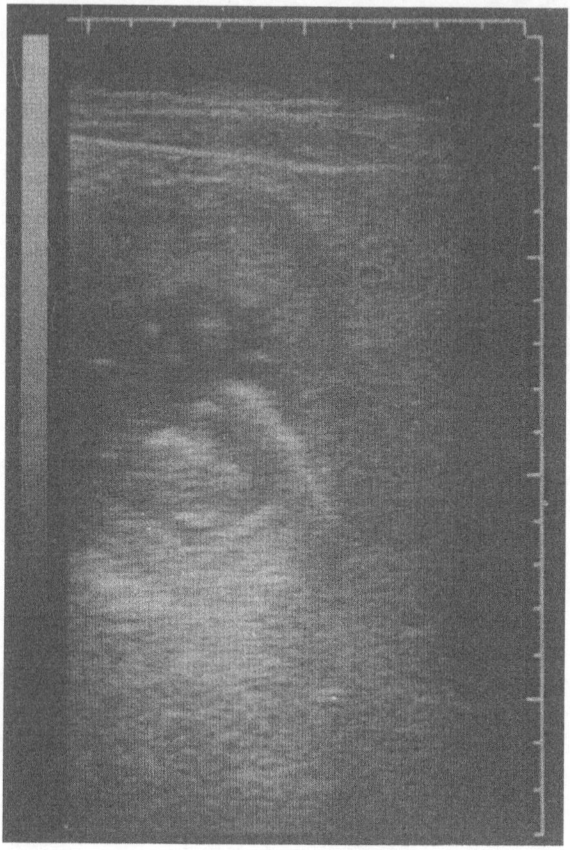

Figure 11.8 Slice width artefact. Cannula appears to be inserted into the sac but in fact lies to one side.

ultrasound beam is produced by firing a series of small transducers separated by small gaps. The transducer array is analogous to a diffraction grating in the optical sense and similar side lobes are produced. The energy in these side lobes is much less than that in the main beam but if the reflector is strong and perpendicular to the propagation direction of the beam an echo of sufficient size will be returned to the probe. This artefact can cause problems in tip localization when a metal cannula is perpendicular to the beam. Fig. 11.10 illustrates this problem. In Fig. 11.10(a) the cannula appears to end in the area shadowed by bowel gas. In Fig. 11.10(b) the cannula has been angled slightly and it can be seen that, in fact, the tip of the cannula is not inserted so far into the patient.

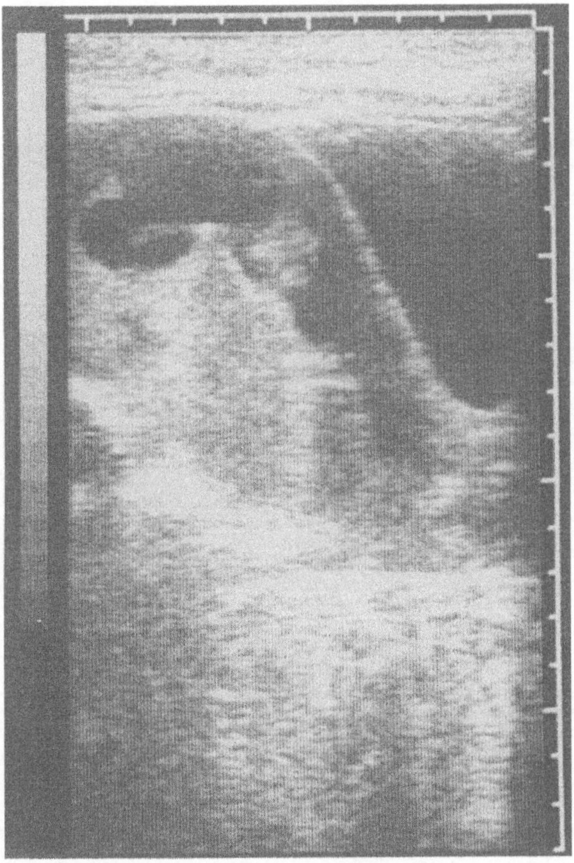

Figure 11.9 Tenting the membranes.

(iii) Reverberation

The cannula we use (a Liu Sampler) has a solid tip and a sampling hole on the side. The solid tip of the cannula sometimes produces a white streak behind the cannula (see Fig. 11.11). This is due to the ultrasound reverberating back and forth in the solid end of the cannula. The artefact appears continuous and does not have the characteristic parallel echoes of reverberation artefacts because the speed of sound in the solid metal is much higher than in soft tissue and therefore the echoes for the front and back surfaces merge into one. Attenuation in metal is fairly low and so the sound echoes back and forth for some time, hence the depth of the streak.

This artefact can be useful for locating the probe tip but is only seen if the parallel sides of the cannula are perpendicular to the beam propagation direction.

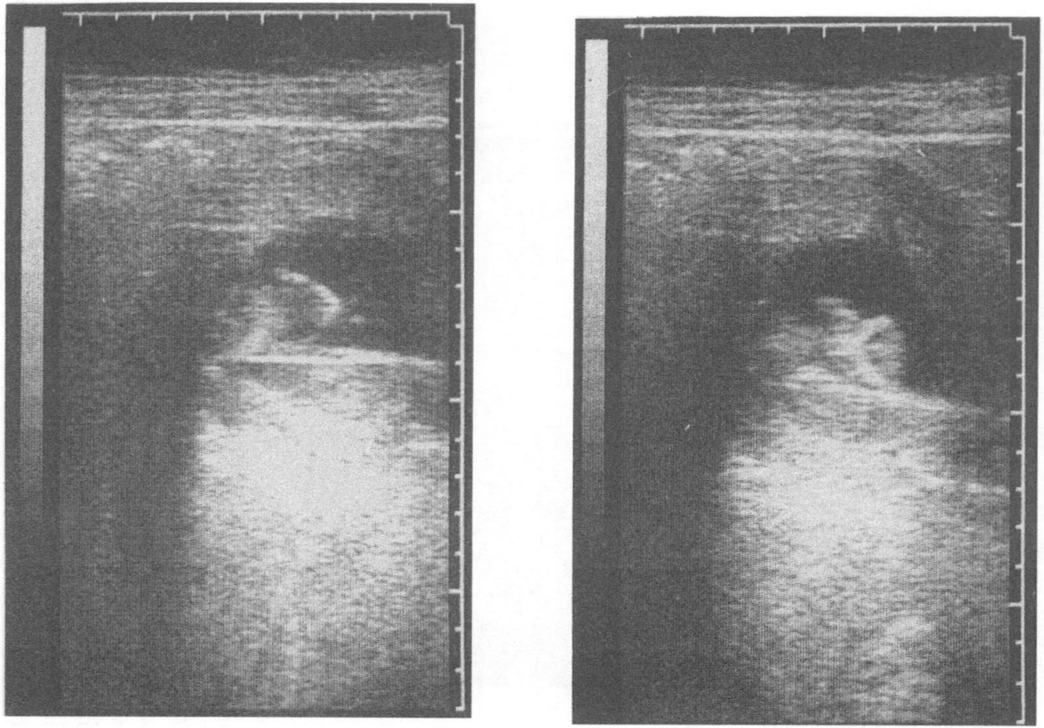

Figure 11.10 (a) Diffraction grating artefact. The tip of the cannula appears to be in the area shadowed by bowel gas. (b) Angling the cannula demonstrates that the cannula is not inserted so far into the patient.

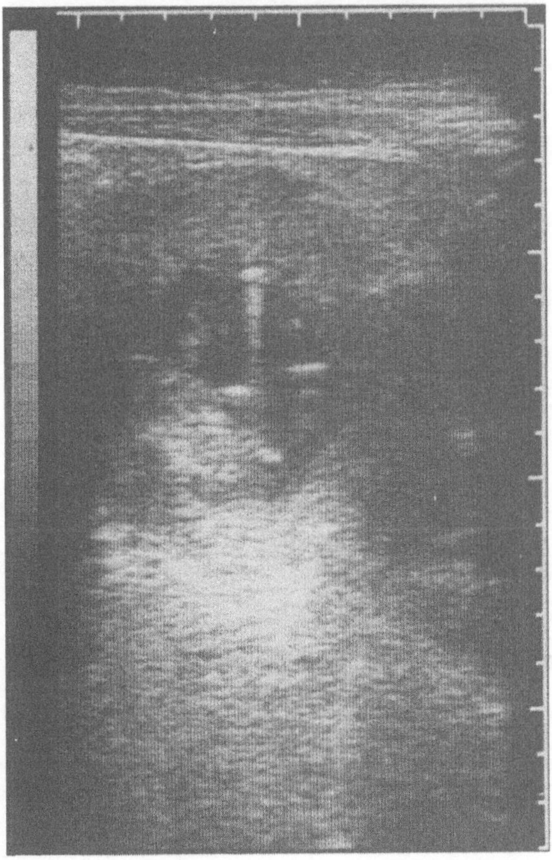

Figure 11.11 Reverberation artefact from the solid end of the cannula.

11.5 PROBLEMS OF ULTRASOUND

Ultrasound is a great help in assisting chorion villus sampling but there are still some situations that cause problems. Some of these have already been mentioned in passing.

For good images it is best if the patient has a full bladder so that the uterus is lifted out of the pelvis and a decent scanning window obtained. However, the patient is probably nervous and it is unreasonable to expect her to have an overfull bladder during the procedure. Compromises between the needs of the ultrasonographer and the comfort of the patient are hard to achieve. It is impossible to fill or empty the bladder to a suitable level without catheterizing the patient, which would be an unwarranted additional intrusion. In some patients the bladder may be empty and in these cases the pubic bone can

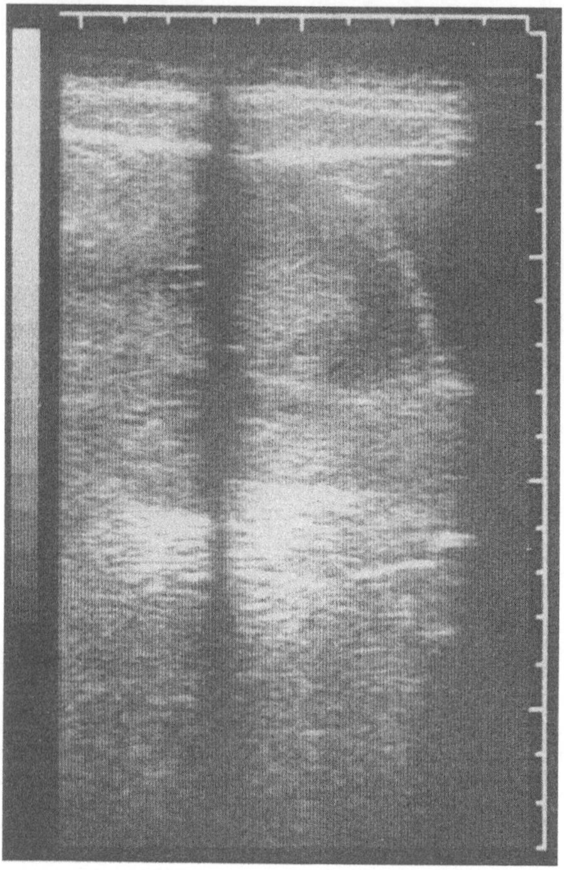

Figure 11.12 Artefact caused by an air bubble under the probe.

shadow the cervix and vagina and even part of the uterus. A sector scanner will minimize this problem because of its facility to direct the beam at an angle under the bone. In clinical practice it may be possible to give the patient a drink and wait until the bladder is suitably full.

Contact problems can be caused by air trapping due to uneven anatomy or an inadequate application of coupling gel. The pubic hair is notorious for trapping air bubbles and should be liberally coated with oil or gel prior to commencing scanning. Fig. 11.12 shows a contact problem with a linear array. The patient was very slender and her pubic bone quite prominent when she was in the lithotomy position. This problem is unlikely to occur with a sector scanner.

Bowel gas can partially or completely obscure the uterus. This can hamper the procedure considerably. A sector scanner can sometimes see under the gas if it is relatively superficial. Fig. 11.13 shows a linear array image and a sector

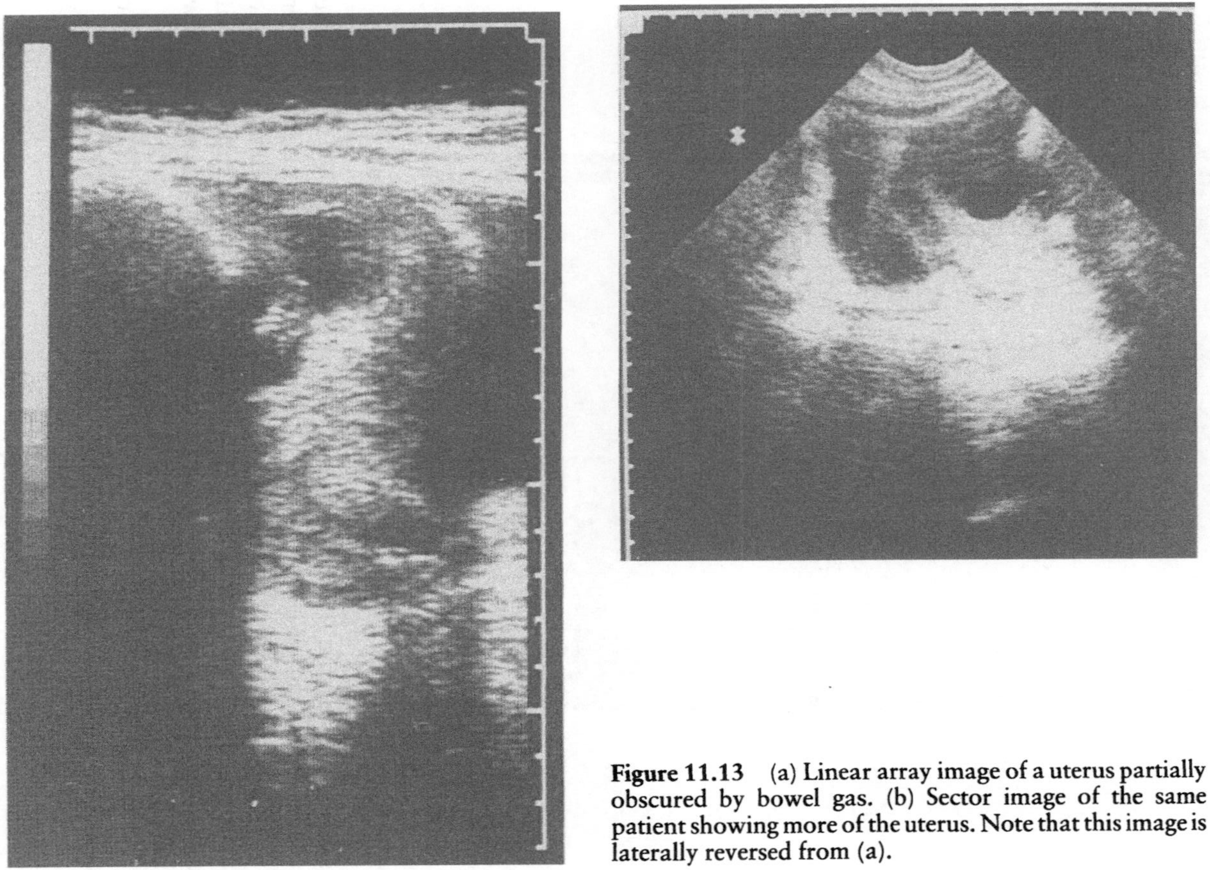

Figure 11.13 (a) Linear array image of a uterus partially obscured by bowel gas. (b) Sector image of the same patient showing more of the uterus. Note that this image is laterally reversed from (a).

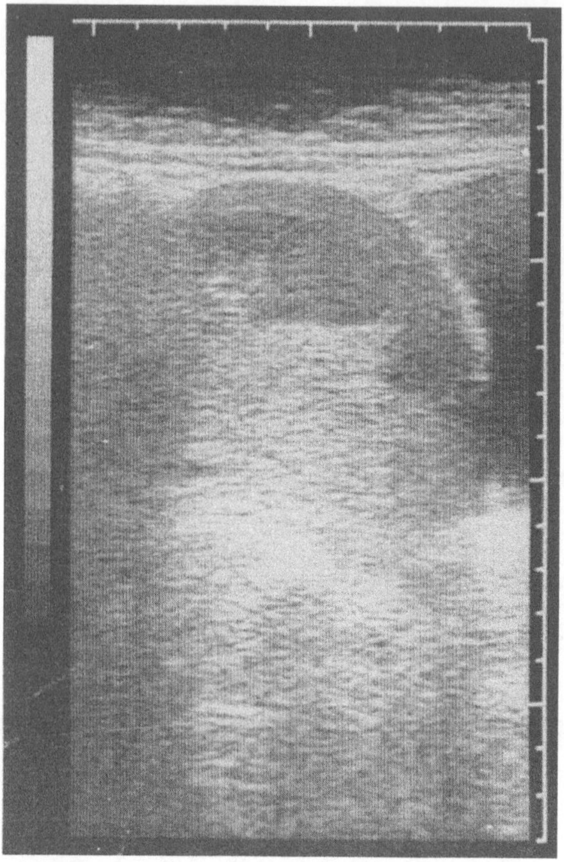

Figure 11.14 Obscuring of the image caused by fat.

scanner image from the same patient. The sector image shows more of the uterus. In most cases it should be possible to see part of the uterus by either scanning obliquely or transversely. In these cases the obstetrician cannot line up the cannula with the direction of the scan and care and patience is needed if sampling is considered. In extreme cases it is best to defer sampling a few hours or days.

Obese patients present problems because fat scatters ultrasound. The image is very snowy and fine detail can be obscured (see Fig. 11.14).

11.5.1 Tip localization

When performing chorion villus sampling location of the position of the tip of the sampling cannula is the most important part of the procedure. Problems such as bowel gas obstruction make this more complicated.

In a straightforward situation when the placenta is nicely placed – posterior positions are best from the imaging point of view – it is relatively easy to see the lie of the cannula and the position of the tip. However, when a straightforward approach is impossible and the cannula has to be inserted at an angle problems can occur. We use a cannula with a curve at the end to assist manipulation to the correct sampling site. The curve in the cannula does, however, introduce problems for tip localization. The cannula will only be completely visualized if the curve lies in the plane of the scan. If the curve lies in some other plane then only part of the cannula can be seen at any one time and it is difficult to be certain that the portion seen is the portion with the tip in it. The solid end of the cannula can be a useful ultrasonic marker if the orientation is good. We have also tried milling a flat surface on one side of the end in an attempt to produce a strong end reflector, but again this relies on suitable orientation. Gentle rocking of the probe frequently produces a flash on the screen as the solid end or reflective surface moves in and out of orientation. Patience and care usually result in accurate tip localization.

Incorporating a small ultrasonic emitter into the end of a catheter clearly demonstrates the position of the tip (Breyer and Cikes, 1984) but unfortunately adds to the complexity and cost of the system.

In conclusion, ultrasound is a valuable tool in achieving successful sampling as long as the operator is well aware of the possible pitfalls.

REFERENCES

Breyer, B. and Cikes, I. (1984) Ultrasonically marked catheter – a method for positive echographic catheter position identification. *Med. Biol. Eng. Comput.*, **22**, 268–71.

Warren, R. C. and Rodeck, C. H. (1985) First trimester prenatal diagnosis. *Hosp. Technol.*, Jan., 26–7.

12

Is ultrasound guidance necessary for successful transcervical chorion villus sampling?

—— I. Z. MacKenzie ——

With the present rate of amniocentesis in England and Wales at 2–3% of all deliveries, there are approximately 15 000 amniocenteses performed annually. The majority are for karyotyping on the grounds of advanced maternal age, and a smaller proportion are performed to investigate raised maternal serum AFP. It is probable that the number seeking karyotyping for advanced maternal age will increase with an increasing awareness within the community of the risks associated with age. Further, the request to know 'if my baby is normal' may well escalate and the use of karyotyping could extend to women in the lower age bracket.

With the development of a possibly safe diagnostic procedure providing the diagnosis of certain fetal abnormalities early in pregnancy permitting abortion within the first three months, the advantages are obvious, but the demands upon resources could be considerable. The need therefore to develop a technique which is safe and reliable is imperative. If that technique is also simple, the possibility of more women seeking or being offered the test is likely to increase. It seems appropriate, therefore, to assess further just how essential is the need for ultrasound guidance of chorion villus sampling.

It is argued that most authors reporting their experience with blind sampling have not approached the procedure using an appropriate technique and have tended to move on to sonar-guided sampling as their experience is just beginning to be gained. If a reliable technique not requiring ultrasound guidance can be developed, then this simpler test could well become available to an even greater number of pregnant women and, further, the chances of the theoretical hazards associated with ultrasound could be reduced. Experience of a non-ultrasound guided technique of chorion villus sampling is presented.

12.1 EQUIPMENT

Two different flexible polyethylene catheters have been tried. The first is a 10-French-gauge (outer diameter 3 mm) soft polyethylene catheter 405 mm long with a spigot holder at the non-operating end (Pharma-Platt, Denmark; see Fig. 12.1). The spigot holder requires modifying using an intravenous cannula to provide a luer fitting to accommodate a 2 or 10 ml syringe. The operating end of the catheter illustrated in Fig. 12.2 has a terminal portal 2.0 mm in diameter with blunt edges and a further side portal 3.0 × 2.0 mm oval diameters situated 10 mm from the tip.

The second catheter is an 8-French-gauge (2.5 mm outer diameter) polyethylene catheter 350 mm long with a capped rubber luer fitting which will accommodate a 2 or 10 ml syringe (Portex, 200/105/080, England; see Fig. 12.3). The catheter has markings originating from the operating tip at 50

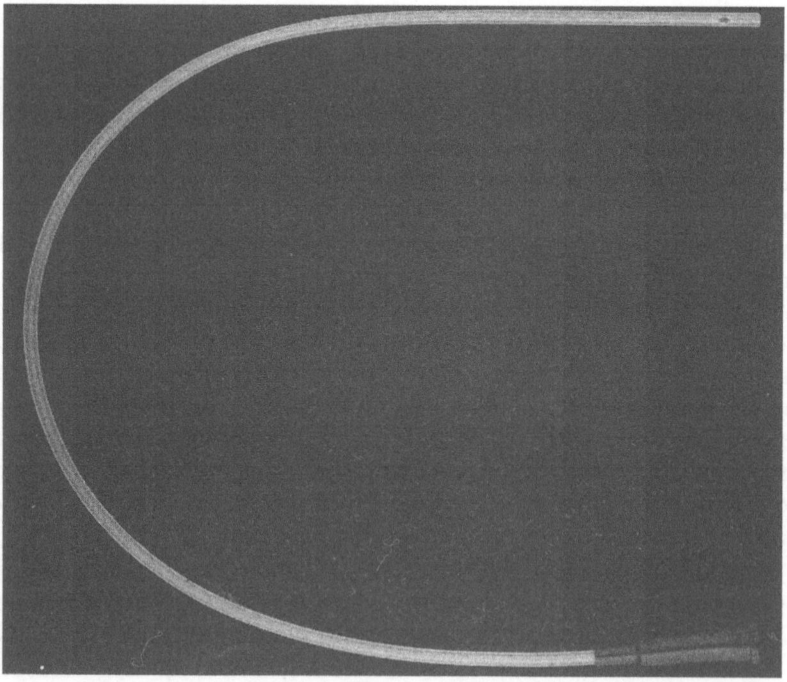

Figure 12.1 10-French-gauge polyethylene catheter with one terminal and side aspirating portal.

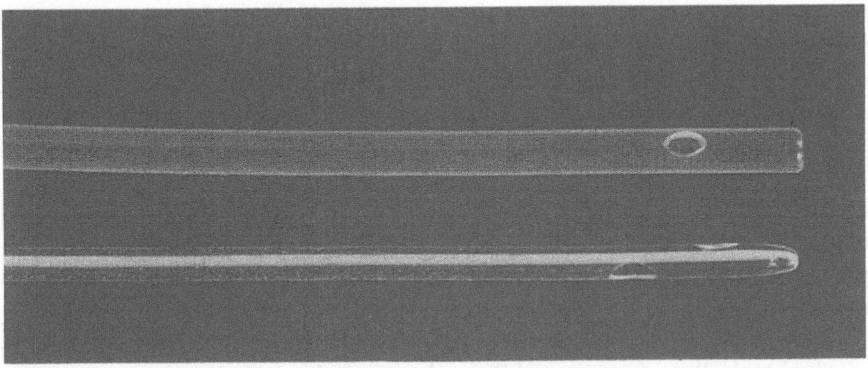

Figure 12.2 Tips of the 10-French-gauge polyethylene catheter with one end with one side portal (upper model) and the 8-French-gauge polyethylene catheter with two side portals (lower model).

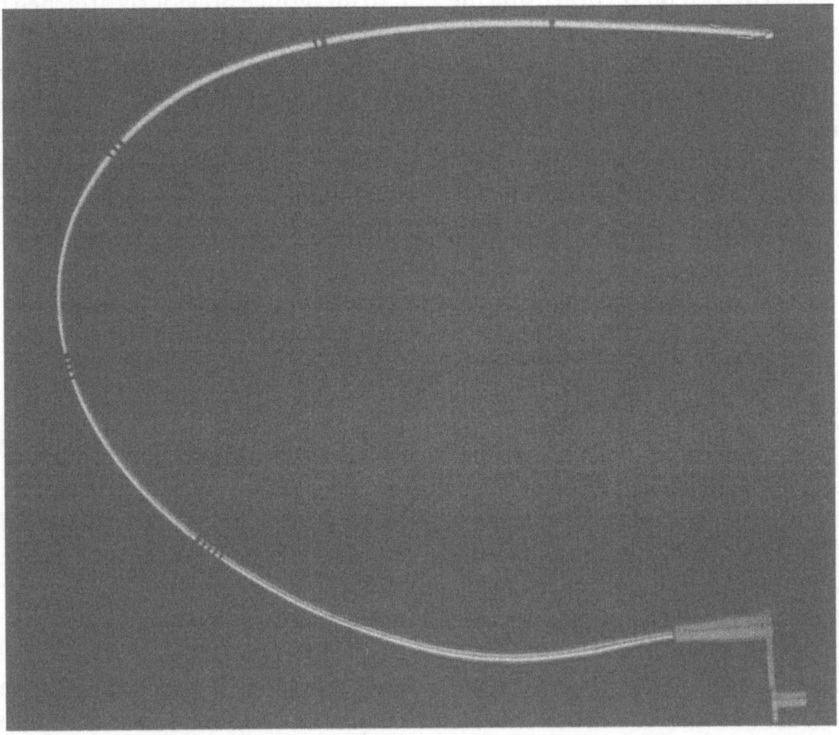

Figure 12.3 8-French-gauge polyethylene catheter with two side aspirating portals.

mm intervals along its length. At the operating end there is no terminal portal but two 3.0 × 2.0 mm diameter side holes, one at 6.5 mm from the tip and the other situated on the opposite side of the catheter 13 mm from the tip. (Fig. 12.2).

12.2 TECHNIQUE

In common with other methods of chorion villus sampling an initial ultrasound examination of the pregnancy is required to confirm that the pregnancy is viable and assess the number of fetuses and the gestation by measurement of the fetal crown rump length.

Using a Sim's speculum, with the patient in the lithotomy position, a single-toothed Volsellum forceps stabilizes the cervix by grasping the anterior lip, the vagina and external cervical os having been carefully cleansed with a solution of povidine iodine in alcohol (Betadine). Without prior probing of the cervical canal, the catheter is inserted 10 cm into the uterus using uterine packing forceps, the distance the same irrespective of gestational age (8–11 weeks range). When in position, pressure within the catheter system is reduced by 2–4 ml suction using the 2 or 10 ml syringe previously attached to the luer fitting at the end of the catheter and without dislodging the site of the catheter, it is rotated through 360° and is slowly withdrawn with continued rotation while maintaining the suction. The contents within the catheter lumen are then flushed through with Eagle's transport medium (containing fetal calf serum, Hepe's buffer, heparin and penicillin and streptomycin) and inspected for the presence of chorionic villi. If none are present, the procedure is repeated to a maximum of four insertions.

12.3 CLINICAL EXPERIENCE

12.3.1 Termination cases

The technique has been developed studying cases admitted for termination, either immediately before or within a few days of the planned procedure (14 cases). A total of 207 cases have been studied; of the 193 performed immediately before termination, 41% were under general anaesthetic and 59% under local anaesthetic using a paracervical block. Altogether 74% of patients were nulliparous, and 26% parous. In the majority the 10-French-gauge catheter was used with the 8-French-gauge catheter being used in a smaller proportion during the latter part of the experience.

In no case was technical difficulty encountered with the passage of the catheter through the endocervical canal. In three cases aspiration of amniotic fluid or extra-coelomic fluid was suspected. The success in obtaining chorionic villi according to the gestation at the time of sampling is shown in Table 12.1. In common with the reports of many others, the early experience (40

Table 12.1 Success in obtaining chorionic villi by blind transcervical aspiration at different gestations

		*Gestation (days since last menstrual period)**							
		–48	*49–55*	*56–62*	*63–69*	*70–76*	*77–83*	*84+*	*Total*
Experimental cases	Total	2	5	9	7	9	4	4	40
(first 40 patients)	N Success	1	2	7	5	7	2	3	27
	% Success	50%	40%	78%	71%	78%	50%	75%	67%
(next 167 patients)	Total	12	19	38	30	41	16	9	167
	N Success	8	18	32	26	37	13	6	140
	% Success	67%	95%	89%	87%	90%	81%	67%	84%
Diagnostic cases	Total	–	–	7	11	7	2	–	27
	N Success	–	–	7	10	7	1	–	25
	% Success	–	–	100%	91%	100%	50%	–	93%

* Gestation in the diagnostic cases has been calculated by measurement of the fetal crown rump length by ultrasound.

cases) has been analysed separately from later experience (167 cases). For the last 167 cases, a suitable sample was obtained on one insertion in 50%, with two insertions in 75% and three insertions in 92%.

In 30 instances, real-time ultrasound scanning using a ATL 100 sector scanner was used to observe the passage of the catheter into the extra-ovular space. In most instances up to 11 weeks gestation the catheter tip passed to the uterine fundus and generally via the anterior aspect of the uterus. It frequently did not come to rest in the main mass of the developing placenta which was commonly noted to be situated near the lower pole of the uterus. Although success did not appear to be related to the precise siting of the catheter tip when fully introduced, success was less readily achieved when the placenta appeared to be developing on the posterior uterine wall. In some cases, failure to obtain villi appeared to be associated with a piece of decidua blocking the catheter aspiration portals but in other instances, there was no obvious explanation, the catheter tip sited in the main placental mass. The catheter with two side aspirating portals was more successful than the catheter with only side portal with only one failed sampling (at 13 weeks gestation) in 22 consecutive attempts.

12.3.2 Diagnostic cases

In a small experience of 27 cases, villus material has been successfully obtained in 25 allowing the karyotype of the pregnancy to be determined. In none was difficulty encountered passing the catheter. One of the two failures occurred in a pregnancy studied at 11 weeks 5 days by both dates and ultrasound examination and the other occurred despite a repeated sampling a week after the first attempt at nine and ten weeks gestation respectively; on both occasions the 10-French-gauge catheter was used and ultrasound observation suggested that the catheter tip was sited in the base of the developing placenta but villi were not aspirated. In all except the first three cases which were successfully sampled, the catheter tip has been observed by ultrasound and as with the termination cases, the success of aspirating villi did not appear to be directly related to the path traversed by the catheter tip.

12.4 DISCUSSION

The majority of published series in which an assessment has been made of blind chorion villus sampling has reached the conclusion that the technique is insufficiently precise to provide a success rate acceptable for diagnostic purposes in clinical practice. If one accepts that mid-trimester amniocentesis is successful in providing a suitable fluid sample in 90.1–98.9% (Goldman *et al.*, 1977; Medical Research Council, 1978; Sant-Cassia *et al.*, 1984) of patients investigated and a result obtained from the cytogenetics laboratory for 97% of the samples provided, then a successful programme of villus sampling should provide tissue for diagnostic purposes in 90% or more of cases studied.

The original series from Tietung Hospital in China (1975) reported 100 cases of blind villus sampling using a 3 mm diameter stiff bent metal cannula advanced for 6–9 cm beyond the external cervical os, either along the anterior or posterior uterine wall. Success in obtaining villi at the first attempt was achieved in 73%, with two attempts in 97% and three attempts 100%. There is, however, no mention in that report of any failures in the series and it is possible that cases which were not successfully sampled have been excluded from the analysis. Furthermore, there is no mention of any experience in villus sampling before the 100 cases reported.

Horwell *et al.* (1983) reported their results with a blind technique in 82 patients at 7–13 weeks gestation using a 16-gauge polyethylene intravenous cannula (Medicut, Sherwood Medical Industries) 6 cm long and a 20 ml syringe. In 19 of their total sample they were unable to negotiate the cervical canal and needed to pass a uterine sound initially. Altogether they were only successful in obtaining chorionic villi in 40% of the patients. The Milan group (Simoni *et al.*, 1983) reported their results using a 14-gauge plastic cannula (Abbocath T) 6.35 cm long in 159 cases, advancing it as far as possible, i.e. a maximum of 6 cm. They were successful in 64% of cases in obtaining villus material with a maximum of three separate insertions. The same authors studied 48 cases using a 1.2 mm diameter flexible catheter (Portex Ltd., England) 15.4 cm long and advanced through the cervix until soft resistance was felt. They succeeded in obtaining villus material in a similar proportion (66%). Using the same technique but with ultrasound guidance their success rate increased to 96%.

The soft resistance mentioned by Simoni *et al.* (1983), however, could not be discerned by Rodeck *et al.* (1983) exploring different methods including endoscopy, believing the resistance referred to was the resistance felt at the internal cervical os. Rodeck and his colleagues dismissed blind sampling in their study when they failed to obtain any villi in 15 patients they investigated using three different short cannulae with diameters ranging from 1.7–4 mm, and a 3 mm diameter 21 cm long polyethylene cannula. Their technique involved advancing the catheter to the resistance they subsequently noted to be the internal cervical os. Liu *et al.* (1983) reported discouraging results using a 14 cm long 14-gauge i.v. cannula (Longdwell) in 130 cases prior to termination. They successfully obtained villi in only 35% of cases, their success being similar at 8–11 weeks gestation to that at 12–14 weeks. As with Simoni *et al.* (1983) and Rodeck *et al.* (1983) they advanced their catheter until an area of resilience was felt, which again could have been the internal cervical os.

The results obtained in the present paper using an 8- or 10-French-gauge polyethylene catheter are better than reports cited above. There are a number of possible explanations for this.

1. Catheter design
Virtually all the series using blind aspiration have concentrated upon catheters or cannulae with a single terminal aspirating portal. Of the two catheters described in the present paper one has two lateral portals, and the other has one lateral and one terminal portal. It is possible therefore that if one portal is against decidua the other one may be against the chorionic villus surface. While data are at present limited, it appears that the catheter with two side portals produces better results.

2. Catheter manipulation
As a result of the ultrasound observations during the sampling it seems probable that at least 6 cm of cannula/catheter need to be introduced past the external cervical os to ensure entering the uterine cavity. If the developing placenta is seen on initial ultrasound examination and its site noted in the lower pole of the uterine cavity then 6 cm may be adequate. However, if it is in the fundal region then advancing the catheter 10 cm will probably be necessary to reach it. The latter distance would seem appropriate, however, since villi from the chorion laeve may also be aspirated on withdrawal of the catheter, thus enhancing the prospects of obtaining suitable tissue for diagnostic purposes. In addition to the distance the catheter is advanced in the uterus it seems possible that there is an advantage in rotating the catheter so increasing the area to which the side portals in the catheter are exposed, thus improving the probability of successfully aspirating villi into the lumen.

3. Vacuum pressure generated
In all the reports quoted above, disposable 2–20 ml syringes were used to reduce pressure in the sampling system. The amount of pressure applied has not always been stated but varied between 1.5–2.0 ml using a 2 ml syringe (Liu *et al.*, 1983) to 'strong suction' using a 20 ml syringe (Horwell *et al.*, 1983). As shown by Liu *et al.* (1984), the volume by which the system is enlarged using the syringe plunger influences the degree of negative pressure within the system, although the precise relationship between syringe size and negative pressure generated withdrawing the plunger an identical volume was not investigated. An optimum negative pressure probably operates, which disrupts villi and allows their transfer into the catheter/cannula lumen but which is insufficient to aspirate decidua. Using a 10 ml syringe in the present study, withdrawal of the plunger 3–4 ml appears to be more successful than a 2 ml syringe withdrawing the plunger 2 ml. Objective data are however presently lacking to confirm this impression.

4. Experience
It is evident that many researchers studying the technique of chorion villus sampling have started with a blind method, and with the low rates of success that are usual when the technique is being developed and learnt, ultrasound guidance is incorporated and success rates improved. The study of Old *et al.* (1982) illustrates the point when ultrasound was used throughout their experience: in the first 26 cases, villi were aspirated in only 30% while in the next 37 cases they were successful in 90%.

Most series reporting transcervical villus aspiration with ultrasound control indicate that the success of getting suitable tissue for cytogenetic studies, biochemical investigation or DNA analyses should be in excess of 90%. The alternative of ultrasound guided transabdominal needle aspiration has a reported success rate of 85% (Smidt-Jensen and Hahnemann, 1984). Indeed, with ultrasound guidance one would expect a successful harvest both transabdominally and transcervically on every occasion and it is not obvious why some sampling procedures are unsuccessful, unless the interpretation of the ultrasound appearances is at fault. Apart from the expected advantage of a virtual 100% success rate of obtaining villi, ultrasound permits the sampling of individual placentae in cases of multiple pregnancy – a situation where blind sampling would be totally unsuitable. Further, there is evidence that villi obtained from the chorion laeve are more difficult to grow in tissue culture than the villi obtained from the chorion frondosum (Gustavii, 1983). In addition, with ultrasound control it should be possible to guide the sampling cannula to the placental tissue in pregnancies beyond 11 weeks gestation when the chorion laeve has largely degenerated. Experience of most workers suggests, however, that success using the transcervical route is reduced beyond this gestation and the results presented accord with that view.

If there are apparent advantages using ultrasound guided sampling, is there any place for sampling blind? Personal experience of sampling with a rigid, malleable metal cannula may cause more trauma in the chorio-decidual space and between the chorion frondosum and decidua basalis, manipulating the cannula to the placental base, than occurs with the blind (ultrasound observed) passage of the soft catheter. This however seems of little consequence as judged by the low 'spontaneous' abortion rates following diagnostic ultrasound guided sampling of continuing pregnancies. Secondly, ultrasound equipment is not readily available in all units around the world and a blind technique may be the only procedure possible. Finally, there remains at present an unanswered question over the safety of sonar during pregnancy. While there is no evidence to indicate a harmful effect from ultrasound as currently used, it is possible that the fetus and placenta are more vulnerable during the first trimester than during later gestations and the least exposure to sonar waves during the early weeks after conception would seem desirable.

To determine the advantages and disadvantages of blind versus ultrasound guided transcervical villus aspiration in the short and long term would require randomized trials comparing the two techniques. It seems probable, however, that such trials would be difficult to mount, even at this relatively early stage in the development of a new diagnostic technique.

ACKNOWLEDGEMENTS

My thanks are due to Dr Jon Jonasson and staff of the Cytogenetics Laboratory, Churchill Hospital, Oxford; Dr Jean Keeling and staff, Paediatric Histology Laboratory, John Radcliffe Hospital; Dr Bruce Castle for ultrasound expertise; and Sister Jane Ferguson for expert nursing care.

REFERENCES

Goldman, B., Mashiah, S., Serr, D. M., Blankstein, J., Chaki, R., Navon, R. and Padeh, B. (1977) A survey of amniocentesis in 925 patients at high risk of fetal genetic disorder. *Br. J. Obstet. Gynaecol.*, **84**, 808–14.

Gustavii, B. (1983) First trimester chromosomal analysis of chorionic villi obtained by direct vision technique. *Lancet*, **ii**, 507–8.

Horwell, D. H., Loeffler, F. E. and Coleman, D. V. (1983) Assessment of a transcervical aspiration technique for chorionic villus biopsy in the first trimester of pregnancy. *Br. J. Obstet. Gynaecol.*, **90**, 196–8.

Liu, D. T. Y., Mitchell, J., Johnson, J. and Wass, D. M. (1983) Trophoblast sampling by blind transcervical aspiration. *Br. J. Obstet. Gynaecol.*, **90**, 1119–23.

Liu, D. T. Y., Slater, E., Norman, S. (1984) Aspiration as a technique for biopsy of chorionic villi. *J. Obstet. Gynecol.*, **5**, 75–7.

Medical Research Council Working Party on Amniocentesis (1978) An assessment of the hazards of amniocentesis. *Br. J. Obstet. Gynaecol.*, **85**, Suppl. 2.

Old, J. M., Ward, R. H. T., Karagozlu, F., Petrou, M., Modell, B. and Weatherall, D. J. (1982) First trimester fetal diagnosis for haemoglobinopathies; three cases. *Lancet*, **ii**, 1413–16.

Rodeck, C. H., Morsman, J. M., Gosden, C. M. and Gosden, J. R. (1983) Development of an improved technique for first-trimester microsampling of chorion. *Br. J. Obstet. Gynaecol.*, **90**, 1113–18.

Sant-Cassia, I. J., MacPherson, M. B. A. and Tyack, A. J. (1984) Midtrimester amniocentesis: is it safe? A single centre controlled prospective study of 517 consecutive amniocenteses. *Br. J. Obstet. Gynaecol.*, **91**, 736–44.

Simoni, G., Brambati, B., Danesino, C., Rossella, F., Terzoli, G. L., Ferrari, M. and Fraccaro, M. (1983) Efficient direct chromosome analyses and enzyme determinations from chorionic villi samples in the first trimester of pregnancy. *Hum. Genet.*, **63**, 349–57.

Smidt-Jensen, S. and Hahnemann, N. (1984) Transabdominal fine needle biopsy from chorionic villi in the first trimester. *Prenat. Diag.*, **4**, 163–9.

Tietung Hospital (1975) Fetal sex prediction by sex chromatin of chorionic villi cells during early pregnancy. *Chin. Med. J.*, **1**, 117–26.

13

Endoscopic chorion villus sampling

—— *Björn Gustavii* ——

13.1 INTRODUCTION

Presented here are the first 100 cases of *completed* pregnancy following chorion villus sampling by the direct vision technique (endoscopic CVS) carried out at Lund University Hospital.

13.2 SAMPLING

Endoscopic CVS, described in detail elsewhere (Gustavii, 1984), involves the transcervical insertion of a fetoscope into the extra-ovular space during continuous infusion of physiologic saline solution (Figs 13.1 and 13.2). The technique gives a clear view of the sampling site.

In an experimental series of cases for first trimester vacuum aspiration abortion, we studied the effect of the extra-ovular saline instillation on intra-uterine pressure (Fig. 13.3) and fetal heart activity (Löfberg *et al.*, 1985). Following the infusion of 150 ml saline, intra-uterine pressure ranged between 16 and 23 mm Hg, thus not more than that during Braxton Hicks contractions. At CVS during continuous saline infusion, fetal heart activity (beats per 15 s) decreased temporarily from about 36 to about 33.

More than 5 mg of tissue and some degree of vascularity were found to be important prerequisites for successfully establishing long-term cultures from the trophoblastic tissue (Gustavii *et al.*, 1985). In clinical practice we try to obtain samples which, besides being vascular, weigh at least 10 mg.

The technique of long-term culturing and the results of the cytogenetic analyses are presented in detail elsewhere (Mandahl *et al.*, 1985; Heim *et al.*, 1985).

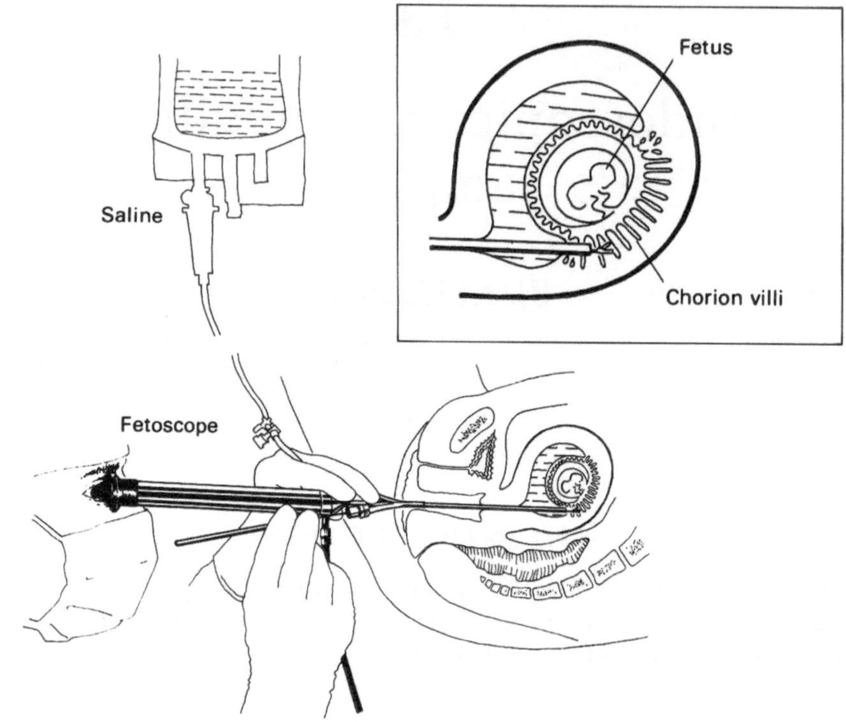

Figure 13.1 Endoscopic CVS during continuous infusion of physiologic saline solution. (Reproduced, with permission, from Gustavii *et al.*, 1984.)

13.3 ONE HUNDRED COMPLETED PREGNANCIES

Table 13.1 lists the indications for CVS in the 100 diagnostic cases. Sampling was done at week eight of pregnancy (one case), week nine (five cases), week ten (35 cases), week 11 (31 cases), week 12 (25 cases), or week 13 (four cases). In one woman, sampling was done twice, in weeks 11 and 12 (see below). No analgesia or anaesthesia was given. Twelve of the women were nulliparous.

Table 13.1 Indications for chorion villus sampling (CVS) in 100 pregnancies

Advanced maternal age	65
Chromosome aberration in a previous child or fetus	13
Balanced translocation in parent	5
Mosaicism in parent	1
Sexing for X-linked disorder	11
Metabolic disease	3
Maternal anxiety	2

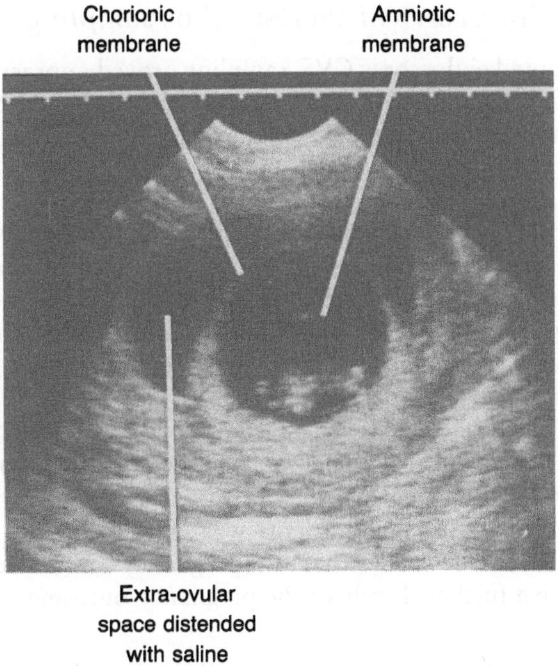

Figure 13.2 Ultrasound scan made at endoscopic CVS in the tenth week of gestation, showing the distension of the extra-ovular space by infused physiologic saline. Note the absence of any change in the outline of the sac. The scan also shows the distance between the chorionic membrane and amniotic membrane that is not yet fused. (Scan: Heléne Edvall.)

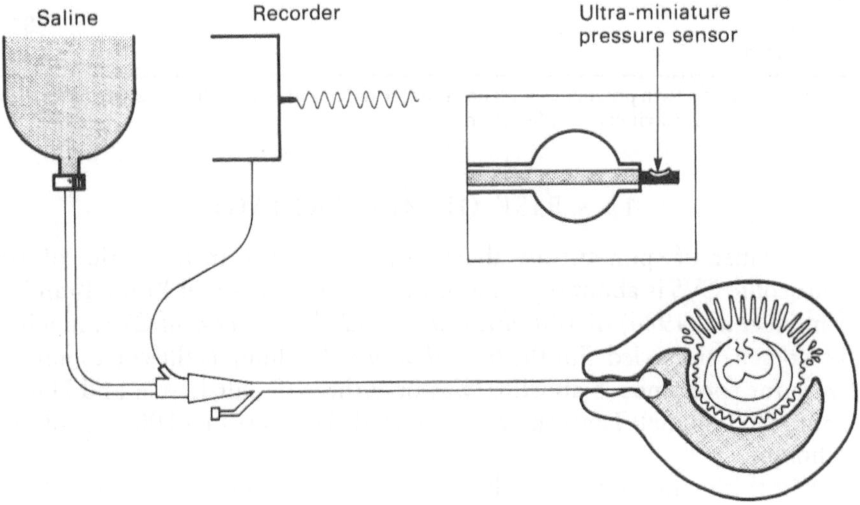

Figure 13.3 Intra-uterine pressure recording during instillation of physiologic saline solution into the extra-ovular space. (Drawing: Ingemar Nilsson.)

Of 101 attempted endoscopic CVS, sampling proved impracticable in one case because of placenta praevia; this case is not included in the presentation. In 100 cases where access to the extra-ovular space was gained, sampling was successful.

Laboratory analysis was successful in 96 of the 100 cases. In the four failures, diagnosis was subsequently established by a further CVS (one case), or by a mid-trimester amniocentesis (three cases). Details of the failures are given elsewhere (Gustavii *et al.*, 1984; Heim *et al.*, 1985).

Pregnancy was terminated because of diagnosis in 14 cases. In five of these cases the reason was an abnormal fetal karyotype; in another four cases, a male fetus was aborted because of the 50% risk of X-linked disease; two fetuses had a metabolic disorder; one fetus had cystic nuchal hygroma combined with hydronephrosis, detected by ultrasound (Gustavii and Edvall, 1984); another fetus had gastroschisis, also detected by ultrasound; and, finally, in one case, although the fetus was chromosomally normal, the woman decided in her 8th week to have the pregnancy terminated. Table 13.2 and Fig. 13.4 give further details of the pregnancy outcome.

Table 13.2 Outcome of pregnancy after endoscopic chorion villus sampling (CVS) in 100 completed pregnancies

Terminated because of diagnosis	14*
Miscarriage	
within 3 weeks of sampling	2
more than 3 weeks after sampling	5
Delivery	
term	78*
pre-term	2

* Figure includes a twin pregnancy with one normal and one affected fetus; selective feticide was carried out (see Gustavii *et al.*, 1984, for details).

13.4 RISK OF MISCARRIAGE

The number of spontaneous abortions, seven cases, in our series of 100 *endoscopic* CVS is about the same as that in the series of Dr Bruno Brambati (Simoni *et al.*, 1984) of 100 *ultrasound-guided transcervical* CVS, in which six women miscarried. For the *transabdominal* technique, the corresponding figure for spontaneous abortion was only three (Smidt-Jensen and Hahnemann, this volume). These three series included the very first 100 cases of each technique.

Since this manuscript was submitted for publication, we have abandoned the endoscopic technique and adopted the *transabdominal* method. The reason for this change of method was the risk of intra-uterine infection with the former (Gustavii *et al.*, 1986a). The risk is shared with other methods using

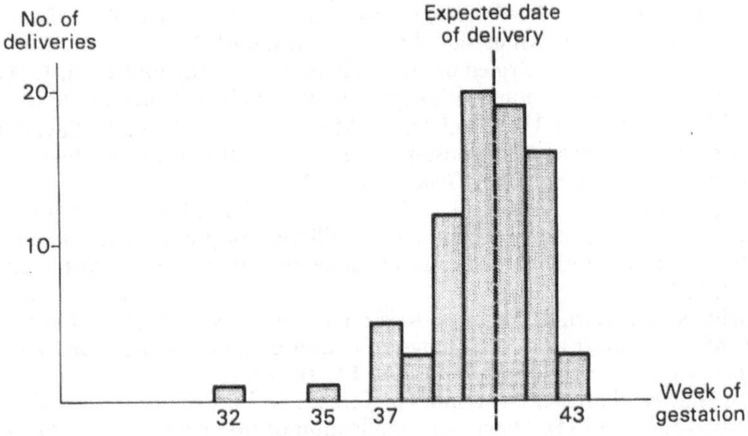

Figure 13.4 Week of delivery in 80 pregnancies subjected to endoscopic CVS in first trimester.

a transcervical approach (Barela *et al.*, 1986). In two of the 134 diagnostic samplings executed with the endoscopic technique, intra-uterine infections subsequently occurred, resulting in miscarriage. The total number of miscarriages in this series was nine.

Up to September 1986, we have carried out 51 diagnostic CV samplings by the transabdominal route: seven of the women have given birth and there has been no case of miscarriage, so far.

One great advantage of the transabdominal procedure is that it is more acceptable to the woman, since it is very similar to amniocentesis. Another advantage is that, with the transabdominal technique, the sampling need not be restricted to the first trimester (Gustavii *et al.*, 1986b).

REFERENCES

Barela, A. I., Kleinman, G. E., Golditch, I. M., Menke, D. J., Hogge, W. A. and Golbus, M. S. (1986) Septic shock with renal failure after chorionic villus sampling. *Am. J. Obstet. Gynecol.*, **154**, 1100–2.

Gustavii, B. (1984) Chorionic villi sampling under direct vision. *Clin. Genet.*, **26**, 297–300.

Gustavii, B., Chester, M. A., Edvall, H., Iosif, S., Kristoffersson, U., Löfberg, L., Mineur, A. and Mitelman, F. (1984) First-trimester diagnosis on chorionic villi obtained by direct vision technique. *Hum. Genet.*, **65**, 373–6.

Gustavii, B. and Edvall, H. (1984) First-trimester diagnosis of cystic nuchal hygroma. *Acta Obstet. Gynecol. Scand.*, **63**, 377–8.

Gustavii, B., Edvall, H., Mineur, A., Heim, S., Mandahl, N., Kristoffersson, U. and Mitelman, F. (1985) Trophoblast samples suitable for long-term culture. *Acta Obstet. Gynecol. Scand.*, **64**, 661–2.

Gustavii, B., Edvall, H., Dahlander, K., Jonsson, N. and Carlén, B. (1986a) Transabdominal chorionic villus sampling. *Lancet*, i, 440–1.

Gustavii, B., Edvall, H., Svalenius, E., Dahlander, K. and Jörgensen, C. (1986b) Second trimester chorionic villus (placental) sampling. *Lancet*, i, 969.

Heim, S., Kristoffersson, U., Mandahl, N., Mineur, A., Mitelman, F., Edvall, H. and Gustavii, B. (1985) Chromosome analysis in 100 cases of first trimester trophoblast sampling. *Clin. Genet.*, **27**, 451–7.

Löfberg, L., Iosif, C. S., Edvall, H. and Gustavii, B. (1985) Direct vision sampling of chorionic villi during extra-amniotic instillation of physiologic saline solution. Effect on intra-uterine pressure and fetal heart activity. *Am. J. Obstet. Gynecol.*, **152**, 591–2.

Mandahl, N., Gustavii, B., Heim, S., Kristoffersson, U., Mineur, A. and Mitelman, F. (1985). Technical aspects of long-term culture and cytogenetic analysis of first trimester chorionic villi. *Karyogram.*, **11**, 10–13.

Simoni, G., Brambati, B., Danesino, C., Terzoli, G. L., Romitti, L., Rosella, F. and Fraccaro, M. (1984). Diagnostic application of first trimester trophoblast sampling in 100 pregnancies. *Hum. Genet.*, **66**, 252–9.

PART THREE

Transabdominal chorion villus sampling

14

Danish experience

— *Steen Smidt-Jensen and Niels Hahnemann* —

14.1 INTRODUCTION

Prenatal fetal diagnosis based on second trimester amniocentesis implies that subsequent measures cannot be taken before the 20th week of pregnancy. However, new obstetric techniques for chorion villus sampling (CVS) combined with modified laboratory methods for genetic diagnosis allow the detection of genetically abnormal fetuses in the first trimester of pregnancy with subsequent early abortion. This new technique also has important implications for maternal and child health because it is likely that it will prove more acceptable to women. Combined with the current increase in understanding of the molecular basis for genetic disease and the increasing usefulness of techniques such as DNA recombinant analysis, this seems to extend both the range and applicability of fetal diagnosis aimed at preventing the birth of infants with serious congenital abnormalities.

Use of CVS is now spreading rapidly and for this reason it is important to define the safety and efficacy of the different techniques. Evaluation of the immediate risk, i.e. the spontaneous abortion rate in sonographically normal first trimester pregnancies, as well as short-term risks, such as premature delivery and fetal malformations, must be defined. Many centres are now trying to define these rates. The long-term risk to infants and society in general must also be considered.

The chorionic villi in the placenta can be reached transabdominally and transcervically. Transabdominal tissue sampling from *in vivo* placentas was originally performed by Alvarez (1966). He reports on 50 cases of chorion villus sampling by transabdominal needle biopsy in diagnosing hydatidiform mole in 10–14 week-old pregnancies. No complication were reported. A total of 215 third trimester transabdominal samples were obtained by Aladjem (1969) for studying morphology of *in vivo* placentas, with no established fetal or maternal complications.

Transabdominal chorion villus sampling (TA-CVS) as a diagnostic method for fetal genetic diagnosis in the 9th, 10th, and 11th week of pregnancy, was introduced by Smidt-Jensen and Hahnemann (1984), and further evaluated (Smidt-Jensen *et al.*, 1984; 1986) as a method of avoiding the risks of contamination of the sample and infection of the fetus by transcervical sampling (Jackson, 1984a).

14.2 MATERIALS

The technique for transabdominal CVS was originally developed at the ultrasonic laboratory, of the Department of Obstetrics at Aalborg Hospital in Denmark. The results presented in this paper are taken from an initial study of women seeking legal abortions and from a continuing study of diagnostic cases (Table 14.1).

Table 14.1 Initial and continuing studies of chorion villus sampling (CVS) and transabdominal chorion villus sampling (TA-CVS)

	Technique	*Number*	*Karyotype*	*Success*	*Rate*
Termination of pregnancy	TA-CVS	72	÷	62	(68%)
	TA-CVS	10	+	10	(100%)
	Transcervical	3	+	3	(100%)
Continuing pregnancy	TA-CVS	170	+	170	(100%)

Before TA-CVS was applied to continuing pregnancies the short-term cytogenetic technique described by Simoni *et al.* (1983) was tested. The cytogenetic work was performed by Professor Aa.J. Therkelsen and co-workers at the Institute of Human Genetics of the University of Aarhus, Denmark.

A total of 670 prenatal genetic investigations took place during 1984 at the ultrasonic laboratory at the Department of Obstetrics in Aalborg. By May 1985, 170 of these investigations had been performed as TA-CVS for genetic analysis.

All women with pregnancies at risk of fetal genetic disease are offered CVS or amniocentesis. To evaluate the fetal loss and the acceptability of TA-CVS, two prospective and randomized studies have been established:

1. Women aged 35 or more are randomized between TA-CVS and amniocentesis.
2. Women aged 30–34 years are randomized between TA-CVS and no CVS, with control measures only.

All the women fulfilled the usual criteria for mid-trimester diagnosis as established by the National Danish Board of Health except for those in the second group. They also all fulfilled the ultrasonic criteria for normal early pregnancy.

Special attention was paid to the first 26 women having TA-CVS (Smidt-Jensen *et al.*, 1986). Each pregnancy was monitored weekly until the 16th week, thereafter monthly by ultrasonography and serum determinations of human placental lactogen (hPL), alpha-fetoprotein (AFP) and blood group antibodies. AFP was also measured before and 10 minutes after sampling in order to evaluate any fetomaternal bleeding. At birth, a careful examination of the baby was performed. This included a registration of the gestational age, birth length and weight and Apgar scores, as well as any perinatal complications and any malformations disclosed at the time of delivery. The examination also included a chromosome study on cultured lymphocytes in umbilical cord blood. The placentas underwent detailed macroscopical and histological examination. They were examined and compared with placentas randomly chosen from a group of pregnancies examined by amniocentesis. Special attention was paid to the cut surface and the maternal surface for the presence of retro-placental impressions and/or haematomas, and any sign of inflamation, infarction or fibrosis.

Post-CVS control measures have now been reduced to screening for neural tube defects (NTD) in 16th week, hPL monthly and determinations of blood group antibodies in 24th and 36th week of pregnancy.

14.3 SAMPLING PROCEDURE

Sonographically normal pregnancy is where fetal heart activity is registered from the seventh week of pregnancy. Normal growth is measured by comparing the gestational age measured from last menstrual period and the sonographically estimated crown rump length. The ability to outline chorionic tissue echoes as a safe target area for fine needle aspiration from the eighth week of pregnancy and the desire to perform a fetal diagnosis before the end of 12th week limits the period for CVS to a gestational age of 8–11 weeks.

Based on our experience from the initial study, TA-CVS is preferentially done in the 9th–10th week of pregnancy (56–77 days). The technique includes the following steps:

1. The woman is carefully informed about the procedure before and during the sample.
2. She is placed in supine position, and the placental region localized by real-time sector sonography. The predetermined needle pathway (Fig. 14.1), achieved by a needle guide attached to the transducer head (Fig. 14.2), is established as a line parallel to the chorionic membrane. For exact alignment the uterine position is adjusted by regulating the bladder contents.

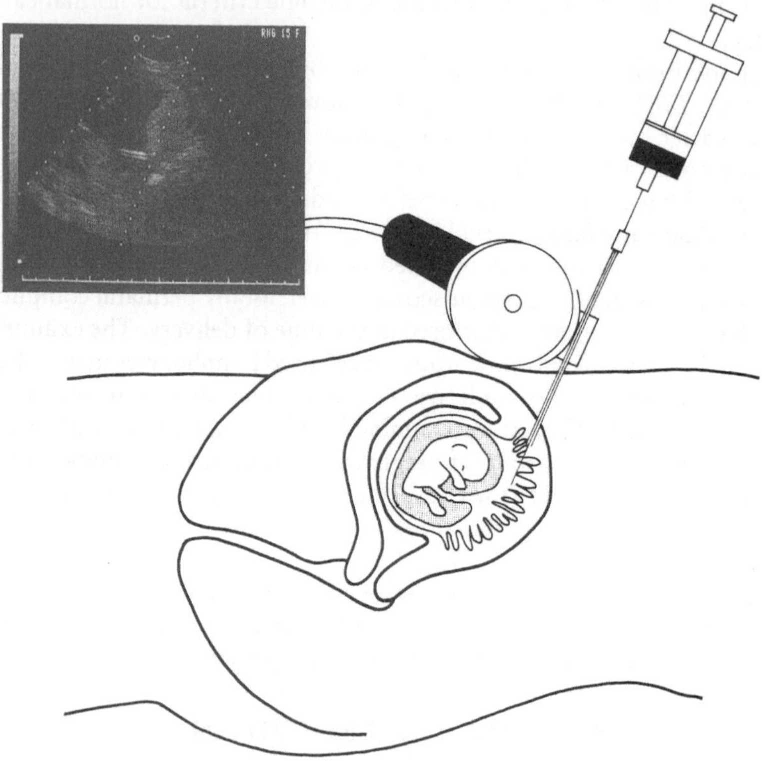

Figure 14.1 Transabdominal CVS guided by on-site real-time ultrasound. The sonographic picture shows the predetermined needle pathway. (Redrawn with permission from Gustavii, 1985.)

3. The skin is cleaned with chlorhexidine 0.5% and the guide needle (length 15 cm, gauge 18) introduced through the uterine wall to the edge of the region for chorionic echoes. The guide needle thus allows a free and painless movement of the aspiration needle (length 20 cm, gauge 22), when suction is performed. Both needles are standard lumbar puncture needles, MEDA, with a cut surface angled at 19 degrees.
4. The chorionic villi are aspirated into a syringe with a few ml of heparinized Hanks buffered saline using repeated aspirations until about 30 mg of tissue is obtained. The time necessary to obtain enough material for a skilled practitioner is about two minutes.
5. The villi are washed repeatedly in Hanks buffered saline, and are carefully selected immediately by naked eye and later using microscopic examination at the cytogenetic laboratory. Any material of suspected maternal origin is discarded.

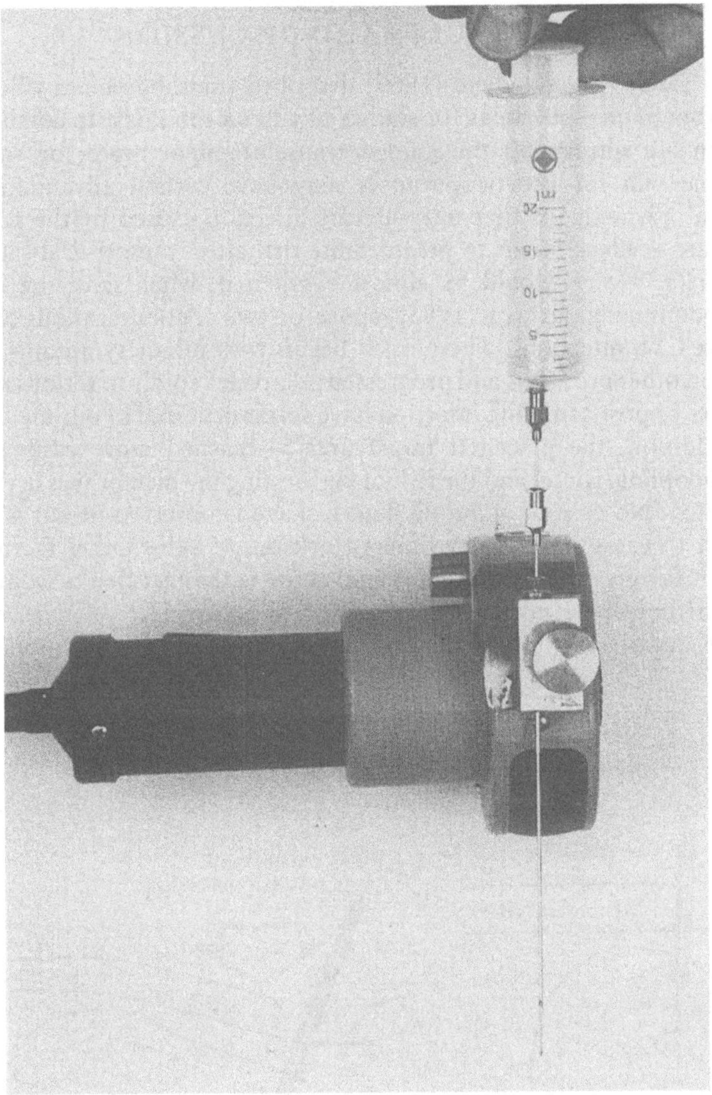

Figure 14.2 The needle guide mounted on the Kretz Combison ultrasound transducer. The guide needle and the aspiration needle are inserted.

6. Finally, the viability of the fetus is monitored by ultrasound, and any alterations in placental morphology, i.e. haematomas or air inlets through the needle, are noted.

The sampling takes place as an out-patient procedure and takes on the average 30 minutes. No anaesthetics are needed.

14.4 RESULTS AND DISCUSSION

Alvarez (1966) and Aladjem (1969) described transabdominal villus sampling from *in vivo* placentas for studies of villi morphology. In combination with on-site ultrasound the guided transabdominal route for sampling chorionic villi for genetic purposes may have certain advantages. The principal advantage is that intra-uterine infection caused by the sampling procedure – which seems to be a definite risk after transcervical sampling, Jackson (1984a) – would be almost eliminated, when sampling is done transabdominally. Jackson (1985) reports on two communications concerning post-CVS infections. These cases began with minor symptoms, minor fever and other problems and progressed relatively rapidly to serious trouble. No cases of post-sampling infection have so far occurred in our material.

In addition, the placental target area is reached more easily by the transabdominal route, and the risk of perforating the membranes is virtually eliminated. No case of amniotic fluid leakage is observed in our study, in contrast to cases reported by others (Jackson, 1984b). Other factors that speak in favour of the transabdominal route is the fact that a woman can relax in the supine position during the procedure. Her relatives may be present, and she can follow the procedure on the sonographic monitor. Of

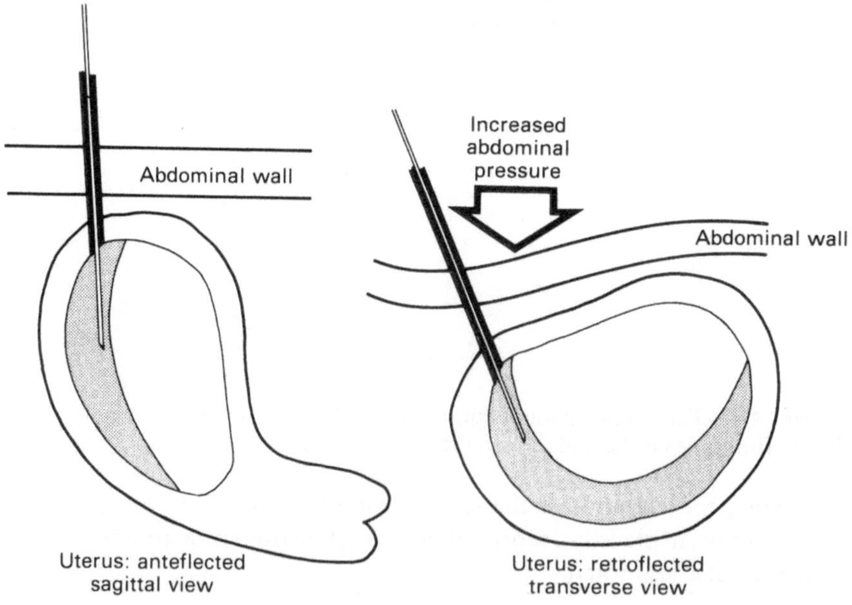

Figure 14.3 Management of transabdominal CVS in cases of posterior localized placentas.

essential importance is also that simultaneous vaginal and abdominal activity is avoided.

Difficulty in sampling might be expected in the case of posterior placentas combined with retroflexion of the uterus, but emptying the urinary bladder and increasing the pressure against the abdominal wall has made sampling possible in all such cases so far. The approach in posterior localized placentas is illustrated in Fig. 14.3.

14.5 SAMPLING RESULTS

One hundred and seventy TA-CVS have been performed, and 73 babies have been delivered to date (Table 14.2). The gestational age at the time of sampling was betweeen the 8th and the 12th week. The mean fetal crown rump length was 3.2 cm (1.6 –5.1 cm).

In 169 cases the quantity of villi aspirated was between 15 mg and 50 mg (mean 30 mg) at the first attempt, which normally include between two and six repeated aspirations. In five cases one additional puncture was necessary to obtain sufficient amounts of villi, as contractions of the abdominal rectus muscle distorted the needle pathway. In one case only 2–3 mg of chorionic villi was extracted at the first attempt. By the CVS one week later the required 30 mg of villi was aspirated without complication. One woman was excluded from our material for two reasons. First, the pregnancy had progressed to the 13th week, which is in excess of our CVS guidelines by two weeks. Secondly, she reacted strongly to the abdominal puncture, and attempts at further puncture were abandoned.

Table 14.2 An overview of 170 transabdominal CVS performed before May 1985 at the Obstetric Department, Aalborg Hospital

		No. of women
TA-CVS in the 8th–11th week of pregnancy*		170
Spontaneous abortions		4
Therapeutic abortions		8
Continuing pregnancies	<28 weeks	48
	28–36 weeks	23
	≥36 weeks	14
Deliveries		73

* One in the 13th week.

14.6 IMMEDIATE COMPLICATIONS

All women were discharged from the ultrasonic laboratory immediately after CVS. A few patients were kept for half an hour to rest, because they experienced some discomfort.

No immediate complications such as vaginal bleeding or infection, intra- or extra-placental haematomas were noted, neither were such abnormalities registered sonographically in the course of the pregnancy. Spotting during the day of CVS was experienced by five women, but they were discharged from hospital after a few days of bed rest. Placental related haematomas was suspected in one of these women. The suspicion was not confirmed by later sonographic investigation or by the placental examination post-partum.

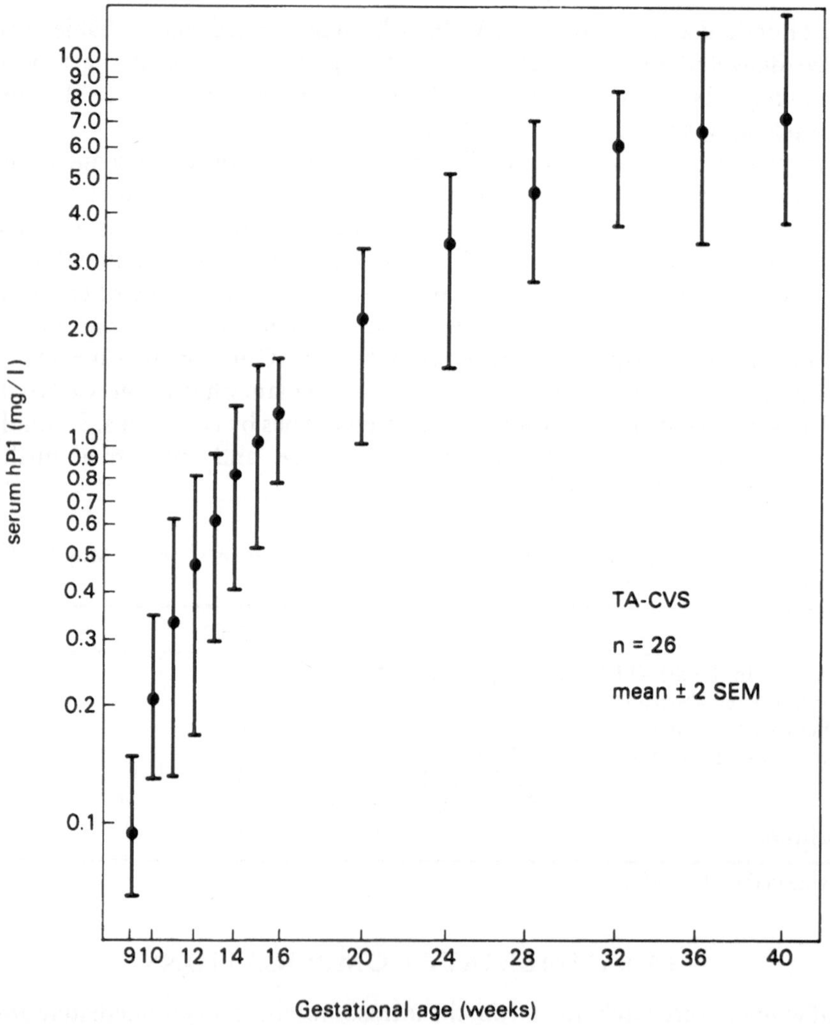

Figure 14.4 Serum determinations of human placental lactogen (hP1) in the first 26 pregnancies followed to term.

14.7 PROGRESS AND OUTCOME OF PREGNANCIES

The results from the first 26 CVS followed to term and the subsequent experience indicate that there are no significant differences in either hPL or biparietal-diameter (BPD) distributions compared with values from a normal population (Figs 14.4 and 14.5). The growth curves for each single pregnancy shows differences from otherwise normal growth curves only in three diagnosed cases and one suspected case of placental insufficiency. The study revealed no placental abnormalities in accordance with the post-CVS sonographic picture. One fetus had a cardiac puncture in the 19th week of pregnancy to determine the level of Factor VIII, which was found to be normal.

Pre-term delivery took place in five of the total cases (6.9%: see Table 14.2), and 13 caesarean sections were performed (17.8%). The perinatal mortality rate was zero. The mean weight for the 73 babies was 3738 grams (1835–5100 grams); 65 scored 9–10 Apgar points and eight scored 6–8 Apgar points at the first minute. None of the babies showed any clinical abnormalities. A major question is whether the CVS pregnancies differ from the amniocentesis pregnancies with respect to the clinical course. Until the results from randomized studies are available, we have compared the CVS pregnancies with those where amniocentesis took place immediately before

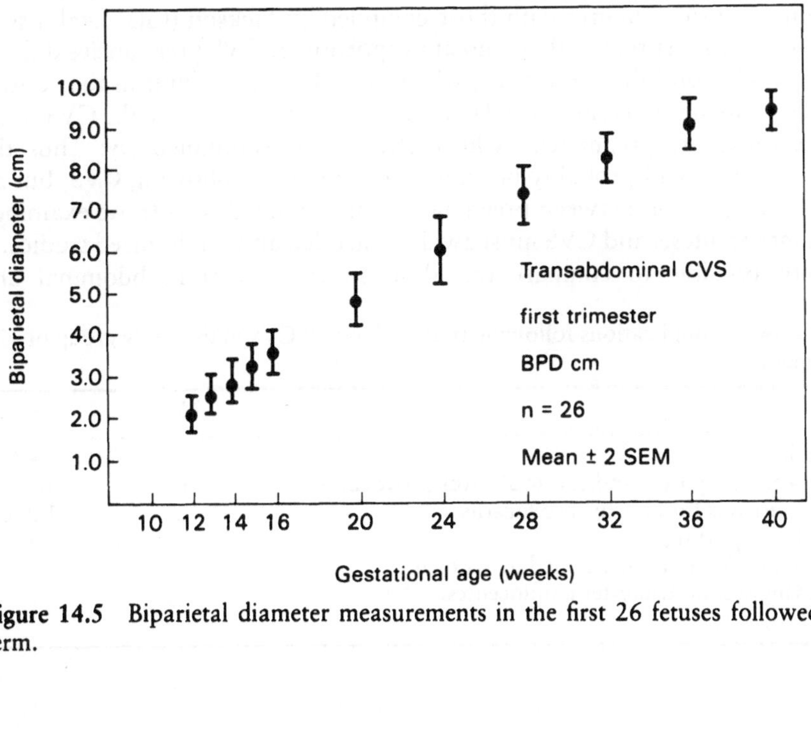

Figure 14.5 Biparietal diameter measurements in the first 26 fetuses followed to term.

each CVS procedure. This very preliminary matched comparison indicates no clinical differences between CVS and amniocentesis with respect to the outcome of pregnancy.

14.8 ABORTIONS

Eight women underwent therapeutic abortion following CVS. Six of these terminations were because of abnormal cytogenetic findings (Table 14.3); one was because of suspected intra-uterine infection with rubella viruses, and the other was for social reasons.

Four women aborted spontaneously before 28th week of pregnancy (2.4%). The karyotypes were normal and fetal demise was detected at 75, 47, 22 and 17 days after CVS.

We have previously introduced the concept of TA-CVS (Smidt-Jensen and Hahnemann, 1984) and also the results from these preliminary trials and present experience support a low abortion rate after TA-CVS. Table 14.4 shows the abortion rates in the largest CVS studies compiled in April 1985 (Jackson, 1985). The evaluation of the real risk of abortion following CVS requires knowledge of the spontaneous abortion rate in first trimester pregnancies aged 9–11 weeks, which are proven normal sonographically. Wilson (1984) and Gilmore and McNay (1985) report on two large series of sonographic normal first trimester pregnancies. The overall abortion rate was 2.1% in both series and 4.0% in both series in women aged 35 or over. Comparing these figures with those compiled by Jackson (total fetal loss = 4.1%), one must realize that a great proportion of CVS pregnancies did not progress beyond the 29th week, which was the cut-off limit in the control studies. Furthermore, abnormal karyotypes are excluded from the CVS study since those are pregnancies which often abort spontaneously. Thus the abortion risk will probably be expected to increase following CVS, but an exact comparison between pregnancies not examined with those examined by amniocentesis and CVS must await controlled and randomized studies. It is not possible to compare the abortion risk for transabdominal and

Table 14.3 Complications following transabdominal CVS in the study group of 170 pregnancies

	No.	*%*
Fetal loss	4	(2.4%)
Abnormal karyotype indicating abortus provocatus	6	(3.5%)
Other reasons for abortus provocatus	2	(1.2%)
Bleeding (spotting)	4	(2.4%)
Discomfort/pain: as mentioned by women having second trimester amniocentesis (n=170)		

Table 14.4 The nine largest CVS series compiled by Jackson (1985)

	Total patients	*Failed sample*	*Abortus provocatus**	*Continued pregnancy*	*Fetal loss**	*Fetal loss%**	*Delivered*
Philadelphia	750	4	54	675	13	1.9	275
Milan	602	9	37	565	12	3.0	250
San Francisco	525	10	37	488	27	5.5	102
Chicago	532	11	36	494	14	2.8	200
Rotterdam	269	21	16	253	9	3.6	53
Genoa	232	9	14	218	14	6.4	57
Alborg	170	0	8	162	4	2.4	73
Paris	140	0	41	99	5	5.5	30
London	140	2	31	109	6	5.5	37

* Total loss % = 4.1.

transcervical CVS on the small numbers of cases available. Table 14.5 depicts details of the four post-CVS abortions in the TA-CVS study. The karyotypes were normal, and only in case 104 do certain facts (two transabdominal punctures and suspicion of fetomaternal bleeding according to the AFP rise) indicate tardive problems. The occurrence of the four abortions 3–10 weeks after CVS procedure is confusing. Would spontaneous abortion have taken place anyway?

Table 14.5 Fetal death following chorion villus sampling (TA-CVS) in the study group of 170 pregnancies

TA-CVS	*No. 82* *34 years* *para 111* *o Rh pos*	*No. 90* *35 years* *para 01* *A Rh pos*	*No. 96* *38 years* *para 1* *A Rh pos*	*No. 104* *38 years* *para 10010* *A Rh pos*
Date, operator	250964, ssj	301084, ssj	131184, ssj	041284, ssj
CRL cm	2.0	2.1	2.2	3.0
Villi mg	50	25	25	40
Needle time	1 min 0 s	3 min 5 s	2 min 0 s	5 min 45 s + 2 min 0 s
se-AFP kU/l	5–7	7–49	10–14	13–290
Karyotype	46,XX	46,XY	46,XX	46,XY
Complications	air bubble	0	0	two attempts
Fetal death detected	79 days	47 days	22 days	17days

14.9 FETOMATERNAL BLEEDING

A total of 32% of the women exhibited serum-AFP values after CVS greater than 2.5 times the mean value for the time of pregnancy concerned, raising suspicion of a fetomaternal bleeding. The mean value for the 161 pre-CVS AFP registered was 8.7 kU/l. Three pre-CVS AFP were greater than the cut-off level. The range in pre-CVS AFP was 4 kU/l and 35 kU/l. Within two or three weeks all values were in normal range. Furthermore, all AFP determinations in the sixteenth week gave values in the normal range, indicating fetuses without open NTD. This was confirmed by ultrasound in 150 cases and at birth in 73 new-born babies.

The rise in post-CVS AFP occurs more frequently compared to the rise following second trimester amniocentesis, which is reported in 8% to 15% of cases of amniocentesis. The significance of this with respect to immunization of rhesus-negative women is still a matter of dispute.

Our study group included 21 rhesus-negative women (17%). With one exception, no abnormal blood group antibodies have been detected. One woman was a para 4, correctly treated with anti-D in her previous pregnancies, as her husband was homozygous rhesus-positive. Following

CVS in the ninth week of pregnancy serum-AFP increased from 6 kU/l to 220 kU/l, and anti-D antibodies were found in increasing amounts from the 27th week of pregnancy. After four late amniocenteses for amniotic fluid bilirubin study, the baby was delivered by a caesarean section in the 37th week. The baby was rhesus-D-positive with a positive direct Coombs' test and with a slight bilirubin elevation, which responded sufficiently to treatment by phototherapy.

In first and second trimester punctures we do not administer anti-D-immunoglobulin to rhesus-negative women. The case described above, however, gives reason for reconsideration, although immunization subsequent to CVS in the first trimester is hardly a likely explanation.

14.10 CYTOGENETIC INVESTIGATION

Chromosome examination following the first 26 TA-CVS were performed on preparations made immediately after sampling (Simoni, 1983), and after incubation for 24 hours in RPMI (Gibco) without serum added. The karyotypes were confirmed by examinations of preparations made after *in vitro* cultivation of chorionic villi, using a slight modification of the technique described by Simoni *et al.* (1983). Chromosome examination of the new-born babies was performed on *in vitro* cultivation of lymphocytes obtained from cord or heel blood.

Cytogenetic examination continued as described with the exception of the immediate chromosome preparation, which had to be excluded from the study as a consequence of organization problems in the laboratory. The cytogenetic examinations revealed 164 normal and six abnormal fetal karyotypes. All pregnancies with abnormal fetal karyotypes were terminated at the parents' request (Table 14.3).

So far there has been agreement between prenatal chromosomal findings and those found post-natally. By short-term methods the mean number of metaphases analysed where 13. In cultured villi a mean of ten metaphases were analysed. Three analyses of twenty-four hour incubations and one culture analysis were not carried out because of laboratory problems. Chromosomal analysis has been carried out in all cases.

Early acquaintance with the fetal sex might raise uncomfortable ethical problems. Therefore information about sex of the fetus is withheld until beyond the 12th week of pregnancy, except in cases of sex-linked diseases.

14.11 CONCLUSIONS

The transabdominal method for chorionic villi sampling is simple and requires only obstetric resources used for amniocentesis and creates cytogenetic problems identical with other methods of CVS. The sampling success rate is high.

There have been few complications resulting from the procedure, and none threatening maternal health. The procedure avoids simultaneous vaginal and abdominal activity, as associated with the transcervical approach, and will certainly appeal to most women. The method is thus highly acceptable, and induces the advantage of the woman remaining conscious during the procedure, and of having relatives present.

The simplicity of the procedure is apparent from its easy adoption by new practitioners. TA-CVS can be applied in existing centres for obstetrical ultrasonography where amniocentesis guided by on-site ultrasound is routine. Thus skilled practitioners trained in ultrasonically guided amniocentesis do not need to practise on women undergoing termination of pregnancy, but could proceed with TA-CVS under initial supervision.

According to the results available at the moment it is our opinion that TA-CVS is a valid alternative to second trimester amniocentesis, and can be used in all pregnancies at risk, not only in high risk pregnancies. However, routine clinical use of the TA-CVS must await further investigation and evaluation of the CVS procedure from studies on randomized groups of pregnancies and studies comparing the different methods for CVS.

REFERENCES

Aladjem, S. (1969) Fetal assessment through biopsy of the human placenta. In *The Fetoplacental Unit* (eds A. Pecile and C. Finzi), Exerpta Medical Foundation, Amsterdam. pp. 392–402.

Alvarez, H. (1966) Diagnosis of hydatidiform mole by transabdominal placental biopsy. *Am. J. Obstet. Gynecol.*, **95**, 538–41.

Gilmore, D. H. and McNay, M. B. (1985) Spontaneous fetal loss rate in early pregnancy. *Lancet*, **i**, 107.

Gustavii, B. (1985) Chorionic villi sampling and miscarriage (in Swedish). *Lakartidningen*, **82**, 1959–60.

Jackson, L. (1984a) *Chorionic villi sampling Newsletter*, 26 August.

Jackson, L. (1984b) *Chorionic villi sampling Newsletter*, 10 December.

Jackson, L. (1985) *Chorionic villi sampling Newsletter*, 17 April.

Simoni, G., Brambati, B., Danesino, C., Rosella, F., Terzoli, G. L., Ferrai, M. and Fraccaro, M. (1983) Efficient direct chromosome analyses and enzyme determinations from the chorionic villi samples in the first trimester of pregnancy. *Hum. Genet.*, **63**, 349–57.

Simoni, G., Brambati, B., Danesino, C., Terzoli, G. L., Romitti, L., Rosella, F. and Fraccaro, M. (1984a) Diagnostic application of first trimester trophoblast sampling in 100 pregnancies. *Hum. Genet.*, **66**, 252–9.

Smidt-Jensen, S. and Hahnemann, N. (1984) Transabdominal fine needle biopsy from chorionic villi in the first trimester. *Prenat. Diag.*, **4**, 163–9.

Smidt-Jensen, S., Hahnemann, N., Jensen, P. K. A. and Therkelsen, Aa. J. (1984) Experience with transabdominal fine needle biopsy from chorionic villi in the first trimester: an alternative to amniocentesis. *Clin. Genet.*, **26**, 272–4.

Smidt-Jensen, S., Hahnemann, N., Hariri, J., Jensen, P. K. A. and Therkelsen, Aa. J. (1986) Transabdominal chorionic villus sampling for first trimester foetal diagnosis. First 26 pregnancies followed to term. *Prenat. Diag.*, **6**, 125–32.
Wilson, R. D., Kendrick, V., Wittmann, B. K. and McGillivray, B. C. (1984). Risk of spontaneous abortion in ultrasonically normal pregnancies. *Lancet*, **ii**, 920–1.

15

Development and clinical application

R. J. Lilford, G. Linton, H. C. Irving, J. Groves, M. K. Mason, A. C. Crompton and D. Maxwell

15.1 INTRODUCTION

The development of a transabdominal technique for chorion villus sampling was inspired by our poor results with the transcervical method. Despite the development of considerable manual skill in the course of our 100 non-diagnostic procedures (Maxwell *et al.*, 1985a), we experienced a high fetal loss rate in our diagnostic series. All our fetal losses occurred a heart-breaking four to five weeks after the procedure. We embarked on the transabdominal route as an alternative procedure for selected cases with fundal or anterior placentas. We now believe that this route is much superior to the transcervical method for essentially all patients. Our technique is very similar to that developed independently and somewhat earlier by Professor Hahnemann's group in Denmark (Smidt-Jensen and Hahnemann, 1984) and they too report favourably on this method.

15.2 THE TECHNIQUE OF TRANSABDOMINAL CHORION VILLUS BIOPSY

Classical teaching states that the uterus is a pelvic organ until twelve weeks gestation. This is not true; the uterus is not abdominally *palpable* until this time but the fundus of the pregnant uterus comes to lie against the abdominal wall after about nine weeks of gestation. The uterus can therefore be reached through the abdominal wall of this point without transversing the bladder or bowel (Fig. 15.1(a)). This route provides access to both the anterior and posterior walls of the placenta but, in order to reach the latter without penetrating the amniotic cavity, an empty bladder is required (see Fig.

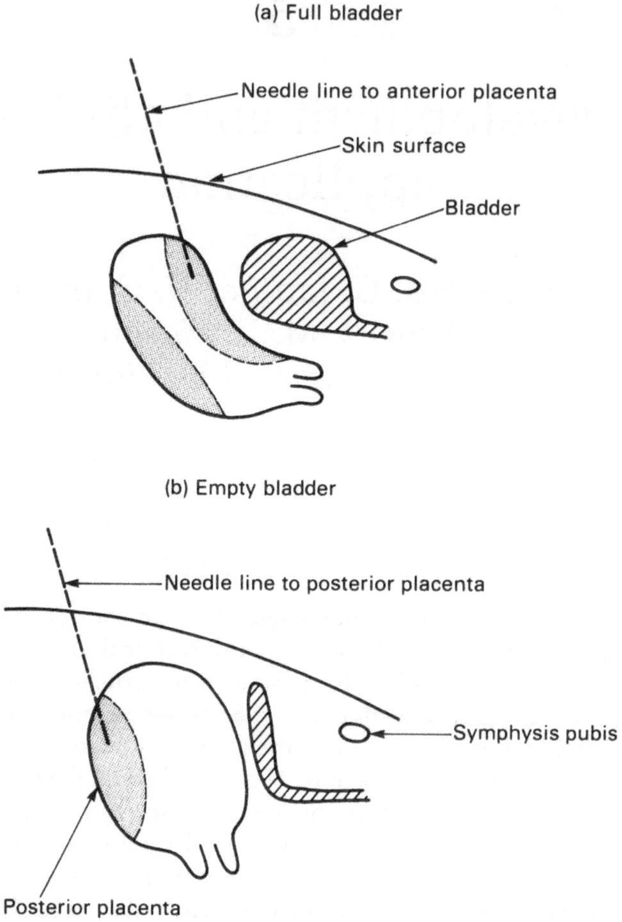

Figure 15.1 Needle path lines for transabdominal chorion villus biopsy showing how the anterior (a) and posterior (b) placenta can be reached through the skin.
These figures show how emptying the bladder anteverts the uterus and enables the posterior placenta to be reached through the skin without traversing the amniotic cavity or bladder.

15.1(b)). In very rare cases, the uterus may still be acutely retroverted before ten weeks of pregnancy but even this can be corrected by vaginal manipulation. Alternatively, the clinician may elect to wait one or two weeks for natural anteversion to occur.

Transabdominal chorion villus sampling has been attempted on 71 patients immediately prior to vaginal termination of pregnancy. Fifty-four of these were carried out at Queen Charlotte's Hospital, London, the remainder at St. James's Hospital, Leeds. Gestational ages ranged from 6–15 weeks of

Table 15.1 Experience in developing the technique of transabdominal chorion villus sampling

Needle/cannula	*No. times used*	*No. successful biopsies*	
Miscellaneous	6	3	
15-gauge Trocar point	6	4	
15-gauge needle point	9	9	Series A
15-gauge + inner 17-gauge aspirating cannula	9	9	
17-gauge needle point + 19-gauge aspirating cannula	45	43	Series B (experimental) and series C (diagnostic)
18-gauge needle point and 20-gauge aspirating cannula	11	11	

pregnancy. In addition, sampling was performed on seven diagnostic cases between 10 and 13 weeks of pregnancy at Queen Charlotte's and a further eight in Leeds.

During the development stages of the technique many different needle combinations were tried and evaluated. These are listed in the order in which they were tested in Table 15.1. The final specification consists of sharp stilette pointed 18-gauge guide cannula with stylet and inner 20-gauge aspirating cannula, which was 1.5 cm longer than the guide (Fig. 15.2) (Rocket of London).

We find it essential to use a very sharp pointed needle to penetrate the skin, rectus sheath and uterus with ease. Trocar-pointed instruments proved to be too blunt for routine use and the force required distorting the tissues. Stilette-pointed instruments allow for easy and smooth entry with constant visualization. It was clear from initial experience that an inadequate aspirate could occur despite accurate localization of the needle tip within the villus mass. It was then realized that more than one aspiration was often required, and that a technique that allowed this while maintaining access to the placenta was to be preferred. We have now come to see this as one of the major advantages of

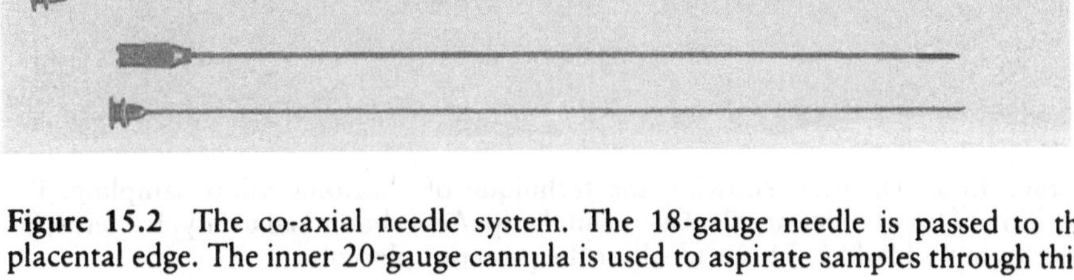

Figure 15.2 The co-axial needle system. The 18-gauge needle is passed to the placental edge. The inner 20-gauge cannula is used to aspirate samples through this.

this technique; namely, that repeated aspirations can be made from a single insertion until sufficient material for analysis is obtained.

Accurate placement of the aspirating cannula within the chorion frondosum was achieved initially by a free-hand method but we now use a needle guided approach. The first needle guide was constructed according to our design in the hospital workshop. At the commencement of each session it was necessary to draw onto the screen of the ultrasound machine the line that the needle would follow. This was done by inserting the needle through the guide and into a water bath. Later, a commercial biopsy attachment was obtained and the machine configured to automatically superimpose the biopsy chart on the image. The transducer is positioned in such a way that the main villus mass was seen lying along the needle path lines on the screen (Fig. 15.3). The 18-gauge needle is inserted into the guide, and passed through the abdominal wall and uterus until its tip can be seen on ultrasound just within the chorion frondosum. The insertion of the needle should take place as a series of sharp movements to ensure that structures such as the rectus sheath and uterus are penetrated cleanly and not distorted or displaced. The stilette is then replaced with the 20-gauge aspirating cannula, to which a 20 ml syringe has been attached. Since this is 1.5 cm longer than the guide, its tip is seen well within the chorion frondosum (Fig. 15.3). The sample is collected by means of suction on the syringe, combined with a gentle up and down

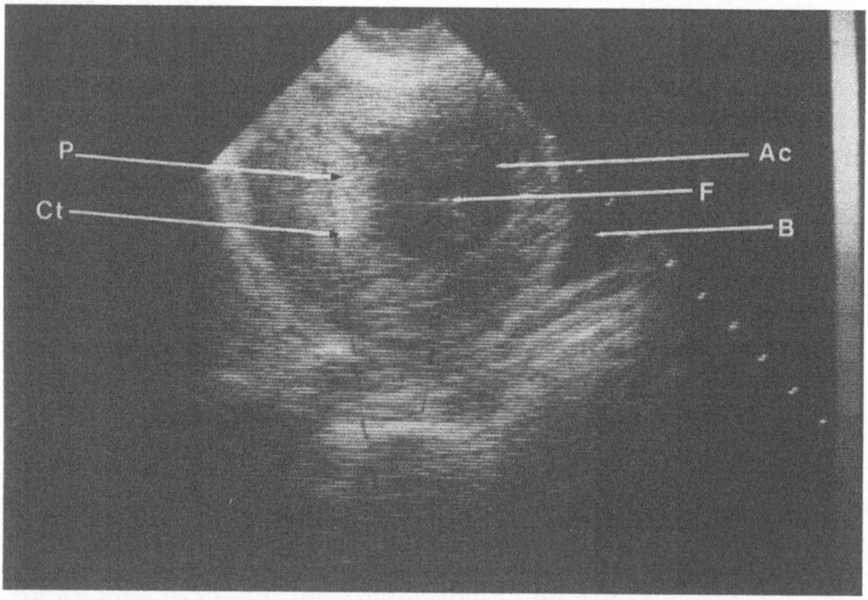

Figure 15.3 Diagram showing the technique of chorionic villus sampling. P – position of tip of outer needle, Ct – cannula tip, Ac – abdominal cavity, F – fetus, B – nearly empty bladder. This is ideal for the posterior placenta.

movement. The inner needle can then be withdrawn and the sample inspected after flushing into a petri dish. The guide cannula is left *in situ* until the specimen is judged adequate. Additional samples, if required, are collected simply by reinserting the inner needle and aspirating again. Aspirates are assessed in theatre for suitability for laboratory analysis.

15.3 RESULTS

Results for all stages of the technique are presented in Table 15.2. Sampling was successful in 78 of the 85 women investigated (92%). In Series A we describe our results during the early development phase. Our results using the definitive technique (with a thin co-axial needle combination) are collected in Series B and C for the experimental and diagnostic series respectively. The sampling success in Series A was 83%, rising to 95% in Series B and 100% in Series C. In Series B we averaged 2.2 aspirations through the inner cannula for an adequate sample to a maximum of four. The two unsuccessful attempts in Series B were both from pregnancies of less than eight weeks gestation.

No maternal trauma was recorded in any of the patients in our developmental series. The amniotic cavity was breached in two cases of Series A. Bloodstained villus aspirates were obtained from three patients in Series A and 4 in Series B. In seven patients, with pregnancies of less than ten weeks gestational age, a retroverted uterus was encountered and a vaginal examination with pressure against the anterior surface of the cervix was required to antevert the uterus prior to successful sampling. Laparoscopic sterilization followed the termination of pregnancy in four cases. A small puncture hole was seen in the anterior surface of the uterus but no further trauma or bleeding was noted.

Karyotypes were attempted in 19 of the 54 non-diagnostic cases from

Table 15.2 Success of transabdominal chorion villus sampling at different stages

Series A	
	attempted – 30
	successful – 25
Series B	
	attempted – 41*
	successful – 39
Series C (diagnostic)	
	attempted – 14
	successful – 14

* There were two sets of twins in these 41 patients. In each case samples were obtained from both placentas.

Queen Charlotte's Hospital. The laboratory was too busy to process all samples and selected these at random as a form of quality control. Successful karyotypes were obtained from 18 cases and those have been reported in detail elsewhere (Maxwell *et al.*, 1986). In four of the five diagnostic cases carried out for cytogenetic indication at Queen Charlotte's Hospital a successful karyotype was obtained by both direct and culture methods. The result was confirmed after delivery or termination of pregnancy. The remaining sample failed to yield adequate metaphases on direct analysis and failed to grow in culture and diagnosis was achieved by amniocentesis in the second trimester. The failure of this diagnostic case to produce a karyotype is more difficult to explain. The sample was judged to be unequivocally adequate by both the obstetric and laboratory staff. The latter now have experience of over 200 chorion samplings and this is the first time that an apparently excellent sample has failed to produce a result. In both patients tested for the diagnosis of sickle-cell disease a heterozygote fetus was detected and this was subsequently confirmed.

Karyotypes were attempted by both direct and culture methods on all non-diagnostic samples at St. James's Hospital. There were 17 patients in this series but this includes two sets of twins. Thus aspirations were attempted from 19 placentae. One aspiration failed at six weeks gestational age. Thus karyotypes were attempted on 18 samples. A karyotype was obtained from all but one of these. The remaining, apparently adequate sample provided no analysable metaphases for direct culture analysis and did not grow in culture. The karyotype was obtained by culture in 17 cases and in all but one of these the direct preparation was successful (Table 15.3).

All diagnostic cases at St. James's Hospital were successful and the indications and outcome of these are shown in Table 15.4. Three terminations of pregnancy have been carried out for abnormal results from the diagnostic series at both hospitals. One pregnancy loss occurred three days after a traumatic sampling. In this patient, a defective transducer was replaced in the middle of the session. The needle path lines were not correct for this transducer and excessive and prolonged manipulation was required to obtain a sample. Five babies have been delivered with no complications and all other pregnancies are continuing normally.

15.4 ADVANTAGES OF TRANSABDOMINAL CHORION VILLUS SAMPLING

Our experience has shown that it is feasible to obtain adequate chorion samples by a transabdominal route. Sampling success rates of essentially 100% bear comparison with those obtained by the transcervical route (Ward *et al.*, 1983). We believe that the transabdominal technique has many advantages. Some of these we have demonstrated; others are theoretical and

Table 15.3 Cytogenetic analysis of chorion samples obtained by the transabdominal route at St James's Hospital

			Direct preparation		*Culture*		
Patient no.	*Gestational age (by crown rump length)*	*Specimen number*	*Karyotype*	*Number of cells counted*	*Karyotype*	*Days to harvest*	*Fetal parts*
1	10	1	46XY	10	46XY	22	Infected
2	11	2	46XX	10	46XX	11	46XX
3	11	3	46XY	8	46XY	13	46XY
4	10	4	46XX	10	46XX	13	Not done
5	6	Unsuccessful sample					
6	11	5	46XY	20	46XY	30	46XY
7	14	6	46XX	8	46XX	15	46XX
8	11	7	46XY	10	46XY	12	46XY
9*	8	8	46XX	7	46XX	18	Not done
		9**	No mitoses		Failed to grow		
10*	12	10	46XX	1	46XX	21	46XX
		11	46XX	4	46XX	10	46XX
11	7	12	46XY	6	46XY	21	Not done
12	11	12					
13	10	14					
14	9	15	Failed		46XY	13	Infected
15	10	16	46XX	4	46XX	17	46XX
16	7	17	46XX	10	46XX	16	46XX
17	8	18	46XX	9	46XX	12	46XX

* Twin pregnancies.
** This was a moderately good sample macroscopically.

Table 15.4 Diagnostic transabdominal chorionic villus sampling at St James's Hospital

Patient number	*Gestational age*	*Indication*	*Outcome*
1	10	β-thalassaemia detection	Heterozygous normal karyotype
2	10.5	Previous Down's syndrome	Normal karyotype
3	11	Non-fragile X, sex-linked mental retardation	Affected – termination of pregnancy – confirmed male fetus
4	10.5	Duchenne carrier for karyotype in first instance	Female fetus
5	11	Maternal age	46XX
6	11	Maternal age	Normal karyotype
7	11	Maternal age	Normal karyotype
8	12	Sickle cell	

await confirmation from several large studies or, ideally (but probably impractically), a randomized trial. The advantages we propose are as follows.

15.4.1 Avoidance of the frequently contaminated cervical canal

The cervix is known to harbour many potentially pathogenic organisms (Charles, 1981; Scialli *et al.*, 1985) and it would not be surprising if a breach of the normally impenetrable cervical mucus plug should lead to ascending infection. This has fetal and maternal implications.

(a) Fetal implications of infection

Acute septic abortion has been recorded after transcervical chorion villus sampling. Other abortions occurring within days of the procedure are probably due to traumatic disruption of the pregnancy and sub-chorial haematoma formation. Many others occur four or five weeks later (Maxwell and Lilford, 1985). It is suggested that these are due to chronic sub-acute infection, possibly with an intracellular parasite. Nearly half of all pregnant patients secrete Listeria or Mycloplasma from the cervical canal during pregnancy (Charles, 1981; Scialli *et al.*, 1985). The most striking feature of the abortion rates reported in Professor Jackson's newsletter (Jackson, 1985) is their extreme variability (from 2% to 30%) among reasonably competent operators. Clearly the successful outcomes are dependent on the most subtle nuances of technique. It would seem that the chances of chronic nonsuppurative infection can be minimized by avoiding tissue trauma and decidual damage. Transcervical aspiration also carries the theoretical risk of innoculating virus into the fetus and it is known that over 10% of pregnant women excrete cytomegalovirus from the cervix (Peckham and Marshall, 1983).

(b) Maternal consequences of infection

In addition to local pelvic sepsis, many cases of which have been reported to the author and a few of which appear in the *Chorion Villus Sampling Newsletter* (Jackson, 1985), there is a risk of endotoxic shock. This clinical picture may precede loss of fetal viability or any clinical signs of abortion. Two of these cases have been described in the newsletter and one patient with renal failure and shock lung did not improve until a hysterectomy was performed. Transabdominal chorion villus sampling is carried out through an area which we know from amniocentesis to be bacteriologically sound. Amnionitis may occur as part of the abortion process following amniocentesis but a series of up to 153 000 cases are reported with no mention of endotoxic shock. Certainly, the picture of endotoxic shock *prior* to the abortion process is typical of ascending infection in pregnancy and comes as no surprise to those of us familiar with the consequences of non-medically induced abortion in developing countries.

15.4.2 Wider gestational age 'window' with the transabdominal technique

Despite current lay and medical emphasis on preconception care, many patients, even in advanced communities such as Leeds in the United Kingdom, do not attend antenatal clinics until 12 or 13 weeks of gestation. The transcervical method is less suitable after 12 weeks of gestation whereas the transabdominal method may be employed until at least 14 weeks. Beyond this time, the 'posterior' placenta becomes truly posterior, even with an empty bladder, and it may therefore be impossible to reach it without passing through the amniotic cavity. Furthermore, in our experience, the number of dividing cytotrophoblast cells suitable for direct analysis declines sharply after 14 weeks.

15.4.3 Multiple sampling may be carried out following a single uterine penetration

The ability to perform multiple sampling through a single cannula is a further advantage of the transabdominal technique with a co-axial needle system. The need for multiple cannula insertions with any methods may increase the possibility of subsequent abortion.

15.4.4 Greater control over sample size

It is often difficult to control the size of the sample obtained transcervically and the alarmingly large specimens which are sometimes inadvertently obtained through the larger, malleable transcervical cannulae are avoided by the use of a fine bore inner needle.

15.4.5 Absence of mucous and decidual contamination

This advantage was reported by both laboratories (Coleman, personal communication).

15.4.6 Technically less demanding

Superficially, the transcervical technique is easier to learn; it is possible within a couple of practice sessions to regularly obtain chorion tissue. The important point, however, is that a successful outcome depends on keeping tissue trauma to an absolute minimum as damage to either membrane or decidua may form a focus for subsequent infection. The learning curves of all centres have shown great improvement in fetal survival rates with experience. While this is true of all techniques in obstetrics it applies to a far greater degree with transcervical chorion villus sampling. The needle guided transabdominal approach is also very easily learnt and we think that, like amniocentesis, it will be more forgiving of inexperience. Certainly, we began our clinical transabdominal series after a smaller number of practice sessions and experienced a much lower fetal loss rate than we encountered with the transcervical method.

15.4.7 Patient comfort

It is difficult to quantify pain but, having practised both methods, we have formed the impression that pain with the transcervical technique has a wider *variance*. In other words, the pain experienced with the transabdominal method is fairly uniform and many patients have said that it is no more painful than amniocentesis. Our referring haematologist, Dr Kay Hunt of Bradford, states that her Moslem patients find the transabdominal technique much preferable to transvaginal procedures.

In conclusion, we have described a technique which would appear to have all the advantages but none of the drawbacks of transcervical chorionic villus aspiration. We believe that this should be evaluated in clinical practice. We would not, however, accept the results of a controlled trial comparing first trimester villus sampling overall with amniocentesis. The type II error (due to inadequate sample size) will preclude such a trial for the transabdominal technique alone, until a larger number of centres adopt this method. We expect that this will soon be possible. A trial comparing two methods of chorion biopsy may be more acceptable.

Since writing this article we have carried out 40 further cases at St James' Hospital. To date we have experienced no miscarriages but one still birth occurred at 29 weeks. We failed to obtain a sample in two cases. Karyotype, gene probe or enzyme diagnosis has proved feasible on all samples.

REFERENCES

Charles, D. (1981) *Infections in Obstetrics and Gynaecology*, Philadelphia, W. B. Saunders. pp. 224–30.

Hammerton, J. L. (1984) Collaborative studies in prenatal diagnosis of chromosome aberrations. *Prenat. Diag.* Special Issue, **4**, 3–4.

Jackson, L. (1985) *Chorion Villus Sampling Newsletter*, 26 July.

Maxwell, D. J. and Lilford, R. J. (1985) An interesting ultrasonic observation following chorionic villus sampling. *J. Clin. Ultrasound*, **13**, 343–4.

Maxwell, D., Czepulkowski, B. H., Heaton, D. E., Coleman, D. V. and Lilford, R. (1985a) A practical assessment of ultrasound-guided transcervical aspiration of chorionic villi and subsequent chromosomal analysis. *Br. J. Obstet. Gynaecol.*, **92**, 660–5.

Maxwell, D., Lilford, R., Morsman, J., Rodeck, C., Old, J. and Thein, S. (1985b) Direct DNA analysis for diagnosing fetal sickle status in first trimester chorion tissue. *J. Obstet. Gynaecol.*, **5**, 133–5.

Maxwell, D., Lilford, R., Czepulkowski, B., Heaton, D. and Coleman, D. (1986) Transabdominal chorion villus sampling; development and clinical application. *Lancet*, i, 123–6.

Peckham, C. S. and Marshall, W. C. (1983) Infections in Pregnancy. In *Obsteric Epidemiology* (eds L. Barron and W. Thomson), Orlando, Academic Press. p. 224.

Scialli, A. R., Neugebauer, D. L. and Fabro, S. (1985) Microbiology of the endocervix in patients undergoing chorionic villi sampling. In *First Trimester Fetal Diagnosis* (eds. M. Fraccaro, G. Simoni and B. Brambati), Springer-Verlag, Berlin, pp. 69–73.

Smidt-Jensen, S. and Hahnemann, N. (1984) Transabdominal fine needle biopsy from chorionic villi in the first trimester. *Prenat. Diagn.*, **4**, 163–9.

Ward, R. H. T., Modell, B., Petrov, M., Karagozlu, F. C. and Dooratsos, E. (1983) Method of sampling chorionic villi in first trimester of pregnancy under guidance of realtime ultrasound. *Br. Med. J.*, **286**, 1542–4.

Section III

CLINICAL APPLICATIONS

16

Pregnancy outcome and the need for centralized data collection in chorion villus sampling

—— *Laird G. Jackson* ——

16.1 INTRODUCTION

The development of first trimester prenatal diagnosis has evolved slowly over the past 16 years since the first reports of Mohr (1968) and other Scandinavian researchers (Hahnemann, 1974; Kullander *et al.*, 1973). Until 1983 there was little collaboration or communication among the few workers interested in this approach. Partly as a result, the relative safety of the Chinese experience of the early 1970s went largely unnoticed until just recently (Department of Obstetrics and Gynaecology, Tietung Hospital, 1975). Wide appreciation of the critical observation of Kazy *et al.* (1979) that real-time ultrasound could greatly improve the sampling procedure, was delayed fully three years from its initial publication. The appearance of his report (Kazy *et al.*, 1982) in an English-language journal finally drew attention to this approach. Even the more recent resurgence of interest in first trimester prenatal diagnosis fostered first by the British (Ward *et al.*, 1983) and then the Italians (Simoni *et al.*, 1983) drew attention only slowly among geneticists and obstetricians. These facts became evident to us in our early exploration of the method in late 1982 when our initial information came entirely from discussions with molecular biologists! Even after our own early work with chorion villus sampling (CVS) it was apparent that a very few pioneers were aware of the significant potential, diagnostic advantages, and unresolved procedural and laboratory risks of this approach. Therefore, after mid-1983 discussions among interested participants in the Fetal Medicine and Surgery Meeting in Aspen, Colorado, a newsletter was initiated to foster communication among CVS investigators. The *Chorionic Villus Sampling Newsletter*, informally dubbed the 'CVS Latest News' was initially circulated to a small group of known active investigators, members of the Fetal Medicine and Surgery Group and members of the International Cooperative Research Group on Prenatal Diagnosis and Fetal Therapy (formerly known as the Fetoscopy Club). The intent was to circulate information on the progress of investigations using the new procedure and to serve as a common international collection point for data on the number of procedures attempted, diagnostic results and problems with either the patients or their pregnancies. All data were contributed voluntarily by the collaborating investigators. The newsletter is compiled by the prenatal diagnosis group at the Division of Medical Genetics, Thomas Jefferson University, Philadelphia, Pennsylvania, USA; and circulated bimonthly to a list of approximately 500 recipients worldwide. It is supported by grants from the World Health Organisation's Heritable Diseases Program and from the March of Dimes Birth Defects Foundation.

Although an important initial function of the newsletter was to circulate a complete and contemporary bibliography and notes on procedural and laboratory protocols, its most important role has been the initiation of a registry of first trimester diagnostic attempts in pregnancies intended to continue. A simple reporting format was used, which documented the total number of patients in which prenatal diagnosis was attempted in the first trimester by chorion villus sampling. The number of patients in whom a successful diagnostic sample was obtained, number of therapeutic pregnancy terminations, number of pregnancies intended to continue after diagnosis, number of fetal losses and total deliveries were also recorded (Table 16.1). The resulting figures are tabulated and listed by individual centre as are the totals for all centres participating. Revised tables are circulated with each newsletter and interim tables are available upon request. In addition, a report format has been devised to record pertinent information about each patient in whom a first trimester prenatal diagnosis is attempted. The form has been

Table 16.1 Fetal loss

Case load/ No. of centres	*Total patients*	*Failed sample*	*Therapeutic abortions*	*Continuing pregnancies*	*Loss max.*	*Loss % max.*	*Delivered*
1–50/40	1048	74	110	938	58	6.2	252
50–100/17	1131	44	92	1039	57	5.5	297
100–200/20	2811	96	203	2608	100	3.8	1151
200–500/11	3129	87	268	2861	127	4.4	1360
7500/6	8591	90	478	8113	264	3.3	4766
Total (92 centres)	16 710	391	1151	15 559	606	3.9	7826

kept as simple as possible and was developed collaboratively by our staff and members of the WHO Working Group on Hereditary Diseases (1983). This form records demographic information about the patient and her past reproductive history, data on the diagnostic sampling procedure, complications including fetal loss, laboratory results and outcome with confirmation of the diagnosis and evaluation of the new-born child. The form uses simple yes/no (+/−) or numerical responses where possible and can be utilized in direct entry in a microcomputer disc format available through the coordinating centre at Jefferson (Fig. 16.1). Response to both the newsletter and the registry has been encouraging. Over 16500 diagnostic cases had been recorded by the end of the third year of the newsletter circulation and a considerable amount of information about fetal loss following the procedure had been accumulated.

16.2 METHOD AND RESULTS

The registry lists the centre doing CVS trials and the investigator performing the procedure, the total number of procedures attempted, the number of failed procedures, terminations of pregnancy for diagnostic reasons, pregnancies intended to continue (total attempted less terminations), number and percentage of fetal losses and the number of delivered pregnancies. A total of 92 centres contributed data to the registry as of September 1986. These centres are located in Australia (5), Canada (3), China (PRC 3, ROC 1), Europe (42), Israel (2), United Kingdom (13), United States (20), and Japan (1). In the total list of contributing centres, there are 17 with 50 or less procedures completed, 25 with 50–100 attempts, ten with 100–200, eight with 200–500 and four with more than 700 procedures in their experience. This represents a fairly wide range of experience among the contributing centres and must be taken into account as the data are reviewed and interpreted. In addition, the data include the experience of each of the investigators from their earliest studies and so reflect the average of that experience with the procedure over a period of learning and probable improvement. This experience is not all with the same method of obtaining the chorionic tissue. The majority of the operators use a fairly standard technique in which a soft 1.5 mm polyethylene cannula, stiffened by a malleable stainless-steel obturator, is gently inserted via the vagina and cervix into the body of the placenta (Ward *et al.*, 1983). This method generally uses the commercially available catheter manufactured by Portex. In addition, three operators use the system pioneered by Dumez in Paris (Goosens, 1983) in which a straight metal sampling forceps of 2.2 mm diameter is inserted transcervically under ultrasound guidance. Gustavii in Lund, Sweden has altered this approach slightly to guide the forceps by inserting them through a sidearm of an optical fetoscope which is inserted transcervically and guided

FETAL DIAGNOSIS REGISTRY
CHORION VILLUS SAMPLING

INTERVIEW-date______ EVAL ULTRASOUND-CRL_____mm RANDOM ALLOCATION????
LMP:MM____DD___YY____ Date:WW___D__ CVS --
Record no.__________ FH? +(2) -(1) Amniocentesis--

REPRODUCTIVE HISTORY

Total prior pregnancies:______
spontaneous abortions___
stillbirths______
therapeutic abortions___
livebirths______
Other preg or delivery problem(list)_______________________

INDICATION FOR PROCEDURE Circle one number(used for computer file)

1. Maternal age
2. Parent chromo rearrangment
4. Prior chromosome anomaly
5. X-linked disease(sexing)
7. Metabolic disease(specify)
8. Hemoglobinopathy(specify)
11. Anxiety
12. Other(specify)

CHORION VILLUS SAMPLING: Use pre-registered sampling method or file current method.
Date: MM___DD___YY___ Bleeding before sampling: No(1) Yes(2)

Uterus position:(circle one)
1.anteverted
2.mid-position
3.retroverted
4.retroflexed

Placental location:
1. Ant 4.low
2. Post 5.lat
3. Fund 6.other

Ultrasound
CRL_____mm
Date: WW___D___
No. fetuses (1) ()1)describe

DESCRIPTION OF PROCEDURE

No. of insertions____
Estimated wt of sample(mg)_______
Difficult procedure? No(1) Yes(2)
Successful procedure? No(1) Yes(2)

SHADE PLACENTA
longitudinal - place X at sample site - transverse

draw uterus, cervix, placental site as necessary

COMPLICATIONS: FOLLOWING SAMPLING

1.bleeding No(1) Yes(2)
2.spotting No(1) Yes(2)
3.discharge No(1) Yes(2)
4.fever NO(1) Yes(2)
5.pain No(1) Yes(2)
6.amnio fl leak No(1) Yes(2)

Describe time and duration if appropriate___________________________

ULTRASOUND AT 16 WEEKS - DATE:MM___DD___YY___ BPD______

DELIVERY: livebirth surviving (1) FETAL LOSS(2)(go below) Neonatal death (3)
date: MM___DD___YY___ Infant:sex: M(1) F(2)
type__________________ weight(gm)_________
Infant abnormalities(describe-0 if none)

Placenta: abnormalities(describe - 0 if none)

FETAL LOSS:(2)

1-miscarriage(SAB)
2-ther abortion(fetal anom)
4-abortion(social etc)
6-intrauterine death(<28wks)
7-stillbirth()28wks)

LABORATORY: - = normal;+ = affected;circle (fail) if failure to obtain result

Fetal Diagnosis: Confirmed? No(1) Yes(2) Comments:(give detail on separate LAB form)-----------(rev 1/86)

Figure 16.1 Patient report form

to the sampling site by ultrasound (Gustavii, 1983). Final selection of the sampling site and sample is done under direct vision. Several investigators are now evaluating a method utilizing transabdominal puncture and ultrasound guidance of a needle through the myometrium to the placental site as pioneered by Hahnemann in Denmark (Smidt-Jensen and Hahnemann, 1984). A smaller sampling needle is then inserted through the guide needle for actual aspiration sampling of the chorion. This method avoids passage through the vagina and the unknown risk of microbial contamination associated with that approach. Finally, although the data include all sampled pregnancies and not just completed ones, all of the pregnancies are beyond the 16th week of gestation and the majority are beyond the 28th gestational week.

The overall registry data show that a total of 16710 patients have had CVS attempted. There have been 391 failed attempts in this total. Of the total, 1151 patients voluntarily terminated their pregnancies leaving 15559 women continuing their pregnancies. Most of the terminations were for confirmed genetic diagnoses although a small number (estimated at less than 1%) were terminated for sex preference or on social grounds. This therapeutic abortion rate for successful sampling is 6.8% and after discounting the terminations for sex preference or social reasons would still be approximately 6%. In the continuing pregnancies, 606 fetuses were lost or 3.9% of the total. There have been 7826 deliveries in the experience of the contributing investigators.

The overall fetal loss figure requires some clarification. In some early procedures cytogenetic assessment was not done when the principal test desired was one of the metabolic enzyme assays. Several instances of fetal loss from cases without diagnostic villus karyotypes have subsequently been shown to be aneuploid at spontaneous abortion. In addition, a few laboratories rely upon tissue culture diagnoses and have experienced loss of aneuploid fetuses at or just prior to completion of karyotyping. Because most parents would have electively terminated such pregnancies when the karyotype result was known within 48 hours, it was decided to eliminate all aneuploid cases from the loss column in the registry and treat them as terminated (diagnostic) cases. The registry data are presented in this manner in Table 16.1.

In attempting to utilize this registry as a tool for evaluation of the CVS procedure a number of questions may be asked. The first concerns the success of the procedure in actually achieving first trimester fetal diagnosis. The registry data do not completely answer this as the data only document failures to achieve any fetal tissue sample. These failures are infrequent, occurring in only 2.4% of attempted samplings. This ranges from a high of 10.6% from one centre with considerable experience to a low of 0.8% in one and nil in another centre with more than 100 cases. The data suggest that the variation is due to the two factors of relative aggressiveness in seeking an analysable sample and the method of sampling used. The highest failure rate comes from a group which adheres to a rule of using no more than two attempted insertions regardless of circumstances, and the nil rate comes from an investigator experienced in the use of the solid sampling forceps. Further information is anecdotal but indicates that few patients are subjected to repeat samplings in a second session (as opposed to repeat insertions of the sampling instrument in the same session) and few patients are rejected for reasons of unsuitable pelvic anatomy (stenosed cervical canal, severely retroflexed uterus, etc.). Thus, the data indicate that the procedure is applicable to almost all candidate patients and that a high percentage of sampling attempts will be successful in experienced hands. The risk of failure therefore appears to be slight.

More significant questions of risk involve the safety of the procedure for the mother, her fetus and her new-born and developing child. For the first two of these questions there appears to be reasonably good assurances from the data collected thus far. It is too early to expect anything but crude information regarding the last issue. Of the nearly 2000 infants delivered, none have been reported to have malformations or problems attributed to the procedure. Less than 1% have had congenital malformation syndromes and these were not conditions that would have been discoverable by prenatal diagnosis. No information is available on the developmental progress of any of these children. The available data on maternal health are also slim. No instances of maternal death have been reported. Although vaginal bleeding is a frequent minor complication, occurring in 30–40% of patients, it is largely confined to spotting or amounts less than usual menstrual flow. Occasionally patients have repeated short periods of heavy bleeding but no one has required treatment other than bed rest and mild sedation. Vaginal infections and chorioamnionitis have been reported in ten patients including at least three receiving antibiotic therapy or intervention. One patient required uterine evacuation to control the infection (Blakemore *et al.*, 1985) and a second required hysterectomy. Most of the patients experienced no more physical difficulties than the usual amniocentesis patient.

The most frequently cited risk of the CVS procedure is the risk of fetal loss by spontaneous abortion. Initial reports suggested that this loss might exceed 10% (Hobbins, 1984) but subsequent data indicates that this estimate was much too high. The registry data reveals a clear preliminary picture of the risk of fetal loss. The rate of fetal loss for a large number of cases is 4.0% and this figure represents an average of those centres with a significant amount of clinical experience. A comparison of those centres with the most experience and those with the least shows a striking difference in rates of fetal loss. The loss rate in the 42 centres with 50 or less procedures each is 6.2%, while in the six centres with more than 700 tests each it is 3.27%, a 50% difference (Table 16.1). There is also some interest in comparing the loss experience with the different methods of sampling (Table 16.2). The most popular method is the use of the soft catheter whose operators show a loss rate of 3.8% (4521 cases). Two operators use an optical instrument similar to a fetoscope, allowing direct vision of the chorion sampling via an inserted sampling forceps with a loss rate of 8.4% (205 cases). Three of the investigators use the thin straight sampling forceps alone with ultrasound guidance and have a 5.1% loss rate (1257 cases). Investigators have used a transabdominal, as opposed to a transcervical approach, and their loss rate is 2.83% (259 cases).

Table 16.2 Fetal loss: alternate sampling methods; 100 or more procedures

Method/ No. of centres	*Total patients*	*Failed sample*	*Therapeutic abortions*	*Continuing pregnancies*	*Loss max.*	*Loss % max.*	*Delivered*
Cannula/79	14 989	364	944	14 045	528	3.8	7049
Forceps/11	1257	18	180	1077	55	5.1	524
Optical + Forceps/2	205	8	15	190	16	8.42	136
Trans-abdominal/3	259	1	12	247	7	2.83	117

16.3 DISCUSSION

The registry data are clearly insufficient to provide a real judgement on the safety of the CVS procedure or a clear assessment of any of the risks. They do show significant trends in at least two areas. These are the risk of failure of the procedure to either obtain a sample of fetal tissue adequate for laboratory analysis or the risk of fetal loss subsequent to the procedure. As stated above, the risk of failure of the procedure appears to be slight. The centres with major experience have less than a 2% failure rate and their more recent experience suggests an even lower rate is achievable. It appears that some patients will have a uterine or placental position (or combination thereof) that will not be safely approached. The percentage of such patients is obviously small and it is likely that it will diminish with further experience.

The fetal loss experience is probably the most important question to be addressed by the registry data. Here the data provide at least a useful early statement of the experience of the investigators which is reassuring for the future development of this procedure. The 4% fetal loss rate would appear to be an extremely low rate of pregnancy loss when compared to predicted rates of pregnancy loss from the 8th–10th week of pregnancy forward (Harlap *et al.*, 1980). However, such rates were obtained from data collected before pregnancy evaluation by ultrasound was possible. More recently, data have been obtained with ultrasound verification of pregnancy viability by determining fetal cardiac activity together with normal crown rump length

(CRL) of the fetus for gestational age with matching gestation sac size (GSS). These data are somewhat difficult to use for comparative purposes as each report provides assessment of the loss experience in different ways, with different populations, and each utilizes different end points of gestation for observation. Nevertheless they provide some insight suggesting a far lower expected rate of pregnancy loss from normal pregnancies than had been previously thought. In one group of women whose pregnancies were evaluated by ultrasound at 8–10 weeks gestation as controls for a collaborative study of diabetic pregnancies, there were two pregnancy losses in the group of 225 women observed through 12 weeks; a 0.9% loss rate. The same group, followed to term, experienced six more losses for an overall rate of 3.7% (Simpson, 1984). In another group from the Netherlands, patients seen at a University Obstetrics Service were followed after ultrasound evaluation of the pregnancy at 8–10 weeks gestation (Christaens and Stoutenbeek, 1984). Two hundred and seventy-four patients were seen with nine pregnancy losses at 16 weeks gestation, a loss rate of 3.3%. Only 236 of these were patients from the normal clinic population, the others having been referred for ultrasound evaluation for (presumably) some suspected difficulty. In the smaller group there were only five losses for a rate of 2.1%. In both of the above studies, the average maternal age was below 35 years. In contrast, the group at the University of British Columbia retrospectively evaluated a large series of ultrasounds and found 796 women having scans at 7–12 weeks gestation whose pregnancies could be evaluated through 20 weeks of gestation (Wilson *et al.*, 1984). There were 17 losses in the group for a rate of 2.13%. These could be further subdivided by maternal age into a group under 30 years (347) with five losses (1.5%), the group from 30–34 years (238) with six losses (2.5%) and a group over 35 years (149) with six losses (4%). Actually the latter group had 133 women between 35 and 39 years of age with 4.5% loss and a group over 40 with no losses that was too small to analyse. In the United Kingdom, Gilmore reported a similar study showing a fetal loss rate in women aged 25–34 of 2.0% and women aged 35–40 or above of 4.0% (Gilmore and McNay, 1984). These latter three studies are therefore consistent in indicating fetal loss rates of 2% in 30–35 year old women and 4% in women over 35 years of age when their pregnancies are found to be normal by ultrasound at 7–12 weeks gestation. Using the reported experience of one large amniocentesis series, another instructive comparison may be made. Golbus *et al.* (1979) in reviewing 3000 amniocenteses (performed mainly for advanced maternal age of 35 and over), noted a combined pregnancy loss in the week prior to the procedure (usually 16–17 gestational weeks) of 2.4%. Following the procedure there was a 1.4% loss of pregnancies through the 28th week of gestation. All of these figures are remarkably close to the loss experience of the larger CVS series and suggest that their losses, especially in the later group of patients where the procedure was performed after the initial learning of these centres, may be largely associated with normal causes of spontaneous abortion and few are directly related to the procedure. Assuming the majority of patients in the CVS registry are 35 and over, the 4% loss figure from the registry data may represent no more than 0.5–1.5% added risk over background loss.

Unfortunately the registry does not provide control data for comparison of fetal loss rates within the same centres performing the CVS procedures. Neither case control nor random or unselected controls are available thus far in any centre reporting. Nevertheless, 100 of the 118 reported CVS losses have been documented with some details of their dates of sampling, data of pregnancy loss, and ultrasound and clinical findings. These data allow some examination of the experience with an intent to find associations between the CVS procedure and the event of fetal loss. Most samples were taken in a narrow time period between the beginning of the ninth week and the middle of the 11th week of gestation. This concentration of the sampling 'window' happened early enough that few losses occurred to patients sampled before or after this time period and so it is not possible to draw conclusions about the safety of the sampling time with any numerical support. It is obviously the conclusion of the investigators that a combination of increased ease of ultrasound visualization of the sampling site, ease of insertion of the sampling device and a perceived lowering of complications led to the choice of this gestational time for sampling. Recent review of data at three large centres supports this assumption (Golbus, Brambati personal communications; Jackson, unpublished data) with fetal losses as low as 1.5% being recorded in procedures done within the 9th–10th gestational week. The reported fetal losses occurred as early as the first 24 hours post-CVS and as late as 38 weeks gestation (these should not be included as fetal loss *per se*). However, all but two losses did occur prior to the completion of 28 weeks. Of these, 75% (or 3.1% fetal loss) occurred by 16 weeks gestation and only 25% (1.1% fetal loss) after 16 weeks and up to 28 weeks. This suggests that few losses after 16 weeks may be attributable to the procedure, but that 1–1.5% of the earlier 3% loss may be affected by the sampling. The distribution in the first six weeks following sampling is of interest, with 19% of the total losses occurring by seven days post CVS, 40% by 14 days, 68% by 28 days and 78% by 42 days. The majority of the losses within the first two weeks may very well be procedurally related. A history of fever or excessive bleeding in these patients occurs more frequently than in those with later losses which also supports this supposition. Of the total of 100 losses, 10–15% had a history of fever or actual infection. Most of these occurred with a history of loss within 15 days of the procedure. In contrast, a history of bleeding was found in later losses as well as in patients with no loss. The transabdominal approach is the only technique in use which completely avoids the possibility of introduction of vaginal contamination into the sampling area by the procedure itself. Clearly the question of infection is one of concern regarding both the potential for fetal loss and maternal morbidity. Further evaluation will need careful development of techniques to monitor the procedure by microbiological and pathological means. In the meantime, care in performance of the procedure appears to offer reasonable safety to the patient and her pregnancy.

In summary, the CVS registry has managed to accumulate a significant amount of information about this new procedure in a short period of time. These data suggest strongly that the procedure has no inherent risks that would preclude its further development. Further assessment of the risks of the procedure to mother, pregnancy and developing child must await the design and implementation of controlled clinical trials involving the collaboration of many investigators.

REFERENCES

Blakemore, K. J., Mahoney, M. J. and Hobbins, J. C. (1985) Infections and chorionic villus sampling. *Lancet*, ii, 338–9.

Christaens, G. C. M. L. and Stountenbeek, P. P. H. (1984) Spontaneous abortion in proven intact pregnancies. *Lancet*, ii, 571.

Department of Obstetrics and Gynecology, Tietung Hospital of Anshan Iron and Steel Co., Anshan, China. (1975) Fetal sex prediction by sex chromatin of chorionic villi cells during early pregnancy. *Chin. Med. Jr.*, **1**, 117–26.

Gilmore, D. H. and McNay, M. B. (1984) Spontaneous fetal loss rate in early pregnancy. *Lancet*, i, 107.

Golbus, M. S., Loughman, W. D., Epstein, C. J., Halbach, G., Stephens, J. D. and Hall, B. D. (1979) Prenatal diagnosis in 3000 amniocenteses. *New Engl. J. Med.*, **300**, 157–63.

Goosens, M., Dumez, Y., Kaplan, L., Lupker, M., Chabret, C., Henrion, R. and Rosa, J. (1983) Prenatal diagnosis of sickle cell anemia in the first trimester of pregnancy. *New Engl. J. Med.*, **309**, 831–3.

Gustavii, B. (1983) First-trimester chromosomal analysis of chorionic villi obtained by direct vision technique. *Lancet*, ii, 507–8.

Hahnemann, N. (1974) Early prenatal diagnosis; a study of biopsy techniques and cell culturing from extra-embryonic membranes. *Clin. Genet.*, **6**, 294–306.

Harlap, S., Shiono, P. H. and Ramrachan, S. (1980) A life table of spontaneous abortions and the effects of age, parity and other variables. In *Human Embryonic and Fetal Death* (eds I. H. Porter and E. B. Hooks), New York, Academic Press. pp. 145–58.

Hobbins, J. C. (1984) Consequences of chorionic biopsy. *New Engl. J. Med.*, **310**, 1121.

Kazy, Z., Bakharev, V. A. and Stygar, A. M. (1979) Value of the ultrasonic studies in biopsy of the chorion, according to genetic indicators. *Akush-Ginekol (Mosk.)*, **8**, 29–31.

Kazy, Z., Rozovsky, I. S. and Bakharev, V. A. (1982) Chorion biopsy in early pregnancy: a method of early prenatal diagnosis for inherited disorders. *Prenat. Diag.*, **2**, 39–45.

Kullander, S. and Sandahl, B. (1973) Fetal chromosome analysis after transcervical placental biopsies during early pregnancy. *Acta Obstet. Gynecol. Scand.*, **52**, 355–9.

Mohr, J. (1968) Foetal genetic diagnosis: development of techniques for early sampling of fetus cells. *Acta Pat. Microbiol. Scandinav.*, **73**, 73–7.

Rodeck, C. H., Morsman, J. M., Nicolaides, K. H., McKenzie, C. M., Gosden, C. M. and Gosden, J. R. (1983) A single-operator technique for first-trimester chorion biopsy. *Lancet*, ii, 1340–1.

Simoni, G., Brambati, B., Danesino, C., Rossela, F., Terzoli, G. L., Ferrari, M. and Fraccaro, M. (1983) Efficient direct chromosome analyses and enzyme determinations from chorionic villi samples in the first trimester of pregnancy. *Hum. Genet.*, **63**, 349–57.

Simpson, J. L. (1984) Low fetal loss after normal ultrasound at 8 weeks gestation. Implications for chorionic villus sampling (CVS). The Diabetes in Early Pregnancy Project NICHD. *Am. J. Hum. Genet.*, **36**, 197S.

Smidt-Jensen, S. and Hahnemann, N. (1984) Transabdominal fine needle biopsy from chorionic villi in the first trimester. *Prenat. Diag.*, **4**, 163–9.

Ward, R. H. T., Modell, B., Petrou, M., Karagozlu, F. and Douratsos E. (1983) A method of chorionic villus sampling in the first trimester of pregnancy under real-time ultrasonic guidance. *Br. Med. Jr.*, **286**, 1542–4.

WHO working group report on fetal diagnosis of hereditary diseases (1983). WHO Document HMG/WG/83.2.

Wilson, R. D., Kendrick, V., Wittman, B. K. and McGillivray, B. C. (1984) Risk of spontaneous abortion in ultrasonically normal pregnancies. *Lancet*, ii, 920–1.

17

Evaluation of the long-term consequences of chorion villus sampling

Iain Chalmers

Prenatal diagnostic activity can be perceived in one of two different ways. On the one hand, it can be seen as a means of identifying *abnormal* fetuses at a stage of pregnancy at which abortion may be considered by parents and society to be more acceptable than the birth and survival of infants with severe impairments. On the other hand, because abnormality will only be diagnosed in a minoriy of fetuses investigated, prenatal diagnostic activity can also be seen as a means of identifying *normal* fetuses so that prospective parents can be reassured that their future child is very unlikely to suffer from the specific conditions sought.

Although these two formulations are obviously opposite sides of the same coin, there is a tendency for the former to dominate in professional discussions of prenatal diagnosis. In the light of the orientation which most medical practitioners have received during their training, this emphasis on abnormality is not surprising. But those involved in prenatal diagnosis may sometimes tend to forget, first, that their activities may have only a modest impact on the birth prevalence of some of the serious conditions which can, in theory, be diagnosed prenatally (Weatherall, 1982); and, secondly, that the successful identification of one abnormal fetus may involve the use of invasive techniques to investigate anything between three and several hundred normal fetuses.

Because such a high proportion of the fetuses they will investigate are normal, those offering prenatal diagnosis have a particularly heavy responsibility to evaluate the safety of their activities in a careful and scientifically credible manner. Normal fetuses can derive no direct benefit from prenatal diagnostic activity, so any adverse effects of the procedures used have to be set against the advantages of correctly identifying other, abnormal fetuses.

The issues can be illustrated by the use of amniocentesis to investigate pregnancies in which there is a higher than average risk that the fetus has Trisomy 21 (Down's syndrome). The majority of babies with Down's syndrome are born to parents in whom there is no risk marker which could have prompted prenatal diagnostic investigation (Weatherall, 1982). A minority of babies with Down's syndrome, however, are born to women for whom a risk marker (maternal age) can be used as a basis for offering amniocentesis selectively. The birth prevalence of Down's syndrome among infants born to women over the age of 35, for example, is about one in 200. Most of the affected fetuses can be identified with acceptable diagnostic precision after culturing fetal cells which have been aspirated at amniocentesis.

The advantages of identifying each fetus which will go on to exhibit Down's syndrome at birth must be set against the disadvantages of using amniocentesis to investigate about 200 normal fetuses. The best available estimate (Tabor *et al.*, 1986) suggests that, even in experienced hands, the procedure will provoke the miscarriage of about two of these two hundred normal fetuses. Perhaps more importantly from a public health perspective, amniocentesis will cause clinically important neonatal respiratory distress, sometimes associated with pneumonia, in a further one of the 200 infants born following the procedure (Tabor *et al.*, 1986), and will probably affect lung function even in some of those babies who are clinically normal (Vyas *et al.*, 1982). In the light of evidence from animal studies that these effects are probably mediated by an irreversible effect of amniocentesis on lung development (Hislop *et al.*, 1984; Finegan, 1984), the possibility that this method of prenatal diagnosis may predispose to chronic lung disease in later life (Hislop and Fairweather, 1982) must be taken seriously. It is the likely scale of this iatrogenic morbidity which is of particular importance: in England alone about 20 000 normal fetuses a year are exposed to amniocentesis in the prenatal search for Down's syndrome.

The introduction of chorion villus sampling (CVS) for prenatal diagnosis during the first trimester of pregnancy must be seen against this background. Even among the fetuses at relatively high risk of abnormality which have so far been investigated using the technique, well over 90% have been normal (*Chorionic Villus Sampling* (*CVS*) *Newsletter*, January 1986). The proportion of normal fetuses among the total number investigated is bound to increase still further as the use of CVS is extended to pregnancies in which the risk of fetal abnormality is much lower. Indeed, some have already begun to hint that the technique should be made available on request, regardless of whether or not the estimated risk of fetal abnormality is above average (*Economist, The*, 1984).

17.1 POSSIBLE ADVANTAGES AND DISADVANTAGES OF CVS

CVS has already proved of considerable value to those families in which couples are at very high genetic risk of conceiving an abnormal fetus. The balance between advantages and disadvantages is much less clear in respect of women and couples at much lower absolute risk (but increased relative risk), such as those women who have a higher than average risk of conceiving a fetus with Trisomy 21. The main impetus behind the introduction of CVS in these circumstances is the assumption (see, for example, Fletcher, 1985) that a policy of prenatal diagnosis during the first trimester will result in less parental anxiety than the current policy of using amniocentesis during the second trimester. Although there are good reasons for challenging this assumption (Wyatt, 1985) there has been phenomenal growth in the use of CVS during the last three years. CVS was introduced during 1982 (Kazy *et al.*, 1982). By the end of 1983, only 240 pregnancies had been investigated with CVS worldwide (*CVS Newsletter*, November 1983). By the end of 1985, the number had risen to over 10 000 (*CVS Newsletter*, January 1986).

So far, the consequences of investigating normal fetuses with CVS has really only been discussed seriously in terms of the risk of unintentionally provoking miscarriage (Hecht *et al.*, 1984). This risk, although important, already appears to be relatively low and seems likely to fall further as experience of CVS accumulates (see Chapter 16). Although it would certainly be wrong to be complacent about the miscarriage of normal fetuses as a result of CVS, the importance of this problem could conceivably pale into insignificance if CVS, like amniocentesis, turns out to affect other fetuses adversely without leading to miscarriage. Extrapolating from present trends it seems likely that, within a few years, hundreds of thousands of children will have been born following pregnancies investigated with CVS. Even if the *incidence* of important long-term adverse consequences of CVS in these children is quite low – say 1% – the actual *numbers* of affected children could be very large indeed.

Marchese and her colleagues (1984) have already begun the speculation about possible long-term consequences of CVS. They point out that between 0.2% and 7.2% of women are asymptomatic carriers of genital herpes simplex virus (Harser *et al.*, 1983) and that fetal infection has been reported following CVS (Kullander and Sandahl, 1983; Ward *et al.*, 1983). Because abortion and severe congenital malformations such as cerebral atrophy, microcephaly and chorioretinitis have been associated with fetal herpes simplex infection in the first trimester (South *et al.*, 1969; Montgomery *et al.*, 1973) there is therefore a possibility that CVS will increase the incidence of these conditions.

It is because the population at risk of long-term adverse effects of CVS like these is likely to be so large, that investigation of the long-term safety of the technique among survivors is by far the most pressing scientific challenge facing those who wish to see an extended use of the technique. As one pioneer of CVS, Bruno Brambati, put it at a WHO Consultation on First Trimester Fetal Diagnosis in Rapallo, Italy in 1984 (HMG/Cons/84.5), those who introduce CVS into clinical practice in such a way that hypotheses about its possible long-term hazards in survivors cannot be tested in a scientifically rigorous manner risk being charged with gross irresponsibility.

17.2 ESTABLISHING A FRAMEWORK FOR FORMULATING HYPOTHESES ABOUT THE EFFECTS OF CVS ON MORBIDITY IN CHILDHOOD

If hypotheses about the possible adverse effects of CVS on morbidity in childhood are to be formulated and tested efficiently, a common language for describing experience with CVS is required as well as a network through which this experience can be disseminated widely and rapidly. Judged by almost any criterion, some of the developments for CVS in these respects has been exemplary. The World Health Organisation took an important and early initiative in bringing together the pioneers of the technique. International scientific journals, notably the *Lancet*, have been playing a crucial role by rapid publication of letters and articles describing experience with CVS. Each of the well-attended meetings in Nottingham, Rapallo and Birmingham has provided an international forum for exchanging information. Above all, the WHO-sponsored register of CVS cases and the series of newsletters for which Dr Laird Jackson of Philadelphia has been responsible have proved to be uniquely valuable in disseminating information efficiently.

All of these activities have contributed to the early recognition of some of the possible short-term adverse consequences of CVS. These include failure to obtain adequate samples for investigation in a proportion of cases (*CVS Newsletter*, February 1985); diagnostic difficulties created both by chromosomal mosaicism (*CVS Newsletter*, June 1984) and maternal cell contamination (Simoni *et al.*, 1983); feto-maternal haemorrhage (Warren *et al.*, 1985); rupture of the amniotic sac (WHO Working Group, 1984); infection of the trophoblast (Garden *et al.*, 1985; McFadyen *et al.*, 1985; Brambati and Varotta, 1985); and the fetus (Ward *et al.*, 1983); miscarriage (Modell, 1985); and, most seriously of all, complications which threatened the lives of some of the women whose pregnancies have been investigated with CVS (*CVS Newsletter*, July 1985; Blakemore *et al.*, 1985).

Although these relatively informal mechanisms have proved efficient in identifying and disseminating information about some of the possible and probable short-term adverse consequences of CVS, they cannot be expected to be so efficient in respect of either subtle short-term effects, or longer-term effects. Because in many places, the clinicians responsible for CVS are frequently not responsible for continuing clinical care during pregnancy and delivery, and because they are almost never responsible for care of children born alive following CVS, the completeness and quality of relevant data collection referring to late pregnancy, infancy and childhood is seriously deficient almost everywhere.

So far, an efficient mechanism for generating and testing hypotheses about long-term adverse consequences of CVS does not exist. Quite simply, the 10 000 or so survivors of CVS remain virtually untouched by scientific investigation. Claims by some (see, for example, Jahoda *et al.*, 1985) that the technique has already been shown to be of acceptable safety should be assessed against this background.

17.3 STRATEGIES FOR TESTING HYPOTHESES ABOUT THE EFFECTS OF CVS ON MORBIDITY IN CHILDHOOD

When the WHO Working Group on Fetal Diagnosis met early in 1983, a variety of possible adverse effects of CVS other than miscarriage were postulated. These included infection, maternal haemorrhage, disruption of placental function, rupture of the amniotic sac and fetal deformities (WHO Working Group, 1984). Case reports and uncontrolled case series reported since the Working Group met suggest that several of these complications may indeed be hazards of CVS (see above). As practical experience of CVS accumulates, the risks of these complications may become less, but they are unlikely to disappear; furthermore other possible adverse effects (both predictable and unpredicted) will certainly be suggested. How should these hypotheses about long-term adverse effects of CVS be tested?

Isolated case reports will sometimes be informative. The available clinical details of the cases of maternal septicaemic shock which have followed CVS, for example, suggest strongly that this is a rare but very serious complication of the procedure (Barela *et al.*, 1986). The features of some fetal abnormalities which become evident for the first time only after delivery may also provide reasonably strong suggestive evidence of adverse effects of CVS. Evidence of causality will obviously be particularly strong if novel expressions of abnormal embryogenesis or damage are observed following CVS – cases comparable to those infants who have exhibited evidence of eye damage following amniocentesis (Cross and Maumenee, 1973; Merin and Beyth, 1980; Fortin and Lemaire, 1975; Isenberg and Heckenlively, 1985).

More probably, however, hypotheses about long-term adverse effects will relate to less specific forms of morbidity (such as increased susceptibility to infection for example) which cannot be confidently ascribed to CVS. Hypotheses related to morbidity of this kind may be prompted by observations made in *uncontrolled case series*. But any hypotheses relating to adverse outcomes which are known to have aetiologies other than CVS can really only be tested satisfactorily by reference to control groups.

Controlled comparisons making use of observational (non-experimental) data will generally take one of two forms. In the first of these – *case-control studies* – children who have the condition representing the postulated adverse effect of CVS (cases) will be compared with others who do not have it (controls) in respect of their prior 'exposure to' CVS. Using the other approach – *cohort studies* – the incidence of the postulated adverse effect will be compared in cohorts of children born after CVS and in other, control cohorts to which CVS has not been applied.

Case-control studies will be of particular value when the postulated adverse outcome of CVS is very rare. Acceptable statistical power can usually be achieved for a relatively modest outlay of research resources. The case-control studies mounted to test the hypotheses that amniocentesis predisposes to dislocation of the hip and talipes (Wald *et al.*, 1983) and neonatal sepsis (Soman *et al.*, 1985) are examples of this approach. As the number of pregnancies investigated with CVS grows, hypotheses about rare long-term adverse effects will gradually accumulate and the case-control method will constitute an important strategy for testing these hypotheses.

Cohort studies mounted to test hypotheses about the short-term effects of CVS are beginning to be reported and some of these will no doubt be extended to explore hypotheses about possible long-term effects as well. Here again, studies mounted to investigate possible long-term effects of amniocentesis provide examples of the methodology in action. In a comparison of a cohort of children born after amniocentesis with a control cohort (MRC Working Party on Amniocentesis, 1978), talipes equinovarus requiring treatment and congenital dislocation of the hip were found more frequently in the amniocentesis cohort. Death from respiratory distress syndrome was also more common among the babies born following amniocentesis than among controls.

Causal inferences based on the observational data derived using these research strategies must always be more tentative than those based on data derived from experiments. More than a decade after the widespread adoption of amniocentesis for prenatal diagnosis, controversy continues to exist about the interpretation of the case-control and cohort analytic studies which have been mounted to assess its possible long-term adverse effects. Essentially, the arguments reflect uncertainties about the adequacy of the control groups in these studies – in other words, whether 'like is being compared with like'. These uncertainties can only be addressed satisfactorily by mounting prospective experiments – *randomized controlled trials.* It is fortunate, even at this advanced stage in the career of amniocentesis, that a randomized trial of amniocentesis has been conducted in Denmark (Tabor *et al.*, 1986). The results suggest that less well-controlled studies using observational data have been misleading in a number of ways. The risks of some complications have been overestimated; the risks of others have been underestimated.

It must seem remarkable to scientists working in other fields that one of science's most powerful weapons, the controlled, prospective experiment, has been used so sparingly by clinical geneticists and obstetricians using invasive fetal diagnostic procedures. To some extent, the failure (until very recently) to employ the risk-minimizing strategy of the experimental method to evaluate amniocentesis must be a reflection of the fact that amniocentesis constituted the only way to obtain certain fetal diagnostic information. This situation does not apply in the case of CVS: amniocentesis is an alternative means of obtaining the same information in almost all circumstances.

Because of the potentially vast number of children who are likely to be born alive following the technique, there is an ethical imperative that evaluative research should use strategies which are scientifically strong. It is against this background that there have been quite unprecedented efforts by the research community to mount randomized trials to compare CVS with amniocentesis, both to minimize bias in the estimates of short-term differences and to establish comparable cohorts for assessing hypotheses concerning longer-term adverse effects. Proposals for randomized comparisons of CVS and amniocentesis have been supported in Denmark, Canada, Finland, the United Kingdom, the Netherlands, and Italy. It is likely that centres in some other countries will collaborate in generating randomized cohorts so that comparisons free of selection bias can be made between these two pre-natal diagnostic strategies. The availability of randomized cohorts for investigation should ensure that the confusion which still reigns concerning the long-term effects of amniocentesis will be avoided or minimized when it comes to assessing the relative safety of CVS.

Some people have suggested that formal evaluation of a new operative technique like CVS should not be attempted until those using it have become experienced in its use. Most of the randomized trials currently recruiting cases require of clinical and laboratory collaborators that they should have demonstrated their ability both to obtain samples and make fetal diagnoses. As this prior experience has usually been derived from sampling pregnancies which were scheduled for termination, however, it has also been suggested that the randomized trials may have been mounted at too early a point on the 'learning curve'. Others have already begun to suggest that it is time that the transcervical approach to CVS was abandoned in favour of the transabdominal approach because the latter seems less likely to be attended by infectious complications. In the face of the considerable uncertainties which these various opinions reflect, the first duty of conscientious practitioners and investigators must be to protect patients as effectively as possible from the unintended adverse consequences of our collective ignorance. The Danes and the Canadians have both behaved in an exemplary way. They have recognized that there is no basis in logic for, on the one hand, limiting the availability of new drugs until their efficacy and safety has been established in controlled trials and, on the other hand, acquiescing in the haphazard dissemination throughout the health services of non-drug interventions like CVS. Accordingly, CVS, as if it were a potentially dangerous new drug, is currently only available within the context of controlled trials. The Danes, in addition, have mounted subsidiary trials to compare transcervical with transabdominal CVS, and to evaluate the role of anti-D administration following CVS. The Danes and the Canadians have set the world an example of how ethical and scientific standards frequently coincide in clinical research and practice.

17.4 SUCCESSFUL IDENTIFICATION OF LONG-TERM ADVERSE EFFECTS OF INTERVENTION DURING PREGNANCY: THE CASE OF DIETHYLSTILBOESTROL

The strategies which can and should be used to evaluate the effects of CVS on morbidity in childhood and possibly adulthood can be illustrated by referring to the research which has uncovered the long-term adverse effects of a previous, widely adopted obstetric intervention – diethylstilboestrol (DES). The possibility that DES had long-term adverse effects was first raised by a mother whose daughter had developed vaginal adenocarcinoma (Ulfelder, 1980). In the 1960s, there had been an increase over expectation in the incidence of this very rare tumour. Case-control studies rapidly confirmed that aetiological role of DES as a transplacental carcinogen (Herbst *et al.*, 1971). These findings led to investigation of the randomized cohorts to look for evidence of more subtle effects which would be unlikely to have given rise to clinical suspicion. The unbiased comparisons made possible by the existence of these randomized cohorts proved to be invaluable in identifying probable and possible adverse effects of DES.

The 25-year follow-up of the randomized trial conducted by Dieckman in Chicago (Bibbo *et al.*, 1977) confirmed that a large proportion of exposed daughters had vaginal adenosis (67% compared with 4% in controls) and also circumferential ridges of the vagina and cervix (40% compared with none in the controls). Exposed daughters also had a higher incidence of irregular menstrual cycles and had had fewer pregnancies. Comparison of the outcome of pregnancies in daughters who had been exposed as fetuses to DES with that of daughters whose mothers had been given a placebo revealed a significantly greater incidence of premature live births, perinatal deaths, spontaneous abortions and ectopic pregnancies in the DES-exposed group (Herbst *et al.*, 1980).

Adverse effects of DES exposure on the reproductive tract were not confined to the female offspring. DES-exposed sons were found to have an increased incidence of epidydimal cysts, hypotrophic testes and capsular induration of the testes (Bibbo *et al.*, 1977). Semen analysis revealed that they also tended to have a low ejaculate volume and impaired sperm motility.

The results of the 27-year follow-up (Beral and Colwell, 1981) of cases entered into the British MRC randomized trial (MRC Conference on Diabetes and Pregnancy, 1955) was in several of the respects mentioned above complementary to the Chicago trial follow-up. In addition, of the men exposed as fetuses to DES, half as many were married or living as married as among the non-exposed men (34% and 62% respectively). Follow up of adults who as fetuses were entered into the other British trial of DES (Swyer and Law, 1954) revealed an unexpected but dramatic excess of psychiatric problems among those exposed to DES *in utero* (Vessey *et al.*, 1983).

Long-term follow-up of the mothers entered into both the Chicago and MRC trials (Bibbo *et al.*, 1978; Beral and Colwell, 1980) indicated that they may have been put at increased risk of serious adverse consequences by DES therapy. In both studies there is a suggestion of an excess number of women with breast cancer in the exposed group. This excess appears to have been confirmed in a larger, non-randomized cohort study (Greenberg and Colton, 1982).

17.5 POTENTIALS AND PROBLEMS IN SCIENTIFIC EVALUATION OF THE EFFECTS OF CVS ON MORBIDITY IN CHILDHOOD

The emergence of CVS as a contender for the role that amniocentesis has come to play in prenatal diagnosis during the last fifteen years has been accompanied by a truly exceptional degree of international consensus that this new technique must be evaluated carefully before it is accepted for widespread dissemination (Modell, 1985). The responsible lead given at the first meeting of the WHO Working Group in 1983 was reflected in recommendations made at subsequent meetings convened under the auspices of the National Institute of Child Health and Development (1983), the Royal College of Obstetricians and Gynaecologists (Rodeck and Nicolaides, 1984), the British Medical Research Council (1984), the Society of Obstetricians and Gynaecologists of Canada (Bryce *et al.*, 1983), the Canadian College of Medical Genetics (Feeny *et al.*, 1985), and the Concerted Action Programme of the European Community (Modell, 1985), among others. The conclusion reached at a second meeting of the WHO Working Group in May 1984 was that the efficacy and safety of CVS should be assessed by mounting randomized comparisons of CVS with amniocentesis. This view has also been reflected in several research proposals developed in Europe and North America.

Because of the widespread acceptance of the scientific strengths of randomized comparisons, research funding bodies have also, in general, responded remarkably effectively to these proposals for mounting trials. By the spring of 1985, at least four randomized trials had begun recruitment. Co-ordination between the groups mounting trials has resulted in informal international agreement on how the basic results of these similar trials can be presented and has thus established the potential for deriving more precise estimates of odds ratios by collaborative analyses of data derived from all comparable trials (Yusuf *et al.*, 1985).

The response of many clinical practitioners to proposals for randomized trials has also been exemplary. The Canadian College of Medical Genetics and the Society of Obstetricians and Gynaecologists of Canada, for example, have both recommended that, because CVS has not yet been adequately investigated, the new diagnostic technique should only be made available within well-designed randomized trials (Feeny *et al.*, 1985). The same decision has been taken by Danish obstetricians and clinical geneticists (Hahnemann, personal communication). In the United Kingdom, the President of the Royal College of Obstetricians and Gynaecologists has written to Fellows and Members encouraging them to participate in the Medical Research Council's trial (Macnaughton, 1985). National meetings of clinicians in both Italy (Brambati, personal communication) and the Netherlands (Gravenhorst, personal communication) have also resolved that widespread collaboration in trials is necessary. The active co-operation of general practitioners in mounting trials in Britain has been solicited both by the Royal College of General Practitioners (Stott, 1985) and at post-graduate meetings at which a commercially sponsored video film about CVS has been shown (Kingswell, personal communication).

It is not only among professionals that support for randomized trials exists however. Press and public responses to the British Medical Research Council's announcement of its randomized trial, for example, have reflected a new appreciation of just how important it is to evaluate new techniques carefully before they become widespread. Responding to an isolated example of an inaccurate and alarmist report of the trial in *The Guardian* newspaper (Veitch, 1985), the co-ordinator of Britain's Maternity Alliance stated that:

> Women have long argued that the efficacy and safety of new techniques, such as ultrasound scans, should be evaluated before they are routinely offered to pregnant women. The Medical Research Council is, therefore, to be congratulated for establishing a randomized controlled trial in order to weigh the advantages and disadvantages of the techniques in terms of fetal loss, side effects for the mother, and short and long term side effects for the fetus (Evans, 1985).

In what must be a quite unprecedented move to promote a randomized trial, the chairman of Britain's Association for Improvements in the

Maternity Services convened a meeting of interested voluntary organizations and consumer groups to encourage them to give public support to the Medical Research Council's (MRC) proposals (Beech, 1986). Representatives of these groups helped to draft the information leaflet for potential participants in the MRC trial and the leaflet will make it clear that seven of these lay organizations have formally and publicly endorsed the trial. The views of a former chairperson of the Patients' Association (currently a lay member of the General Medical Council) were of particular interest. Like the Canadian professionals quoted earlier, she felt that requests by women for investigation with CVS should not be entertained by clinicians unless the procedure was offered to them as informed participants within a randomized controlled trial (Robinson, 1985). A survey of patients who had been investigated with amniocentesis in one London hospital has confirmed that the majority would consider this restriction reasonable (Barby and Bobrow, unpublished observations).

Given this broadly-based consensus that randomized comparisons of CVS and amniocentesis are highly desirable for both scientific and ethical reasons, it is to be hoped that the evaluation of CVS may stand as an example of how medical innovation should occur. Unfortunately, the future of the trials which have been mounted is uncertain because there is both passive and active resistance to these studies from at least three sources.

First, some women are demanding CVS from those clinicians whom they know are in a position to offer it to them. It is easy to sympathize with these demands when they come from women who have had a previous pregnancy terminated during the second trimester, or from others who are at very high risk of carrying an abnormal fetus. But a growing demand is coming in addition from women who fall outside these very high risk groups (*Lancet*, 1985). As this demand is met by those who remain unconvinced by the case for careful evaluation, it will become increasingly difficult to recruit women to controlled trials. Yet another technique will have become part of routine medical practice without having been adequately evaluated. Although women are being made aware of this possibility by some of those attempting to represent their interests at national level (Micklethwait, 1985), they have been encouraged by others to exercise their 'right to choose' the method by which prenatal diagnosis is made despite the lack of evidence on long-term effects which might inform their choice (National Childbirth Trust, 1985).

Commercial interests have also contributed to the difficulties faced by those trying to mount randomized comparisons of CVS and amniocentesis. Prenatal diagnosis is already big business in entrepreneurial health care systems in which payment is by item of service, like those in the United States and Italy. If the income of practitioners, hospitals and research groups can be promoted by acquiescing in the growing public demand for prenatal diagnosis during the first trimester rather than the second trimester of pregnancy, then it is not surprising that scientific evaluation of this new technique will receive a low priority in some quarters. Manufacturers of equipment for chorion villus sampling and analysis also have a vested interest in promoting rapid dissemination of first trimester fetal diagnosis. Their promotional literature certainly does not dwell on current ignorance of the short-term and possible long-term adverse effects of CVS.

In addition to passive resistance to randomized trials motivated by commercial interests, however, some clinicians are actively obstructing scientific evaluation of CVS because they feel that the new technique has so many advantages that it should be adopted as soon as possible (*The Economist*, 1984; Jahoda *et al.*, 1985; Schulman, 1985).

The DES story, cited earlier, is just one of a number of salutory reminders that it has often not been possible to predict the adverse consequences of well-intentioned interventions like CVS. Formal clinical experiments (randomized trials) constitute 'a guided step into the unknown' (Silverman, 1985) through which the adverse consequences of our ignorance can be recognized efficiently and contained. Clinicians and others who, in their enthusiasm for innovation, propose dispensing with this risk-limiting step will be judged by at least some people to be acting in an unscientific, reckless and fundamentally unethical manner (Keirse *et al.*, 1985).

Those involved in the evaluation of CVS still have an opportunity to set an example of how to behave more responsibly. As an article (Muller *et al.*, 1981) in the *New England Journal of Medicine* put it: 'Let's not let the genie escape from the bottle – again'.

REFERENCES

Barela, A. I., Kleinman, G. E., Golditch, I. M., Menke, D. J., Hogge, W. A., Golbus, M. S. (1986) Septic shock with renal failure after chorionic villus sampling. *Am. J. Obstet Gynecol.* **154**, 1100–12.

Beech, B. A. (1986) Consumer view of randomised trials of chorionic villus sampling, *Lancet*, i, 1157.

Beral, V. and Colwell, L. (1980) Randomised trial of high doses of stilboestrol and ethisterone therapy in pregnancy: long term follow-up of the mothers. *Br. Med. J.*, **281**, 1098–101.

Beral, V. and Colwell, L. (1981) Randomised trial of high doses of stilboestrol and ethisterone therapy in pregnancy: long-term follow-up of the children. *J. Epidemiol. Commun. Health*, **35**, 155–6.

Bibbo, M., Gill, W. B., Azizi, F., Blough, R., Fang, V. S., Rosenfield, R. L. *et al.* (1977) Follow-up study of male and female offspring of DES-exposed mothers. *Obstet. Gynaecol.*, **49**, 1–8.

Bibbo, M., Haenzel, W. M., Wied, G. L., Hubby, M. and Herbst, A. L. (1978) A twenty-five year follow-up study of women exposed to diethylstilbestrol during pregnancy. *New Engl. J. Med.*, **298**, 763–7.

Blakemore, K. J., Mahoney, M. J. and Hobbins, J. C. (1985) Infection and chorionic villus sampling. *Lancet*, **ii**, 339.

Brambati, B. and Varotta, F. (1985) Infection and chorionic villus sampling. *Lancet*, **ii**, 609.

Bryce, R., Fuller, P., Mohide, P. *et al.* (1983) Clinical trial of chorion biopsy. *Can. Med. Assoc. J.*, **63**, 349–57.

Cross, H. E. and Maumenee, A. E. (1973) Ocular trauma during amniocentesis. *Arch. Ophthalmol.*, **90**, 303–4.

Economist, The (1984) The Birthpangs of a New Science. 14 July, pp. 81–5.

Evans, R. (1985) Unpublished letter submitted to *The Guardian*, 15 May.

Feeny, D., Fuller, P. J., Milner, R., Mohide, P. T., Tomkins, D. J. and Torrance G. W. (1985) Chorionic villus sampling. *Lancet*, **i**, 1269–70.

Finegan, J. K. (1984) Amniotic fluid and midtrimester amniocentesis: a review. *Br. J. Obstet. Gynaecol.*, **91**, 745–50.

Fletcher, J. C. (1985) Ethical aspects of a controlled clinical trial of chorion biopsy approach to prenatal diagnosis. *Prog. Clin. Biol. Res.*, **177**, 213–48.

Fortin, J. G. and Lemaire, J. (1975) Une complication oculaire de l'amniocentese. *Can. J. Ophthalmol.*, **10**, 511–13.

Garden, A. S., Reid, G., Benzie, R. J. (1985) Chorionic villus sampling. *Lancet*, **i**, 1270.

Greenberg, E. R. and Colton, T. (1982) Epidemiologic evidence for adverse effects of DES exposure during pregnancy. *Am. Statist.*, **36**, 268–72.

Harser, J. H., Pazin, G. J., Armstrong, J. A., Breinig, M. C. and Ho, M. (1983) Characteristics and management of pregnancy in women with genital herpes simplex virus infection. *Am. J. Obstet. Gynecol.*, **145**, 784–91.

Hecht, F., Hecht, B. K. and Bixenman, H. A. (1984) Caution about chorionic villi sampling in the first trimester. *New Engl. J. Med.*, **311**(21), 1388.

Herbst, A. L., Hubby, M. M., Blough, R. R. and Azizi, F. (1980) A comparison of pregnancy experience in DES-exposed and DES-unexposed daughters. *J. Reprod. Med.*, **24**, 62–9.

Herbst, A. L., Ulfelder, H. and Poskanzer, D. C. (1971) Adenocarcinoma of the vagina. Association of maternal stilbestrol therapy with tumour appearance in young women. *New Engl. J. Med.*, **284**, 878–81.

Hislop, A. and Fairweather, D. V. I. (1982) Amniocenteses and lung growth: an animal experiment with clinical implications. *Lancet*, **ii**, 1271–2.

Hislop, A., Fairweather, D. V. I., Blackwell, R. J. and Howard, S. (1984) The effect of amniocentesis and drainage of amniotic fluid on lung development in Macana fascicularis. *Br. J. Obstet. Gynaecol.*, **91**, 835–42.

Isenberg, S. J. and Heckenlively, J. R. (1985) Traumatized eye with retinal damage from amniocentesis. *J. Pediatr. Ophthalmol. Strabismus*, **22**, 65–7.

Jahoda, M. G. J., Vosters, R. P. L., Sachs, E. S. and Galjaard, H. (1985) Safety of chorionic villus sampling. *Lancet*, **ii**, 941–2.

Kazy, Z., Rozofsky, I. S. and Bakharer, V. A. (1982) Chorion biopsy in early pregnancy: a method of early prenatal diagnosis for inherited disorders *Prenat. Diag.*, **2**, 39–45.

Keirse, M. J. N. C., Kanhai, H. H. H. and Bennebroek Gravenhorst, J. (1985) Safety of chorionic villus sampling. *Lancet*, **ii**, 1312.

Kullander, S. and Sandahl, B. (1983) Fetal chromosome analysis after transcervical placental biopsies during early pregnancy. *Acta Obstet. Gynecol. Scand.*, **52**, 355–9.

Lancet editorial (1985) Can first-trimester fetal diagnosis be reliably evaluated? *Lancet*, i, 735–6.

Macnaughton, M. C. (1985) President's Newsletter, Royal College of Obstetricians and Gynaecologists. February.

Marchese, C. A., Carbonara, Viora E., La Prova A. and Campogrande, M. (1984) Biopsy of Chorionic Villi for Prenatal Diagnosis, *Acta. Obstet. Gynecol. Scand.*, **63**, 737.

McFadyen, I. R., Taylor-Robinson, D., Furr, P. M. and Bounstouller, Y. L. (1985) Infection and chorionic villus sampling. *Lancet*, ii, 610.

Medical Research Council (1984) Meeting to discuss the evaluation of the safety of chorion biopsy techniques, London, 30 March.

Merin, S. and Beyth, Y. (1980) Uniocular congenital blindness as a complication of midtrimester amniocentesis. *Am. J. Ophthalmol.*, **89**, 299–301.

Micklethwait, P. (1985) NCT and Medical Research. *New Generation*, **4**(2), 5–6.

Modell, B. (1985) Chorion Villus Sampling: evaluating safety and efficacy. *Lancet*, i, 737–40.

Montgomery, J. R., Flanders, R. W. and Yow, M. D. (1973) Congenital anomalies and herpesvirus infection. *Am. J. Dis. Child.*, **126**, 364–6.

Muller, J. E., Stone, P. H., Markis, J. E. and Braunwald, E. (1981) Let's not let the genie escape from the bottle – again. *New Engl. J. Med.*, **304**, 1294–6.

National Childbirth Trust (1985) A need to know. *New Generation*, **4**(2), 6.

National Institute of Child Health and Human Development (1983) Summary of an *ad hoc* advisory meeting on chorion villus sampling, 18 October.

Report to the Medical Research Council by their Working Party on Amniocentesis. *Br. J. Obstet. Gynaecol.*, **85**, supplement no. 2.

Rodeck, C. H. and Nicolaides, K. H. (1984) *Prenatal Diagnosis*, Royal College of Obstetricians and Gynaecologists/John Wiley and Sons, London.

Robinson, J. (1985) Contribution to meeting held at Friends Meeting House, Euston Road, London, 17 June.

Schulman, J. D. (1985) Safety of Chorionic Villus Sampling. *Lancet*, i, 1164.

Silverman, W. A. (1985) *Human experimentation: a Guided Step Into the Unknown*, Oxford University Press.

Simoni, G., Brambati, B., Danesino, C. *et al.* (1983) Efficient direct chromosome analysis and enzyme determination from chorionic villi samples in the first trimester of pregnancy. *Hum. Genet.*, **63**, 349–57.

Soman, M., Green, B. and Daling, J. (1985) Risk factors for early neonatal sepsis. *Am. J. Epidemiol.*, **121**, 712–19.

South, M. A., Rompkins, W. A. F., Morris, C. R. and Rawls, W. E. (1969) Congenital malformation of the central nervous system associated with genital type (type 2) herpesvirus. *J. Pediat.*, **75**, 13–18.

Stott, P. (1985) Sampling of the chorionic villi: a technique to complement amniocentesis. *J. Royal Coll. Gen. Pract.*, **35**(274), 316–17.

Swyer, G. I. M., Law, R. G. (1954) An evaluation of the prophylactic antenatal use of stilboestrol. Preliminary report. Proceedings of the Society for Endocrinology. *J. Endocrinol.*, **10**, vi–vii.

Tabor, A., Philip, J., Madsen, M., Bang, J., Obel, E. B., Nordgaard-Pedersen, B. (1986) Randomized controlled trial of genetic amniocentesis in 4,606 low-risk women. *Lancet*, i, 1287–93.

Time (1983) 29 August, p. 77.

Ulfelder, H. (1980) The stilbestrol disorder in historical perspective. *Cancer*, **45**, 3008–11.

Veitch, A. (1985) Abortion risk for medical trials women. *The Guardian*. 15 May.

Vessey, M. P., Fairweather, D. V. I. and Norman-Smith, B. (1983) Adverse effects of stilboestrol treatment in pregnancy on mothers and offspring. *J. Obstet. Gynaecol.*, **3**, 55–7.

Vyas, H., Milner, A. D. and Hopkin, I. E. (1982) Amniocentesis and fetal lung development. *Arch. Dis. Child.*, **57**, 627–8.

Ward, R. H. T., Modell, B., Petrou, M., Karagozlu, F. and Douratsos, E. (1983) Method of sampling chorionic villi in first trimester of pregnancy under guidance of real time ultrasound. *Br. Med. J.*, **286**, 1542–4.

Wald, N. J., Terzian, E. and Vickers, P. A. (1983) Congenital talipes and hip malformation in relation to amniocentesis: a case control study. *Lancet*, **ii**, 246–9.

Warren, R. C., Butler, J., McKenzie, F. C., Morsman, J. M. and Rodeck, C. H. (1985) Does chorion villus sampling cause fetomaternal haemorrhage? *Lancet*, **i**, 691.

Weatherall, J. A. C. (1982) A review of some affects of recent medical practices in reducing the numbers of children born with congenital abnormalities. *Health Trends*, **14**, 85–8.

WHO Working Group (1984) Fetal diagnosis of hereditary diseases. *Bull. World Health Org.*, **62**, 345–5.

Wyatt, P. R. (1985) Chorionic biopsy and increased anxiety. *Lancet*, **ii**, 1312–13.

Yusuf, S., Peto, R., Lewis, T., Collins, R. and Sleight, P. (1985) Beta blockade during and after myocardial infarction: an overview of the randomised trials. *Progr. Cardiovasc. Diseases*, **XXVII**(5), 336–71.

18

Early prenatal diagnosis and therapeutic potentials for the fetus

—— *W. Allen Hogge and Mitchell S. Golbus* ——

Despite the remarkable advances in the prenatal detection of congenital abnormalities over the last decade, the ultimate goal of the reproductive geneticist continues to be the development of techniques for fetal therapy to complement these diagnostic capabilities. The emergence of chorion villus sampling as a method for prenatal diagnosis in the first trimester should have benefits for fetal treatment efforts by making possible earlier intervention. Ultimately, it may be possible to not only treat, but also prevent certain fetal diseases in ways analogous to those used for postnatal diseases.

18.1 MEDICAL DISORDERS POTENTIALLY AMENABLE TO PRENATAL THERAPY

18.1.1 Fetal metabolic disorders

Advances in the postnatal treatment of inherited metabolic conditions coupled with improved and earlier techniques for the prenatal detection of these disorders have raised the possibility that early (prenatal) treatment might be indicated for the optimal management of some fetuses. To date there has been limited experience with this approach to management, but the results have been encouraging. Ampola *et al.* (1975) reported the prenatal diagnosis and subsequent therapy of a fetus with a B_{12}-responsive form of methylmalonic acidemia. This disorder is known to be treatable postnatally with a pharmacological dose of B_{12} which is converted to 5′-deoxy-adenosylcobalamin, a necessary co-factor in the enzyme reaction that catalyses the conversion of *L*-methylmalonyl CoA to succinyl CoA. Initial therapy with 10 mg/day cyanocobalamin was not begun until 32 weeks gestation, and only a marginal increase in maternal B_{12} level occurred. However, at approximately 34 weeks gestation the method of administration was changed to 5 mg/day intravenously, and the maternal serum B_{12} level rose to six times normal accompanied by a progressive decrease in maternal urinary methylmalonic acid excretion. Despite this clinical evidence of a therapeutic effect, the concentration of amniotic fluid methylmalonic acid at delivery (41 weeks gestation) was four times normal. Postnatally, the infant did well requiring only protein restriction, without vitamin supplemention, for metabolic control. There was clear evidence of improved fetal biochemical status; however, it is impossible to assess the benefits to the fetus of *in utero* therapy. It seems likely that reducing the level of methylmalonic acid might have had some beneficial effect on fetal development, but, of course, a controlled study is impossible to perform.

A second case of prenatal vitamin therapy has been reported, and appears to suggest the beneficial effects of this form of therapy. Packman *et al.* (1982) described the prenatal diagnosis and treatment of a fetus with biotin-responsive multiple carboxylase deficiency, an inborn error of metabolism causing a clinical picture of severe metabolic acidosis, dermatitis, and abnormal organic acid excretion. In this case oral administration of 10 mg/day of biotin was begun at approximately 23 weeks gestation and continued to term. Following birth, the diagnosis was confirmed by enzyme assay on cultured skin fibroblasts. The infant was continued on biotin, and postnatal development has been normal. In this case the evidence suggests that biotin administration effectively prevented the neonatal complications associated with this disorder, and no significant toxicity from the treatment was observed. More recently, a report of the prenatal therapy of vitamin B_{12} responsive homocystinuria was published (Rosenblatt *et al.*, 1985). This case, like those above, demonstrates the effectiveness of antenatal treatment, but does not demonstrate its advantages compared to prompt postnatal therapy.

18.1.2 Fetal endocrine disorders

Two recently reported cases demonstrate the possibility of successful *in utero* therapy of disorders resulting from alterations in fetal hormone concentration. To prevent masculinization of fetuses at risk for congenital adrenal hyperplasia David and Forest (1984) attempted to suppress the fetal adrenal gland by maternal administration of steroids. In the first case treatment was begun at 6.4 menstrual weeks with 40 mg per day of hydrocortisone. Amniocentesis at 17 weeks suggested only partial fetal adrenal suppression with abnormally high levels of 17 alpha-hydroxyprogesterone, androstenedione, and testosterone. The karyotype was 46XX with HLA typing predictive of an affected fetus. At birth the infant had clitoral hypertrophy and slight posterior labial fusion. However, in the second case 0.5 mg b.i.d. of dexamethasone was begun at five menstrual weeks, with amniocentesis at 15 weeks confirming adrenal suppression and predicting an affected female fetus. Neonatal evaluation confirmed 21-hydroxylase deficiency, but there was no evidence of masculinization.

18.2 THE FUTURE OF FETAL THERAPY

An era has begun when basic and clinical research will be increasingly turned to the management of the fetus with a correctable congenital defect. But instead of attempts at temporary management, attention will be turned to the permanent correction of genetic disorders and other birth defects.

18.2.1 Stem cell transplantation

The management of childhood immunodeficiency diseases and a number of hematologic disorders involves the intravenous transplantation of bone marrow cells that reach a target organ (the recipient bone marrow) where they multiply and function to supplement the deficient cell type. There have been similar techniques used in attempts to supplement deficient enzyme production in a number of inherited metabolic disorders (Krivit *et al.*, 1984; Rappeport and Ginns, 1984). Despite the success of bone marrow transplantation a number of problems remain, including graft rejection and graft versus host disease. In the case of metabolic disorders there are other problems that have prevented clinical application of postnatal bone marrow transplantation as a mode of therapy. Although there has been some success in raising levels of the deficient enzymes, only minimal success has been reported in reversing the clinical signs and symptoms of the various disorders, and there has been no success in getting the enzymes across the blood-brain barrier to affect neurologic status (Krivit *et al.*, 1984; Moser *et al.*, 1984). Finally, in the majority of allogeneic bone marrow transplants the recipient is immunocompetent and must be pre-treated with radiation and/or chemotherapy to prevent host versus graft rejection.

For these reasons and because the fetus appears more tolerant of foreign cells (Silverstein, 1964), in theory, one approach to therapy would be *in utero* transplantation. It may be a relatively easy step to translate the methods utilized in animal models to the human fetus because of the established experience with the provision of cells to the fetus with erythroblastosis fetalis, traditionally by an intraperitoneal approach, but more recently by direct intravascular transfusions (Bang *et al.*, 1982; Rodeck *et al.*, 1984). In addition, it has been shown that a fetal liver cell suspension injected into the umbilical vessels can be transferred across the placental microcirculation as well as directly into the fetus (Gustavii *et al.*, 1982). Because the fetal liver is the major hematopoietic organ in the second-trimester fetus, it may be possible to seed both the fetal liver and fetal bone marrow using hematopoietic stem cells (that is, cells that have not yet differentiated into specific cell types, and which divide as needed to maintain the marrow population). The best source of donor cells may in fact be fetal liver cells because these stem cells are those which normally seed the bone marrow during gestation. Likewise, the optimal time to transplant should be prior to the 20th week of gestation, the time during which the fetus usually would be seeding its bone marrow with hematopoietic cells from the liver.

If the fetus is more tolerant of a graft, it also follows that the engrafted stem cells should be immunotolerant of the recipient because the fetal lymphocytes which respond to specific foreign antigens are still 'naive'. There is clinical support for this concept in those cases where human fetal liver has been used for postnatal transplant purposes. There appears to be considerably less graft versus host disease in these patients. Therefore, for the fetal recipient the fetal liver may be the ideal source of stem cells.

This mutual immunotolerance would allow the use of allogeneic stem cell grafts from unmatched donors, and, possibly, even pooled donor cells, obviating the need for HLA typing and a specific donor search as is generally required for postnatal bone marrow transplantation. It also would remove the need for pre-treatment with radiation and/or chemotherapy as is necessary with immunocompetent recipients who have the capacity to reject an allogeneic graft. Pre-treatment may be unnecessary as well because the human fetus has a receptive stromal environment, and is programmed for the reception of hematopoietic stem cells.

18.2.2 Gene therapy

More ideal than replacement of the deficient protein or enzyme by donor cells would be the correction of the mechanism responsible for the disorder. The rapid advances in molecular genetics have brought much closer to reality the possibility of inserting normal genes into an individual to correct a genetic defect. The first successful gene therapy in mammals was reported by Hammer *et al.* (1984) who successfully corrected autosomally inherited dwarfism in mice. This strain of mice, called 'little', has a mutation that results in reduced levels of growth hormone, and is a model for human isolated growth hormone deficiency. By micro-injection of a rat hormone gene into mouse oocytes these investigators produced transgenic mice that expressed the growth hormone gene at a high level. Unfortunately, this expression not only restored growth, but also changed the phenotype from dwarfs to giants. In addition to the problem of control of the inserted gene the authors pointed out several reasons why these techniques were not applicable to humans. First, only 1% of the injected eggs developed into mice that expressed the gene. Secondly, the mutant sequence is not replaced with a normal DNA sequence because the integration site of the foreign DNA is unpredictable. Finally, because the integration is unpredictable, the foreign DNA could disrupt a normal gene, creating a new mutation, or alter the regulation of adjacent genes leading to potentially greater harm.

For these reasons more attention has been turned to other delivery systems for inserting DNA into donor cells, usually bone marrow cells. The system with the most potential appears to be the RNA viruses (retroviruses). With a retrovirus vector up to 100% of the cells could be infected and express the integrated gene. A large number of cells can be infected simultaneously, and the integration is of a single copy (vector plus foreign DNA) at a single, although random, site. Using this technique Miller *et al.* (1984) successfully infected mouse bone marrow cells *in vitro* with retroviruses encoding human hypoxanthine phosphoribosyltransferase (HPRT). These infected cells were transplanted into irradiated mice and expression of human HPRT protein was detected in hematopoietic tissue of the mice. Despite this success, a number of potential problems must be overcome. First, unless the transplanted cells have a selective advantage over the mutant endogenous cells, partial or complete bone marrow destruction is necessary. Secondly, although the transcriptional signals of the retrovirus cause expression of the foreign DNA, the level of expression remains low. In the future it may be possible to construct DNA sequences containing enhancer genes. These DNA sequences of 50–150 base-pairs in length can increase the expression of an adjacent gene up to 1000-fold. Finally, a major disadvantage to this vector system is the requirement for cell replication for integration of the donor sequences. The result is that non-dividing tissue, such as the brain, could not be infected.

For the reasons discussed above, there are a limited number of disorders potentially amenable to gene therapy with presently available techniques. In general, diseases where therapy might be possible are those where the missing enzyme functions in the cell that makes it, or where there is a deficiency of a circulating protein that is not under tight regulation. Two possible candidates are adenosine deaminase deficiency (severe combined immunodeficiency disease) and purine nucleoside phosphorylase deficiency (also causing a severe immunodeficiency disease). Both are presently treated by postnatal bone marrow transplant from a normal donor. Although HPRT deficiency also is a potential candidate, there are two possible limitations: (a) the gene could be inserted into bone marrow cells, but not brain cells, (b) the effects of the enzyme deficiency may not be reversible.

Before these techniques can be transferred to human genetic disorders on a larger scale, a number of problems must be solved. There must be methods to package the DNA and make it cell-type specific. This DNA will have to be efficiently transferred into the donor cells, and the donor cells efficiently delivered to the host. Methods to regulate the expression of transferred genes must be found, and when all these obstacles are overcome, a final criterion must be met; the delivery-expression system must be safe in humans. If these problems can be solved, the clinical application of human gene therapy has the potential to be a powerful therapeutic tool (Anderson, 1984).

18.3 CONCLUSION

In utero fetal therapy is an experimental form of fetal medicine, and, thus, should be applied only in those centres in which ongoing research is being done, and where a multidisciplinary team is assembled to address all the issues involved. Innovative fetal intervention must be fully tested in the laboratory, carefully and continually evaluated in light of current knowledge of the disorder in question, and honesty presented to the family before it is undertaken. Fetal therapy must be based on sound genetic principles and a clear understanding of the disorders in question, and must be the logical extension of knowledge gained from thoughtful research in genetics and developmental biology.

REFERENCES

Ampola, M. G., Mahoney, M. J., Nakamura, E. and Tanaka, K. (1975) Prenatal therapy of a patient with vitamin B_{12}-responsive methylmalonic acidemia. *New Engl. J. Med.*, **293**, 313–17.

Anderson, W. F. (1984) Prospects for human gene therapy. *Science*, **226**, 401–9.

Bang, J., Bock, J. E. and Trolle, D. (1982) Ultrasound-guided fetal intravenous transfusion for severe rhesus hemolytic disease. *Br. Med. J.*, **284**, 373–4.

David, M. and Forest, M. G. (1984) Prenatal treatment of congenital adrenal hyperplasia resulting from 21-hydroxylase deficiency. *J. Pediatr.*, **105**, 799–803.

Gustavii, B., Lofberg, L. and Olofsson, T. (1982) Transfer of tissue cells to the fetus. *Acta Obstet. Gynecol. Scand.*, **61**, 361–5.

Krivit, W., Pierpont, M. E., Ayaz, K. *et al.* (1984) Bone marrow transplantation in the Maroteaux-Lamy Syndrome (mucopolysaccharidosis Type VI): Biochemical and clinical status 24 months after transplantation. *New Engl. J. Med.*, **311**, 1606–11.

Hammer, R. E., Palmiter, R. D. and Brinster, R. L. (1984) Partial correction of murine hereditary growth disorder by germ-line incorporation of a new gene. *Nature*, **311**, 65–7.

Miller, A. D., Eckner, R. J. Jolly, D. J., *et al.* (1984) Expression of a retrovirus encoding human HPRT in mice. *Science*, **225**, 630–2.

Moser, H. W., Tutschka, P. J., Brown, F. R. III *et al.* (1984) Bone marrow transplant in adrenoleukodystrophy. *Neurology*, **34**, 1410–17.

Packman, S., Cowan, M. J., Golbus, M. S. *et al.* (1982) Prenatal treatment of biotin-responsive multiple carboxylase deficiency. *Lancet*, i, 1435–9.

Rappeport, J. M. and Ginns, E. I. (1984) Bone marrow transplantation in severe Gaucher's disease. *New Engl. J. Med.* **311**, 84–8.

Rodeck, C. H., Nicolaides, K. H., Warsof, S. L. *et al.* (1984) The management of

severe rhesus isoimmunization by fetoscopic intravascular transfusions. *Am. J. Obstet. Gynecol.*, **150**, 769–74.
Rosenblatt, D. S., Cooper, B. A. and Schmutz, S. M. (1985) Prenatal vitamin B_{12} therapy of a fetus with methylcobalamin deficiency (cobalamin E disease). *Lancet* **i**, 1127–9.
Silverstein, A. M. (1964) Ontogeny of the immune response. *Science*, **144**, 1423–8.

19

Early prenatal diagnosis and fetal surgery

—— *K. H. Nicolaides and C. H. Rodeck* ——

Prenatal diagnosis of congenital abnormalities provides those couples who choose to have such knowledge with a more informed basis upon which to make reproductive decisions. While abortion is presently the main option in the prevention of severe abnormalities, in a few selected cases *in utero* fetal therapy may be a realistic alternative. Potentially correctable fetal malformations usually have a multifactorial mode of inheritance and are therefore unlikely to be amenable to first trimester diagnosis by placental biopsy. However, early second trimester diagnosis by ultrasonography may be beneficial, because *in utero* surgical correction has the potential of arresting the progressive destructive consequences of the underlying defect while allowing further fetal development.

In the future, first trimester prenatal diagnosis followed by *in utero* marrow transplantation, at a stage of pregnancy before the development of fetal immune competence, could result in correction of inherited haematologic and metabolic disease. The feasibility of this approach is currently under investigation in animal models.

This chapter reviews the experience with animal and human studies in the surgical correction of fetal malformations.

19.1 HYDROCEPHALUS

Congenital hydrocephalus, with a birth incidence of 5–25 per 10 000 births (Stein *et al.*, 1981; Williamson, 1965), may result from genetic aberrations such as autosomal trisomies, chromosomal deletions and translocations, or infectious agents including cytomegalovirus, toxoplasmosis, or rubella. However, the majority of cases have no clear-cut aetiology and are probably due to a combination of genetic and environmental factors. The risk of recurrence in subsequent pregnancies is in the range of 2–5%, but a minority of cases are inherited as X-linked or autosomal recessive traits (Editorial, 1962; Burton, 1979; Habib, 1981).

19.1.1 Associated abnormalities

Spina bifida is found postnatally in 25–30% of patients with congenital hydrocephalus, and conversely hydrocephalus is present in over 80% of the cases of spina bifida. In a combined series of 114 fetuses with the antenatal sonographic diagnosis of ventriculomegaly, other abnormalities were present in 76% of the cases (Glick *et al.*, 1984; Chervenak *et al.*, 1984; Pretorius *et al.*, 1985).

19.1.2 Prognosis

The outlook in cases of congenital hydrocephalus is poor with high fetal wastage, perinatal death or chronic handicap. In the three series of antenatally diagnosed ventriculomegaly, referred to above, 30 (26%) of the 114 fetuses survived and on short-term follow-up only half of these were free of handicap.

19.1.3 Prenatal diagnosis

Fetal hydrocephalus is diagnosed from 16 weeks gestation, by the ultrasonographic demonstration of abnormally dilated cerebral ventricles (Campbell, 1977). A transverse axial scan of the fetal head at the level of the cavum septum pellucidum will demonstrate the lateral borders of the anterior horns, the medial and lateral borders of the posterior horns of the lateral ventricles, the choroid plexuses, the third ventricle and the Sylvian fissures. In hydrocephalus (Fig. 19.1) there is an increase in the distance from the lateral wall of the anterior horn to the mid-line (V) compared to the width of the hemisphere (V/H). The level of the obstruction is defined by examining the aqueduct of Sylvius and third and fourth ventricles.

19.1.4 Prenatal therapy: animal studies

Michejda and Hodgen (1981) inserted a ventriculo-amniotic shunt with a one-way mechanism in a group of rhesus fetal monkeys with corticosteroid induced hydrocephalus. Whereas untreated hydrocephalic neonates rarely survived more than 14 days, manifesting progressive muscular weakness and frequent epileptic seizures, the treated fetuses seldom died and the neonates showed normal growth rates and motor development. This data suggests that when progressive hydrocephalus is arrested by intrauterine treatment, fetal

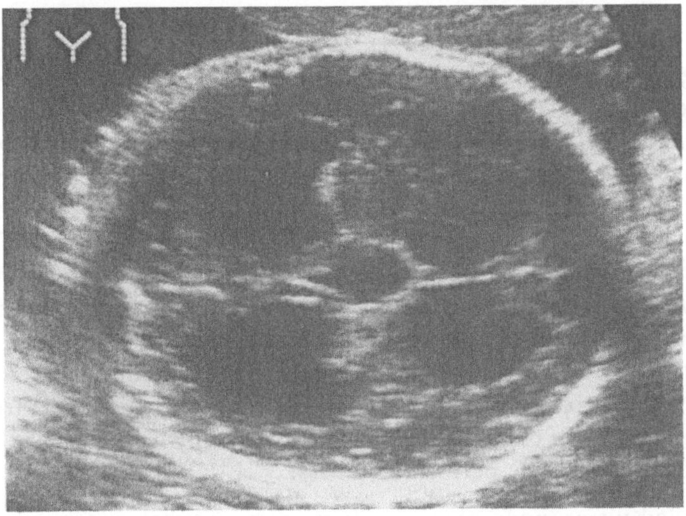

Figure 19.1 Transverse section of the fetal head at the level of the septum cavum pellucidum in a hydrocephalic fetus demonstrating the dilated third and lateral cerebral ventricles.

brain tissue resumes its ability to grow rapidly and reorganize its cyto-architecture (Michejda, 1985). Similar encouraging results from prenatal shunting were obtained in fetal lambs and monkeys where hydrocephalus was induced by the injection of kaolin into the cisterna magna (Edwards *et al.*, 1984).

19.1.5 Prenatal therapy: human studies

On the basis of the encouraging results from animal studies and experience with cerebrospinal fluid diversion procedures in human neonates, which in selected cases are known to be beneficial (Foltz and Shurtleff, 1963; McCullough and Balzer-Martin, 1982), investigators have treated hydrocephalic fetuses *in utero* by ultrasound guided cephalocenteses or ventriculo-amniotic shunting (Osathanondh *et al.*, 1980; Birnholz and Frigoletto, 1981; Clewell *et al.*, 1981, 1982; Frigoletto *et al.*, 1982). The total world experience of the treatment of hydrocephalus recorded in the International Fetal Surgery Registry consists of 39 cases (F. Manning, personal communication). No significant maternal morbidity was reported, but there were 7 fetal or neonatal deaths (18%) due either to the procedure or to other associated abnormalities. Although detailed developmental data is not available, of the 32 survivors only 11 are reported as having essentially normal development at 1–18 months, whilst 18 (56%) are severely handicapped.

19.1.6 Conclusions and recommendations

The higher incidence of handicap amongst survivors of *in utero*-shunted fetuses compared to those that survived under a policy of selective abortion emphasizes the danger that therapeutic intervention may allow survival in a vegetative state of what would have been a non viable fetus. Furthermore, the efficacy of treatment cannot be determined until long-term postnatal neurological follow-up is available and we gain a better understanding of the natural history of the disease. Although the theoretical advantage of ventricular decompression at the earliest possible opportunity is compelling, there is no method at present of assessing brain function *in utero* or of excluding an associated intrinsic central nervous system malformation, therefore some infants will be grossly retarded even with apparently successful treatment.

The consensus of centres involved in fetal therapy is that prenatal decompression should not be performed unless:

1. Detailed ultrasonographic examination is undertaken to exclude other anatomical defects.
2. Fetal chromosomal abnormalities or infection has been excluded.
3. There is evidence of progressive dilation and cortical thinning on serial sonographs.
4. The fetus is too immature to be delivered for postnatal shunting.
5. The parents are fully counselled as to the experimental nature of the procedure prior to obtaining their informed consent.

Very few cases will fulfil these criteria. Thus, the place for this procedure is very limited.

19.2 NEURAL TUBE DEFECTS

Neural tube defects (NTDs) resulting from failure to close the neural tube during the third to fourth weeks of gestation, are among the most common serious congenital malformations. The birth incidence in the UK, at 4–5 per 1000, is subject to large geographical and temporal variations (Alberman, 1978). Anencephaly and spina bifida, with an approximately equal prevalence, account for 95% of the cases and encephalocoele for the remaining 5%.

19.2.1 Prognosis

While anencephaly is fatal at or within hours of birth, the natural history of spina bifida is variable. Surviving infants are often severely handicapped and require frequent surgical interventions (Frank and Fixsen, 1980) and institutional care. Handicap typically consists of weakness of the lower limbs, urinary and faecal incontinence and hydrocephalus with mental retardation.

Without surgical treatment only 20% of infants survive to the age of two years (Laurence, 1964), whereas if active surgical intervention within 24 hours of birth is undertaken for all infants, 40% will survive for more than 7 years but only 1% will be free of handicap (Lorber, 1971). At present the most widely adopted approach is to withhold active treatment from those infants with unfavourable prognostic signs present at birth (other major malformations, gross paralysis of the legs, extensive spinal lesions, kyphosis or scoliosis and moderate or severe hydrocephalus; Lorber, 1971, 1972). With this approach, the five year survival for infants with open spina bifida is 30%, and 95% of these are moderately to severely handicapped. The corresponding figures for infants with closed lesions are 60% and 70% respectively (Althouse and Wald, 1980).

19.2.2 Prenatal diagnosis

The presence of open spina bifida can be inferred by the demonstration of elevated levels of amniotic fluid alpha fetoprotein (AFP) in pregnant women undergoing amniocentesis because of maternal serum AFP (Wald and Cuckle, 1984). More directly, the diagnosis can be made ultrasonographically by visualization of the spinal lesion (Figs 19.2 and 19.3), which is commonly associated with hydrocephalus and the Arnold–Chiari malformation.

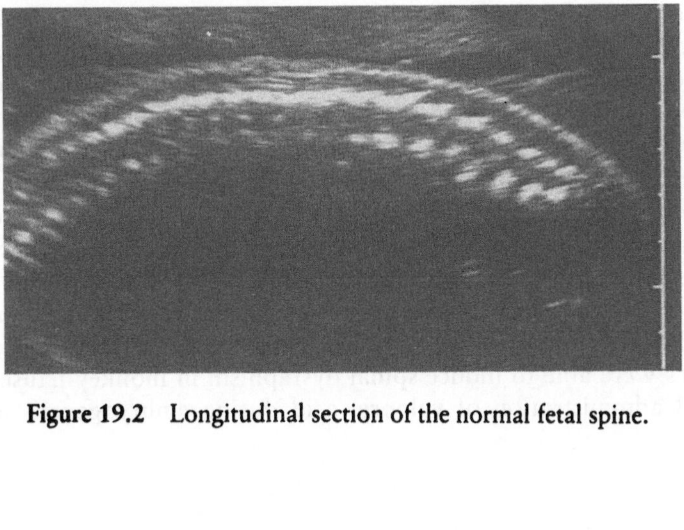

Figure 19.2 Longitudinal section of the normal fetal spine.

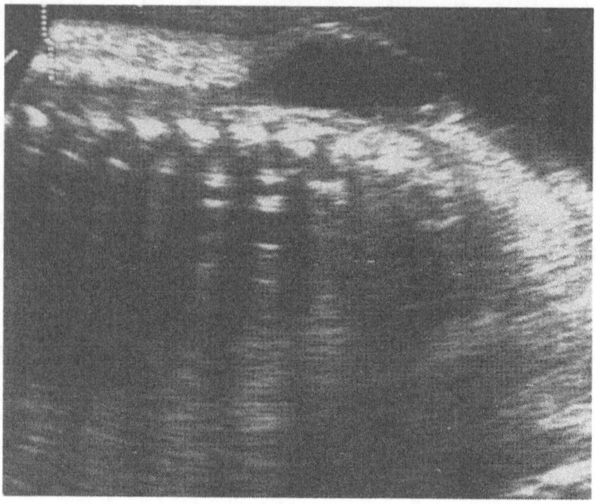

Figure 19.3 Lonigitudinal section of the fetal spine demonstrating a sacral myelomeningocoele.

19.2.3 Prevention

Although supplementation of the maternal diet with vitamins may have a protective effect on the development of NTDs (Smithells, 1983; Laurence, 1984), more definitive evidence is awaited from a multicentre study which is currently being performed by the Medical Research Council.

19.2.4 In utero closure: animal studies

Michejda (1985) induced a spina bifida-like condition in eight monkey fetuses at 110–125 days gestation by intrauterine lumbar laminectomy, followed by manual displacement of the spinal cord from the central canal. The defect was subsequently closed in five cases with an allogeneic bone paste. On neurological assessment after delivery at term (160–165 days), the three untreated animals showed severe abnormalities including paraplegia, incontinence and somatosensory loss below the induced lesion. On histological examination of the vertebral column, there was no significant new bone formation or healing, while the exposed spinal cord showed degenerative changes. In contrast, the *in ŭtero* treated animals had completely normal neurological development, complete restoration and remodelling of bone and morphologically normal spinal cords. More recently Michejda and her associates were able to induce spinal dysraphism in monkey fetuses by the maternal administration of valporic acid during embryogenesis and succeeded in producing complete cure by *in utero* closure in later pregnancy (personal communication).

19.2.5 Human therapy

To date, no attempt has been made to treat spina bifida in human fetuses. The high mortality and morbidity associated with both open and closed lesions in the human demand extreme caution in extrapolating from the findings of the animal studies.

19.3 CONGENITAL DIAPHRAGMATIC HERNIA

Congenital diaphragmatic hernia (CDH), with a birth incidence of 2–5 per 10 000, results from failure to close of the posterolateral pleuroperitoneal fold at 8–9 weeks gestation.

19.3.1 Associated abnormalities

Associated lethal non-pulmonary malformations are found in 95% of the stillbirths and in up to 60% of those that die within 24 hours of delivery; craniospinal and cardiac anomalies predominate (Butler and Claireaux, 1962; Puri and Gorman, 1984). Thus, although in the paediatric literature the incidence of associated defects is quoted at approximately 20%, the true incidence at birth is more like 60%.

19.3.2 Prognosis

One third of the infants are stillborn (Butler and Claireaux, 1962; Touloukian and Cole, 1975; Harrison *et al.*, 1978; Puri and Gorman, 1984). More than 50% of the liveborn neonates die before surgery is undertaken, either as a result of associated malformations or due to pulmonary hypoplasia and hypertension. The mortality for those infants that develop respiratory distress requiring operative repair within the first 24 hours of life remains at 50–80% (Raphaely and Downes, 1973; Mishalany *et al.*, 1979; Ruff, 1980; Wiener, 1982; Hansen *et al.*, 1984; Reynolds *et al.*, 1984). By contrast the survival for infants that first develop symptoms after the first 24 hours of life is nearly 100% (Marshall and Sumner, 1982; Wiener, 1982).

19.3.3 Prenatal diagnosis

CDH can be diagnosed by the ultrasonographic demonstration of stomach and intestines (90% of the cases) or liver (50%) in the thorax and the

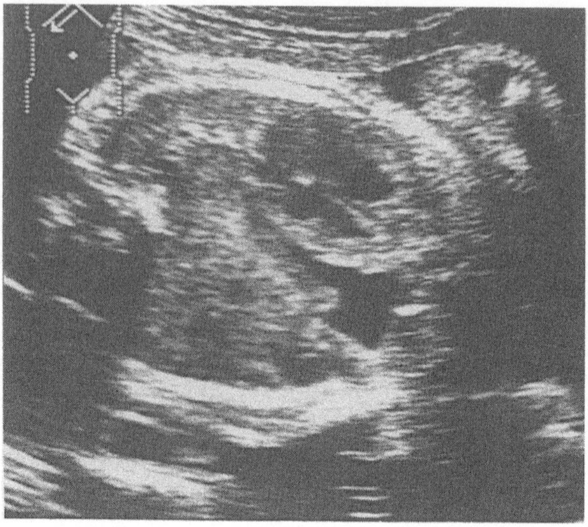

Figure 19.4 Transverse section of the thorax demonstrating the presence of stomach and intestines in the chest and the associated mediastinal shift in a fetus with diaphragmatic hernia.

associated mediastinal shift to the opposite side (Fig. 19.4). Polyhydramnios, ascites and other malformations are often present.

19.3.4 Pulmonary development

The bronchial tree is fully developed by the 16th week of gestation at which time the full adult number of airways is established. The alveoli continue to develop even after birth, increasing in number and size until the growth of the chest wall is completed in adulthood. The growth of blood vessels supplying the acinus (intra-acinar vessels) parallels alveolar development, while the growth of pre-acinar vessels follows the development of the airways (Reid, 1984).

In CDH the reduced thoracic space available to the developing lung leads to reduction in airways, aveoli and arteries. Furthermore, there is an increase in arterial medial wall thickness and extension of muscle peripherally into the small pre-acinar arteries (Kitigawa *et al.*, 1971) offering an explanation for the pulmonary hypertension and persistent fetal circulation observed after neonatal repair.

19.3.5 *In utero* correction: animal studies

With the use of a fetal lamb model in which diaphragmatic hernias were created by making a hole in the diaphragm at 100 days of gestation, Harrison and associates (1981) developed a successful *in utero* surgical technique which involved reduction of the viscera from the thoracic cavity into the peritoneal cavity and repair of the diaphragmatic defect. The abdominal contents were accommodated without increased intra-abdominal pressure, which would compromise blood flow in the umbilical vein, by enlarging the abdominal cavity with abdominoplasty. This involved the incorporation of an oval silicone rubber patch into the abdominal wall. The repair was performed on 10 lambs at 120 days gestation; four died postoperatively and six were viable after term delivery (140 days). In autopsied lambs, the lungs were larger, well expanded and histologically more mature than non-repaired controls.

19.3.6 Human fetal therapy

There are no reported cases of *in utero* correction of human CDH. For a fetus with an ultrasonographically demonstrable large CDH at 16–18 weeks gestation, irreversible maldevelopment of the bronchial tree and vasculature is likely and therefore *in utero* surgical correction at some later gestation is physiologically irrational. However in fetuses with a diaphragmatic defect which allows the intrathoracic herniation of abdominal viscera only after midgestation (when the bronchial tree and pre-acinar vessels are fully developed), prenatal correction, by allowing further development of the alveoli and intra-acinar vessels, may well prevent pulmonary hypoplasia and neonatal death.

19.4 OBSTRUCTIVE UROPATHY

Urinary tract anomalies occur in approximately 2 per 1000 births and they can be broadly classified into dysgenetic and obstructive. Dysgenetic disorders include renal agenesis and infantile (Potter type I) or adult (Potter type III) polycystic kidney disease. The term 'obstructive uropathy' encompasses a wide variety of different pathological conditions characterized by dilatation of part or all of the urinary tract.

19.4.1 Prognosis

When the obstruction is complete and occurs early in fetal life, renal hypoplasia (deficiency in total nephron population) and dysplasia (formation of abnormal nephrons and mesenchymal stroma) ensue (Potter type II renal disease). On the other hand, where intermittent obstruction allows for normal renal development, or when it occurs in the second half of pregnancy, hydronephrosis will result (Potter type IV) and the severity of the renal damage will depend on the degree and duration of the obstruction (Beck, 1971; Tanagho, 1972).

19.4.2 Multicystic dysplasia

Potter type II renal disease results from inhibition of the action of the ampulla of the ureteric bud, with consequent hypodysplasia of collecting tubules and nephrons. The collecting tubules become cystic and the diameter of the cysts determines the size of the kidneys, which may be enlarged (type IIA) or small (type IIB). Ultrasonographically, the former are recognized as large multicystic and the latter as shrunken and hyperechogenic. Occasionally only one of a few adjacent collecting tubules are involved so that only a segment of the kidney is abnormal. The condition, which is not familial, is associated with urethral or ureteric atresia. Malformations in other parts of the body occur in up to 50% of the cases. If renal involvement is bilateral, which is the commonest presentation, the condition is always fatal in the perinatal period. If only one kidney is abnormal, nephrectomy after delivery is usually necessary but otherwise the prognosis is good.

19.4.3 Ureteropelvic junction obstruction

Prenatal diagnosis of ureteropelvic junction obstruction (UPJ) is based on the demonstration of hydronephrosis in the absence of dilated ureters and bladder; amniotic fluid volume is usually normal (Garrett *et al.*, 1975; Kay *et al.*, 1979; Matturri, 1980). Both kidneys are affected in approximately 40% of the cases. Serial scans should be performed and early delivery undertaken, for postnatal therapy, if there is evidence of progressive bilateral pelvicalyceal dilatation and decreasing amniotic fluid volume. Postnatally, renal function is assessed by serial isotope imaging and pyeloplasty is performed if there is evidence of deteriorating function. Up to two thirds of the infants have moderate or good function and can be managed conservatively (Thomas, 1984).

19.4.4 Urethral obstruction

Incomplete or intermittent urethral obstruction, due to posterior urethral valves, is associated with enlargement and hypertrophy of the bladder and varying degrees of hydroureters, hydronephrosis (Fig. 19.5), oligohydramnios and pulmonary hypoplasia. It is suggested that early renal development is normal and the renal damage, observed in severe cases, is due to the back pressure effect of obstruction (Osathanondh and Potter, 1964; Beck, 1971; Tanagho, 1972; Fetterman *et al.*, 1974; Harrison *et al.*, 1982). An alternative hypothesis is that the quality of the renal parenchyma, in cases of posterior urethral valves, is determined by the position of origin of the ureteric bud from the Walfian duct (Henneberg and Stephens, 1980). The bud arising from the normal position on the duct achieves a normal location in the

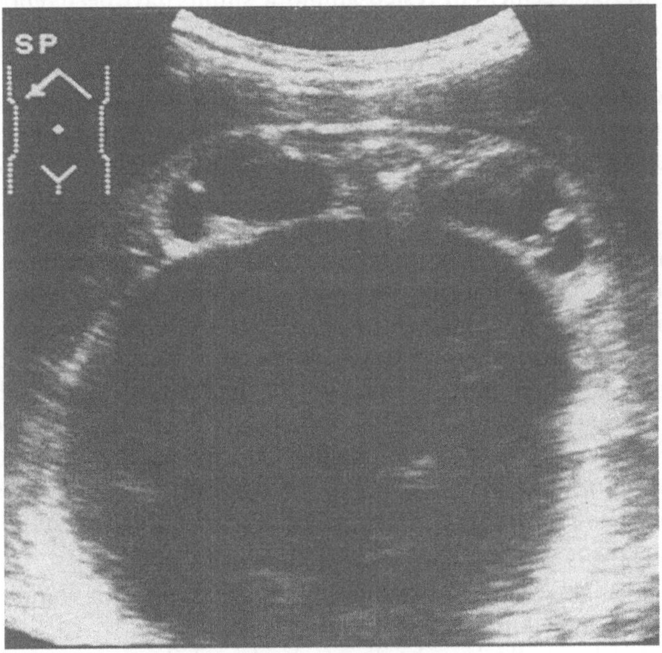

Figure 19.5 Transverse section of the fetal trunk demonstrating the dilated bladder and hydronephrotic kidneys in a fetus with urethral obstruction.

bladder and penetrates the normal metanephric mesenchyme forming a normal kidney. The buds arising more caudally from the duct acquire more lateral locations on the bladder and penetrate the tail end of the nephrogenic cord, producing a spectrum of renal hypoplasia and dysplasia that is progressively more severe the more laterally the ureteral orifice is sited. Similarly, there is controversy as to whether the associated pulmonary hypoplasia is secondary to oligohydramnios and thoracic compression (Thomas and Smith, 1974) or due to a primary pulmonary malformation (Reid, 1984).

19.4.5 In utero therapy

On the assumption that unrelieved obstruction causes progressive renal and pulmonary damage, several investigators have performed *in utero* decompression of the urinary tract, either by open surgical diversion (Harrison *et al.*, 1982) or by the ultrasound-guided insertion of suprapubic vesico-amniotic catheters (Berkowitz *et al.*, 1982; Golbus *et al.*, 1982; Rodeck and Nicolaides, 1983). To date a total of 72 cases of obstructive uropathy treated by the *in utero* placement of vesico-amniotic shunts have been reported to the International Fetal Surgery Registry (F. Manning, personal communication). There were three procedure-related perinatal deaths, 11 elective abortions because of associated abnormalities or poor renal function, one intrauterine death due to multiple defects and 28 neontal deaths mainly due to pulmonary hypoplasia. The remaining 30 (42%) survived and apparently only in two is there long term morbidity. The oldest child is five years. The underlying pathology was posterior urethral valves in 20 cases and urethral atresia in three, multicystic kidneys in one, 'Prune Belly' syndrome in three, multiple non-renal defects and chromosomal abnormalities in 11, and no diagnosis was made or proven in 34 cases.

These results fail to demonstrate conclusively that *in utero* intervention improves renal or pulmonary function beyond what can be achieved by postnatal surgery. However, they expose the need firstly for the investigation of these fetuses with the aim of excluding associated non-renal abnormalities and secondly for the development of reliable criteria in the assessment of renal function or irreversible renal and pulmonary damage. Our approach to the management of fetal urethral obstruction includes:

1. Detailed high resolution sonographic examination for the detection of associated malformations.
2. Fetal blood sampling for the diagnosis of fetal chromosomal abnormalities (Nicolaides *et al.*, 1986).
3. Insertion of a vesico-amniotic shunt.

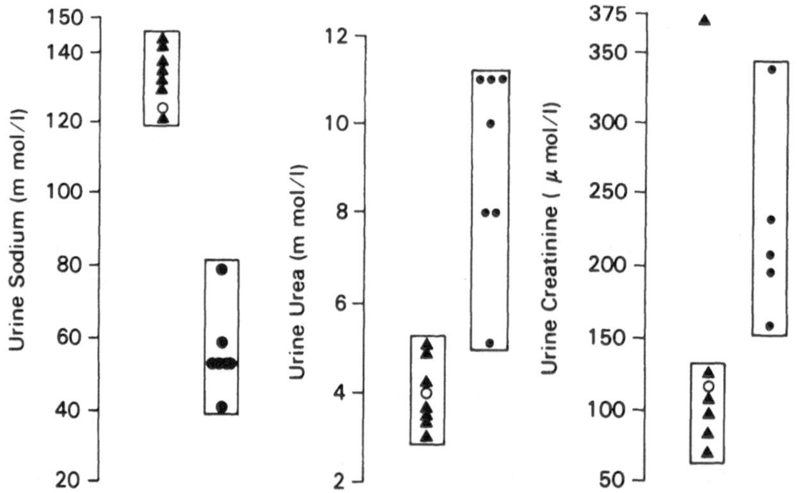

Figure 19.6 Urine biochemistry in 15 fetuses with obstructive uropathy. Seven survived with moderately good renal function (●), seven died in the neonatal period (▲), primarily due to pulmonary hypoplasia, and one is surviving with poor renal function (○).

We consider this to be both diagnostic and therapeutic. Poor renal function is inferred from the ultrasonic findings of severe oligohydramnios, increased renal parenchymal echogenicity, and more accurately defined by a fetal urinary sodium of more than 100 mmol/l, creatinine of less than 150 µmol/l and urea of less than 6 mmol/l (Fig. 19.6) and by failure to increase the amniotic fluid volume over a seven day period after insertion of the shunt.

REFERENCES

Alberman, E. (1978) Epidemiology of neural tube defects. In *The Diagnosis and Management of Neural Tube Defects* (eds J. A. Jordan and E. M. Symonds), Royal College of Obstetricians and Gynaecologists, London, RCOC, p. 1.

Althouse, R. and Wald, N. J. (1980) Survival and handicap of infants with spina bifida. *Archs. Dis. Childh.*, **55**, 845.

Beck, A. D. (1971) The effect of intrauterine urinary obstruction upon the development of the fetal kidney. *J. Urol.*, **105**, 784.

Berkowitz, R. L., Glickman, M. G., Smith, G. J. W. *et al.* (1982) Fetal urinary tract obstruction: what is the role of surgical intervention in utero? *Am. J. Obstet. Gynecol.*, **144**, 367.

Birnholtz, J. C. and Frigoletto, F. D. (1981) Antenatal treatment of hydrocephalus. *New Engl. J. Med.*, **303**, 1021.

Burton, B. K. (1979) Recurrence risks for congenital hydrocephalus. *Clin. Genet.*, **16**, 47.

Butler, N. and Claireaux, A. E. (1962) Congenital diaphragmatic hernia as a cause of perinatal mortality. *Lancet*, **i**, 659.

Campbell, S. (1977) Early prenatal diagnosis of neural tube defects by ultrasound. *Clin. Obstet. Gynecol.*, **20**, 351.

Chervenak, F. A., Duncan, C., Ment, L. R. *et al.* (1984) Outcome of fetal ventriculomegaly. *Lancet*, **ii**, 179.

Clewell, W. H., Johnson, M. L., Meier, P. R. *et al.* (1981) Placement of ventriculoamniotic shunt for hydrocephalus in a fetus. *New Engl. J. Med.*, **305**, 955.

Clewell, W. H., Johnson, M. L. and Meier, P. R. (1982) A surgical approach to the treatment of fetal hydrocephalus. *New Engl. J. Med.*, **306**, 1320.

Editorial (1962). Sex-linked hydrocephalus with severe mental defect. *Br. Med. J.*, **1**, 168.

Edwards, M., Harrison, M., Holks *et al.* (1984) Kaolin induced congenital hydrocephalus in utero in fetal lambs and rhesus monkeys. *J. Neurosurg.*, **60**, 115.

Fetterman, G. H., Ravitch, M. M. and Sherman, F. E. (1974) Cystic changes in fetal kidneys following urethral ligation: studies by microdissection. *Kidney Int.*, **5**, 111.

Foltz, E. L. and Shurtleff, D. B. (1963) Five year comparative study of hydrocephalus in children with and without operations (113 cases). *J. Neurosurg.*, **20**, 1064.

Frank, J. D. and Fixsen, J. A. (1980) Spina bifida. *Br. J. Hosp. Med.*, **24**, 422.

Frigoletto, F. D., Birnholz, J. and Greene, M. F. (1982) Antenatal treatment of hydrocephalus by ventriculoamniotic shunting. *JAMA*, **248**, 2496.

Garrett, W. J., Kossoff, G. and Osborn, R. A. (1975) The diagnosis of fetal hydronephrosis, megaureter and urethral obstruction by ultrasonic echography. *Br. J. Obstet. Gynaecol.*, **82**, 115.

Golbus, M. S., Harrison, M. R., Filly, R. A. *et al.* (1982) In utero treatment of urinary tract obstruction. *Am. J. Obstet. Gynecol.*, **142**, 383.

Glick, P. L., Nakayama, D. K., Harrison, M. R. *et al.*, (1984) Management of the fetus with ventriculomegaly, *J. Pediatr.* **105**,

Habib, Z. (1981) Genetics and genetic counselling in neonatal hydrocephalus. *Obstet. Gynecol. Survey*, **36**, 529.

Hansen, J., James, S., Burrington, J. *et al.* (1984) The decreasing incidence of pneumothorax and improving survival of infants with congenital diaphragmatic hernia. *J. Pediatr. Surg.*, **19**, 385.

Harrison, M. R., Bjordal, R. I., Langmark, F. *et al.* (1978) Congenital diaphragmatic hernia: the hidden mortality. *J. Pediatr. Surg.*, **13**, 227.

Harrison, M. R., Golbus, M. S., Filly, R. A. *et al.* (1982) Fetal surgery for congenital hydronephrosis. *New Engl. J. Med.*, **54**, 32.

Harrison, M. R., Nakayama, D. K., Noall, R. *et al.* (1982) Correction of congenital hydronephrosis in utero. II, Decompression reverses the effects of obstruction on the fetal lung and urinary tract. *J. Pediatr. Surg.*, **17**, 965.

Harrison, M. R., Ross, N. A. and deLorimier, A. A. (1981) Correction of congenital diaphragmatic hernia in utero. III, Development of a successful surgical technique using abdominoplasty to avoid compromise of umbilical blood flow. *J. Pediatr. Surg.*, **16**, 934.

Henneberg, M. O. and Stephens, F. D. (1980) Renal hypoplasia and dysplasia in infants with posterior urethral valves. *J. Urol.*, **123**, 912.

Kay, R., Lee, T. G. and Tank, E. S. (1979) Ultrasonographic diagnosis of fetal hydronephrosis in utero. *Urology*, **13**, 286.

Kitigawa, M., Hislop, A., Boyden, E. A. *et al.*, (1971) Long hypoplasia in congenital diaphragmatic hernia. A quantitative study of airway, artery and alveolar development. *Br. J. Surg.*, **58**, 342.

Laurence, K. M. (1964) The natural history of spina bifida cystica: detailed analysis of 407 cases. *Archs. Dis. Childh.*, **39**, 41.

Laurence, K. M. (1984) Prevention of neural tube defects. In *Prenatal Diagnosis* (eds C. H. Rodeck and K. H. Nicolaides). Proceedings of the 11th Study Group of the Royal College of Obstetricians and Gynaecologists, London, RCOG, p. 261.

Lorber, J. (1971) Results of treatment of myelomeningocele. An analysis of 524 unselected cases, with special reference to possible selection for treatment. *Dev. Med. Chid. Neurol.*, **13**, 279.

Lorber, J. (1972) Spina bifida cystica. Results of treatment of 270 consecutive cases with criteria for selection for the future. *Arch. Dis. Child.*, **854**, 47.

Marshall, A. and Sumner, E. (1982) Improved prognosis in congenital diaphragmatic hernia: Experience of 62 cases over 2 year period. *J. Roy, Soc. Med.*, **75**, 607.

Matturri, M., Peters, B. E. and Kedziora, J. A. (1980) Prenatal and postnatal sonographic demonstration of bilateral ureteropelvic junction obstruction. *Med. US*, **4**, 94.

McCullough, D. C. and Balzer-Martin, L. A. (1982) Current prognosis in overt neonatal hydrocephalus. *J. Neurosurg.*, **57**, 378.

Michejda, M. (1985) Antenatal treatment of neural tube defects. In *The Fetus as a Patient* (ed. Asim Kurjak), Elsevier Science Publishers BV, p. 131.

Michejda, M. and Hodgen, G. D. (1981) In utero diagnosis and treatment of non-human primate fetal skeletal anomalies. I, Hydrocephalus. *J. Am. Med. Ass.*, **246**, 1093.

Mishalany, H. G., Nakada, K. and Woolley, M. M. (1979) Congenital diaphragmatic hernias: eleven years' experience. *Arch. Surg.*, **114**, 1118.

Nicolaides, K. H., Rodeck, C. H. and Gosden, C. M. (1986) Fetal malformations should have rapid antenatal karyotyping. (in press)

Osathanondh, R., Birnholz, J., Altman, A. M. *et al.* (1980) Ultrasonically guided transabdominal encephalocentesis. *J. Reprod. Med.*, **25**, 125.

Osathanondh, V. and Potter, E. L. (1964) Pathogenesis of polycystic kidneys. *Arch. Pathol.*, 77, 459.

Pretorius, D. H., Davis, K., Manco-Johnson, M. L. *et al.* (1985) Clinical course of fetal hydrocephalus: 40 cases. *AJR*, **144**, 827.

Puri, P. and Gorman, F. (1984) Lethal non pulmonary anomalies associated with congenital diaphragmatic hernia; implications for early intrauterine surgery. *J. Pediatr. Surg.*, **19**, 29.

Raphaely, R. C. and Downes, J. J. (1973) Congenital diaphragmatic hernia: prediction of survival. *J. Pediatr. Surg.*, **8**, 815.

Reid, L. M. (1984) Lung growth in health and disease. *Br. J. Dis. Chest*, **78**, 105.

Reynolds, M., Luck, S. R. and Lappen, R. (1984) The 'critical' neonate with diaphragmatic hernia: a 21-year perspective. *J. Pediatr. Surg.*, **19**, 364.

Rodeck, C. H. and Nicolaides, K. H. (1983) Ultrasound guided invasive procedures in obstetrics. *Clin. Obstet. Gynaecol.*, **10**, 515.

Ruff, S. J., Campbell, J. R., Harrison, M. W. *et al* (1980) Pediatric diaphragmatic hernias: an 11 year experience. *Am. J. Surg.*, **139**, 641.

Smithells, R. W. (1983) Diet and congenital malformation. In *Nutrition in Pregnancy* (eds D. M. Campbell and M. D. G. Gillmer). Proceedings of the 10th study group of the Royal College of Obstetricians and Gynaecologists, London, RCOG, p. 155.

Stein, S. C., Feldman, J. G., Apjel, S. *et al.* (1981) The epidemiology of congenital hydrocephalus. *Child's Brain*, **8**, 253.

Tanagho, E. A. (1972) Surgically induced partial urinary obstruction in the fetal lamb. II, Urethral obstruction. *Invest. Urol.*, **10**, 35.

Thomas, D. F. M. (1984) Urological diagnosis in utero. *Arch. Dis. Childh.*, **59**, 913.

Thomas, I. T. and Smith, D. W. (1974) Oligohydramnios, cause of the non-renal features of Potters syndrome, including pulmonary hypoplasia. *J. Pediatr.*, **84**, 811.

Touloukian, R. J. and Cole, D. A. (1975) A state-wide survey of index pediatric surgical conditions. *J. Pediatr. Surg.*, **10**, 725.

Wald, N. J. and Cuckle, H. S. (1984) Neural tube defects: screening and biochemical diagnosis. In *Prenatal Diagnosis* (eds C. H. Rodeck and K. H. Nicolaides). Proceedings of the 11th Study Group of the Royal College of Obstetricians and Gynaecologists, London, RCOG, p. 219.

Wiener, E. S. (1982) Congenital posterolateral diaphragmatic hernia: new dimensions in management. *Surgery*, **92**, 670.

Williamson, E. M. (1965) Incidence and family aggregation of major congenital malformations of the central nervous system. *J. Med. Genet.*, **2**, 161.

20

Towards a chorion villus sampling service

David T. Y. Liu

The advantages of chorion villus sampling for prenatal diagnosis are becoming increasingly obvious and indicate that this is a technique which is here to stay. Furthermore, it is essentially a simple procedure and unlike fetoscopy which is best developed in specialized centres, chorion villus sampling should be well within the capability of all obstetricians. It is, however, slightly more intricate than amniocentesis and as with all new techniques certain preparation and training will be required. The following steps are considered essential to development of our clinical service and are presented here as possible guidelines for those intending to become similarly involved.

20.1 APPROACH

The first consideration is to determine which of all the various approaches for obtaining chorionic tissue is the most appealing. If chorion villus sampling is expected to replace the majority of amniocentesis tests, the approach chosen should be one which is comparable in terms of ready acceptance by patients, diagnostic reliability, economy in all aspects and ease in acquiring the necessary expertise. Obstetricians are familiar with the transcervical route to the uterine cavity hence the popularity of this approach in current practice. This approach is shown by us to be well accepted by patients and compared favourably with amniocentesis performed under similar conditions. When asked to indicate on a longitudinal scale between one and ten the degree of discomfort experienced during villus sampling, most patients selected a score of around three. Furthermore, upon recall patients remembered the episode as significantly less unpleasant (Tables 20.1 and 20.2).

A further advantage of the transcervical approach is the range of available techniques which can be entertained. The spectrum includes blind aspiration,

Table 20.1 The level of pain indicated on a linear scale between 1 and 10 by studied patients from each stage of the sampling procedure during and after the event

	Mean response immediately	*Mean response on recall*	*Mean difference*	*P*
Insertion of speculum	3.27 ± 2.3	2.5 ± 1.6	0.77 ± 1.59	<.001
Pelvic scan	1.11 ± 0.4	1.05 ± 0.3	0.06 ± 0.04	ns*
Insertion of cannula	1.98 ± 1.6	1.85 ± 1.5	0.13 ± 0.96	<0.05
Aspiration of trophoblast	1.76 ± 1.1	1.48 ± 0.8	0.28 ± 0.64	<0.002
Is the procedure painful	2.69 ± 1.6	2.26 ± 1.1	0.43 ± 0.90	<0.002

* Not significant.

Table 20.2 The level of pain indicated on a linear scale between 1 to 10 by studied patients from each stage of amniocentesis during and after the event

	Mean response during procedure	*Mean response on recall*	*P**
Insertion of needle	2.6 ± 1.9	2.6 ± 1.8	ns†
Aspiration of fluid	1.9 ± 1.5	1.9 ± 1.6	ns†
Pain	3.4 ± 2.8	3.2 ± 2.1	ns†

* Differences not significant using Wilcoxon signed rank sum test, n=25.
† Not significant.

which is simple and economical, and extends to ultrasound guided endoscopic directed sampling, which can be costly both in terms of time and expense. Though blind aspiration is practised successfully in China (Tietung Hospital, 1975) two independent studies found chorionic villi can only be obtained from a third of sampling attempts and thus is unlikely to attract much clinical application (Horwell *et al.*, 1983; Liu *et al.*, 1983).

Ultrasound examination is essential to determine the number of pregnancies, stage of gestation and to exclude abnormalities. Ultrasound machines are becoming increasingly more sophisticated. A portable version with a 3.5 or 5 mega-Hertz probe, which is adequate for villus sampling, is within financial reach of most obstetric departments. When ultrasound facility is available, it makes sense to employ scanning to identify and direct the implement safely to the appropriate sampling site. Whether linear array, convex or a sector probe is used can be a matter of individual preference. Investigators, however, would agree that the introduction of ultrasound significantly improved the rate of successful villus sampling and allows clinical application (Ward *et al.*, 1983; Simoni *et al.*, 1983). Though ultrasound guided transcervical chorion villus sampling commands current interest, the slight risk of introducing infection remains a valid consideration for all transcervical approaches and is the main reason why some investigators prefer a transabdominal approach (see relevant chapters).

20.2 IMPLEMENT

This is governed by the choice of approach which is selected. If ultrasound guided transcervical sampling with a disposable implement such as the Nottingham brush, a plastic cannula (Portex, England) or a malleable hollow metal tube is used, ready identification by sonar or high echogenicity is an obvious advantage. A limit of only two and at most three sampling attempts for adequate diagnostic material is suggested as ideal. Any need for repeated intervention invariably increases the risk of trauma and infection. The implement selected should satisfy these requirements. Understandably, personal preference will be a major determinant. An ideal sampling implement has not yet been identified. In the meantime, we have found it useful to use our own design (The Sampler) which incorporates many features of acknowledged value for the transcervical approach.

20.3 TRAINING

Patients who intend pregnancies to continue must not be used to develop expertise in chorion villus sampling. It is, therefore, necessary and logical to seek co-operation from patients requesting first trimester therapeutic abortions. Any research with the fetus is a sensitive issue. Ethical clearance must be obtained and both local and international guidelines (e.g. the Peel Report) should be stringently adhered to. All levels of medical staff likely to be associated with this category of patient should be fully informed of the purpose and aim of the additional intervention. Conscientious objectors to these procedures can then be re-deployed to mutual advantage. Discussion with our local hospital chaplaincy committee suggests no real reason why obstetricians who object to termination of pregnancies cannot train with this category of patients provided they do not carry out the therapeutic abortion. The following steps were adopted for recruitment of patients to participate in our training programmes.

1. We approached patients only after they have been accepted for therapeutic abortion. This avoids the question of coercion of patients to participate.
2. Only patients over 16 years of age, able to communicate and not unduly distressed were considered suitable. These issues are of particular importance when out-patient studies are conducted.
3. Participating patients were fully informed and provided notated consent.

Following the above guidelines over 90% of the 1000 patients we approached agreed to support our studies. Furthermore, many volunteered the pleasing comment that they would like to contribute to scientific advance rather than waste their pregnancies.

Expertise is best acquired in two stages. Sampling is easier when the patient is anaesthetized because she is relaxed and manipulations will not cause distress. An ideal training time is immediately before the anaesthetized patient has her pregnancy terminated in the operating theatre.

Obstetricians must become familiar with the use of ultrasound and appreciate the significance of the scan findings in the first trimester. Although it is perfectly feasible for the obstetrician to both scan and perform the sampling it is better when an assistant is there to help. The operator will then have both hands free and a trained assistant can immediately examine collected samples by phase-contrast microscopy and determine the quality of the sample. A second sampling attempt is then only necessary if inadequate diagnostic material is obtained.

A total of fifty patients has been suggested as a useful number to develop skills. It is, however, true that a we all learn at different rates. A definitive number of training sessions is not meaningful. A better criterion is to practise until the operator is assured of successful adequate sampling more than 90% of the time. When confidence and expertise is obtained with anaesthetized patients only then should the second stage of training with conscious patients begin. If 90% successful samplings is the training target to aim for, one rapidly appreciates that a training programme would involve over 200 patients. The learning curve for chorion villus sampling is undoubtedly longer than that for amniocentesis. Self-discipline at this stage of training is essential to protect the interests of clinical patients.

20.4 DEVELOPMENT OF SUPPORT SERVICES

Before a clinical service for chorion villus sampling can be offered the cytogenetic, genetic and biochemical departments must be encouraged to adapt their techniques with amniocytes to chorionic villi. Results from these departments' feasibility trials with the new material are important to the obstetrician who may need to select the most appropriate diagnostic technique. Some indication of the diagnostic capabilities from these departments is also required when clinical patients present for counselling.

Not all obstetric departments have access to all the above facilities in their hospital nor can it be expected that a single centre can command expertise in all recognized diseases which can be diagnosed prenatally. Chorionic villi, however, can be despatched by special post to departments with recognized expertise. If local facilities are lacking, provision should be made to ensure close liaison with centres offering the required services (see Chapter 21).

20.5 CLINICAL PATIENTS

Like amniocentesis, demand for chorion villus sampling will be principally for age related karyotyping. Less common inheritable diseases are usually referred to centres with special interests where counselling by clinical geneticists will be conducted to establish among other things the degree of inheritable risk. Patients seeking villus sampling for diagnosis of chromosome abnormalities must be afforded detailed counselling too. The obstetrician must examine with patients and their attendant partners the risk of inheritable problems, the incidence and type of risk of the diagnostic procedure, the failure rate from the laboratories and the risk compared with and need to resort to amniocentesis. The advantages of early diagnosis should be discussed. It is the prerogative of the informed patient to make the eventual choice.

True 'risk' of chorionic villus sampling will not be known for some time. It is not too difficult for patients to contemplate this diagnostic approach if the risk of inheritable disease is high or where amniocentesis is known to have certain limitations. Early diagnosis with chorionic villi and the prospect of easier resolution, or in the foreseeable future a prospect for therapy, more than outweighs any potential risk. The situation for age-related karyotyping is a different matter. The figure of about 0.5–2% interference risk for the fetus is generally accepted and is used for counselling when amniocentesis is discussed. The incidence of miscarriage in the first trimester is understood to be around 10%. Fetal loss is however not as high subsequent to ultrasound verification of normality (Christiaens and Stoutenbeek, 1984; Wilson *et al.*, 1984). Our own study also lends support to this fact. From the first trimester to 28th week the spontaneous miscarriage rate is between 2 and 3% after ultrasound confirmation of normality (Table 20.3). Currently fetal loss following chorion villus sampling is considered to be about 2% over and above the background spontaneous fetal loss rate. The miscarriage rate is higher for the older women and where there is a family history of inheritable disorders (Gustavii, 1984; Lauritsen, 1976). Furthermore, the quote of 0–2% interference fetal loss is calculated from results of the first ten thousand or so diagnostic samples by an international cohort of investigators who are still examining the technique (see Chapter 16). A figure similar to that for amniocentesis is a realistic anticipation. However, until this is achieved, counselling must be directed to provide patients with the choice between earlier diagnosis with possibly a higher risk to the fetus and the tried

Table 20.3 A prospective study of spontaneous miscarriage after ultrasound verification of gestational normality. Patients are followed from scan dates in the first trimester until 28 weeks.

Total patients studied	1068
Miscarried	
(a) total	29 (2.7%)
(b) within 16 weeks	16 (1.5%)
(c) 16–28 weeks	13 (1.25%)

amniocentesis at mid-trimester. Patients must also appreciate that amniocentesis is necessary if chorion villus sampling is not achieved or fails to provide the diagnosis.

The following routine adopted by us is presented as a guide for patients considering transcervical chorion villus sampling.

1. All patients are offered the opportunity for detailed counselling and discussion. This includes counselling by a clinical geneticist and obstetricians.
2. An ultrasound examination of the fetus is considered mandatory. Twin pregnancies and where abnormal fetal development is suspected will require alternative management.
3. The cervix is examined to exclude infections and appropriate swabs are taken for culture. This is best performed sometime before sampling is attempted.
4. The patient and her partner's blood groups are determined.
5. Sampling under ultrasound guidance is performed as an out-patient procedure. Patients are encouraged to maintain a full bladder. Sedatives are usually not prescribed.
6. If the situation is not suitable for sampling or if difficulty is encountered, further discussion with the patient is conducted. A later time or date is set for another attempt. We impose the realistic limit of conducting only two sampling attempts.
7. The fetus is re-scanned immediately after sampling to reassure both the patient and doctor. Where indicated, anti-D immunoglobin (50 μg) is given. Our own study suggests there was no alteration in the kleihauer count after sampling (Liu *et al.*, 1983). However, because the kleihauer test may not be sufficiently sensitive at this stage of pregnancy, we introduced serum alpha-fetoprotein (AFP) estimation as being possibly more reliable. Four per cent of samples evoke a rise in maternal serum levels of this protein. We have continued using maternal serum AFP as an indicator of the degree of fetal disturbance following sampling. Whether this procedure is useful remains to be seen.
8. Patients are discharged after the sample has been taken. They are advised to report all complications.
9. Provisions must be made for admission of patients into hospital when complications such as excessive bleeding are encountered. If perforation of the gestation sac occurs, patients must be retained in hospital to consider evacuation of the uterus. Formal admission is also required if the occasional sampling under general anaesthesia is required.
10. All relevant aspects of the sampling procedure must be fully documented. International guidelines are being formulated to obtain core data to facilitate continuous audit of this new technique. Patients' progress

throughout pregnancy will be followed. It is anticipated that a full paediatric assessment will be conducted when the child born after chorion villus sampling is 16 months of age.

11. Patients are instructed to retain aborted material for cytogenetic examination.

All indications suggest chorion villus sampling for prenatal diagnosis is welcomed and will become of increasing importance. Understandably, many more obstetricians will be attracted to this technique. A strict training protocol, correct patient management and adequate documentation will contribute to allow expression of the benefits of chorion villus sampling without the hindrance of iatrogenic bias. We hope the above discussion will promote this ethos.

REFERENCES

Christiaens, G. C. M. L. and Stoutenbeek, P. L. (1984) Spontaneous abortions in proven intact pregnancies. *Lancet*, i, 571–2.

Gustavii, B. (1984) Chorionic biopsy and miscarriage in first trimester. *Lancet*, i, 562.

Horwell, D. H., Loeffler, T. E. and Coleman, D. V. (1983) Assessment of a transcervical aspiration technique for chorionic villus biopsy in the first trimester of pregnancy. *Br. J. Obstet. Gynaecol.*, **90**, 196–8.

Lauritsen, J. G. (1976) Aetiology of spontaneous abortion. A cytogenetics and epidemiological study of 288 abortuses and their parents. *Acta Obstet. Gynecol. Scand.* Supplement 52, 3–29.

Liu, D. T. Y., Mitchell, J., Johnson, J. and Wass, D. M. (1983) Trophoblast biopsy by blind transcervical aspiration. *British Journal of Obstetrics and Gynaecology*, **90**, 1119–23.

Simoni, G., Brambati, B., Danesino, C., Rossella, F., Terzoli, G. L., Ferrari, M. and Fraccaro, M. (1983) Efficient direct chromosome analysis and enzyme determinations from chorionic villi samples in the first trimester of pregnancy. *Hum. Genet.*, **63**, 349–57.

Tietung Hospital, Department of Obstetrics (1975) Fetal sex predication by sex chromatin of chorionic villi cells during early pregnancy. *Chin. Med. J.*, **1**, 117–26.

Ward, R. H. T., Modell, B., Petrou, M., Karagozlu, F. and Douratsos, E. (1983) Method of sampling chorionic villi in first trimester of pregnancy under guidance of real-time ultrasound. *Br. Med. J.*, **286**, 1542–4.

Wilson, R. D., Kendrick, V., Wittmann, B. K. and McGillivray, B. C. (1984) Risk of spontaneous abortion in ultrasonically normal pregnancies. *Lancet*, **ii**, 920.

21

Chorion villus sampling for direct chromosomal analysis in a non-teaching hospital

—— *John W. Eddy* ——

The present method of diagnosing chromosomal abnormalities in pregnancy consists of amniocentesis at 16 weeks when desquamated fetal cells are obtained from the liquor and cultured; a chromosome analysis is possible on the cultured cells in 3–4 weeks. This is a well tried method with a low morbidity, the miscarriage rate in experienced hands being as low as 0.3%. The drawback is the gestational age at which it is done and the delay in producing a result. Patients diagnosed as having an abnormality are faced with a termination at 19–20 weeks when the pregnancy is obvious to all and the material mortality of termination may be as high as 0.26 per 1000 as compared to 0.01 per 1000 when performed before 12 weeks (Report on Confidential Enquiries into Maternal Death, 1982). There is also the emotional strain on the patient waiting for the result during the 3–4 weeks as well as the psychological trauma of the termination. Thus, collection of fetal material with chromosome analysis before 12 weeks would greatly reduce the physical as well as mental morbidity to the patient. The development of chorion villus sampling in the United Kingdom at centres like University College (UCH), Kings College Hospital (KCH) and Glasgow for the extraction of DNA for analysis using DNA markers demonstrated the possibility of obtaining early fetal tissue which could be the basis for a direct chromosome analysis and therefore an alternative test to amniocentesis.

In the United Kingdom in 1983 some 17 000 amniocenteses were performed for chromosome analysis (Dr L. Butler, personal communications) to exclude 'mongolism' (Down's syndrome) in patients over 37 years. Most of these were collected from non-teaching hospitals, the amniotic fluid being transported to the appropriate regional genetic laboratory for processing. If the majority of these 17 000 patients are to benefit from an earlier, quicker test like chorion villus sampling at 8–12 weeks, such a test must be practicable within the concept of the present amniocentesis service and be available within all district general hospitals.

In 1983, the author, in collaboration with Dr Leslie Butler, Director of Cytogenetic Services at Queen Elizabeth Hospital Hackney, set out to see if such a service was possible between Colchester, a district general hospital some 60 miles from London, and the Regional Laboratory in London.

21.2 COLLECTION OF VILLUS MATERIAL FROM ONGOING PREGNANCY

The techniques used were worked out by trial and error on patients undergoing therapeutic abortion and any unit considering this technique must practise on terminations prior to performing this test on ongoing pregnancies. Some fifty attempts were made to collect samples from terminations before an ongoing pregnancy was sampled. This is probably too small a number but patient demand resulted in earlier attempts in ongoing pregnancies than had originally been intended.

In theatre, under full sterile precautions, the patient with a full bladder is placed in the lithotomy position. No pre-medication is given, the abdomen is scanned and the gestational age is estimated and viability of the pregnancy confirmed. The cervix is grasped with a tenaculum and a malleable Portex cannula, 2 mm in diameter, is passed through the cervix under ultrasound guidance (it was not necessary to sound the endocervix). The cannulae are malleable so that they may be bent to reach anterior or posterior areas of placental thickening. Straight cannulae occasionally cause ultrasound artefact which suggest the tip may not be as far in as the ultrasound picture suggests, so bending the tip is recommended. Once the tip is in the centre of the placental mass the metal trocar is removed and a syringe attached.

Aspiration to 2–3 ml is applied and the cannula moved back and forward over 3–4 mm distance in a 'hovering' technique reminiscent of that described by Steen Smidt-Jenson (Chapter 14) in his transabdominal approach. With good ultrasound control tissue can be seen passing down the cannula and with experience the volume of tissue obtained can be estimated. The cannula is then removed, still under negative pressure, and emptied into tissue culture medium. Unlike the University College Hospital (London) method of Ward and Modell (1983) the aspirating syringe does not contain tissue culture medium so as to prevent accidental contamination of the uterine cavity. Ideally at this point, the sample is examined under a dissecting microscope to confirm the presence of villus material.

A simple, if less scientific method, is to hold the bottle of tissue culture medium containing possible villi, up to a spotlight and provided there is not a lot of blood present, villi will be visible to the naked eye as fine white frondular structures. If a reasonable amount of villi is present nothing further need be done but if little tissue is seen a second attempt to obtain villi is made. No more than two attempts were ever made on one day. Failure to obtain adequate tissue on two passes with the cannula meant the patient either opted for amniocentesis or returned in one week for a further attempt.

21.2 ULTRASOUND

For successful collection of villi material high quality ultrasound scanning is necessary. This means good equipment and trained personnel. In Colchester a number of machines have been tried, the best was the Picker 7000 but at £35 000 it is not available to every hospital. Its disadvantage was its potential vulnerability to frequent movement round the hospital from the ultrasound department to the operating theatre. A cheaper alternative was found in the Toshiba Sonylayer at £6000 which is well within any hospital budget. The other option is collecting the specimen in an ultrasound procedure room which unfortunately was not available to the author.

All the six ultrasound technicians in the district were trained in this scanning technique to avoid any problems of availability due to leave or illness.

The technique of scanning has already been described elsewhere in this book by Richardson and Liu (Chapter 11) but the main point which is worth emphasizing is that the tip of the cannula must be visible at all times; if not it is better to remove and re-insert rather than risk inadvertently puncturing the sac. However, this is not common as at 8–9 weeks the sac wall is very strong and can be pushed in by the cannula to meet the other wall without puncturing. In this series only one sac was punctured in the termination group and no ongoing pregnancy was perforated.

21.3 TRANSPORT

A number of culture media were used as transport media for the villi. The most successful was Hamms F10 with colchicine. The media has a refrigeration life of about four weeks in this district general hospital. It should be removed one hour before use to allow it to warm to room temperature. Once the villi have been collected the culture media bottle is packed in a plastic cocoon and placed in a padded bag which was sent via British Rail Red Star service to London arriving in the cytogenetic laboratory some three hours after collection. Experience showed that delays of up to six hours between collection and handling in the laboratory were acceptable but longer delays, especially overnight, resulted in a marked drop in viable cells for direct chromosome analysis. It would, therefore, appear that hospitals intending to use this technique need to arrange transport so that specimens are received and laboratory procedures started within the same working day as collection of the villi.

21.4 CHROMOSOME ANALYSIS

In this series it had been decided that direct chromosome analysis would be performed rather than culture of the tissue with secondary chromosome analysis hence the presence of colchicine in the transport media.

Chorionic villi undergo very active multiplication, if the outer cell layer of the villi is removed; the second and more actively dividing layer should contain numerous cells in metaphase. The technique is to isolate these cells and produce a chromosome photograph of them which allows chromosome analysis. The most successful method used on the latter samples was that described by Simoni *et al.*, 1983. As far as possible handling of the villus material was done within the normal work pattern of the laboratory so that results are available after approximately 48–72 hours.

The standard of chromosome analysis from the point of view of G-banding was not up to blood lymphocyte analysis where 800–1200 bands are possible, but it did compare favourably with culture from amniocentesis with 400 bands, which is quite adequate for the diagnostic reasons the test was performed.

Some centres have preferred to culture the villi before performing chromosome analysis. This takes about 11 days and is still quicker than following amniocentesis and produces slightly better results from the point of view of G-bands. The problem is that occasionally clones of abnormal cells may grow making accurate analysis difficult. The great advantage of the direct method, as well as its speed, is that the origin of the cells is obvious so that maternal contamination is virtually impossible.

21.5 RESULTS

21.5.1 First series: 34 cases performed prior to termination (see Table 21.1)

This was our first attempt at villi collection. A Diagnostic Sonar XL machine was used which was not up to the definition required and the scanners had difficulty locating the cannula tip, hence the poor rate of villi collection – 53%. The transport of the villi was in locally produced tissue culture media which we now feel was suspected as poor blood chromosome analysis was experienced at that time. When villi were present chromosome analysis was possible in 61%. Following collection of the samples, two attempts only being made, the pregnancy was immediately terminated. The products were collected for independent chromosome analysis which confirmed the results of the villus analysis.

Table 21.1 First series: direct process without preselection of villus material

Mass of tissue	*No. of samples*	*Villi present*	*Chromosome analysis*
<1 mg	7	1	zero
1–5 mg	11	5	2
5–10 mg	12	8	6
>10 mg	4	4	3
Total	34	18 (53%)	11 (32%)

The results, although disappointing, did show that the procedure was technically possible within the limits of a non-teaching hospital, 60 miles from the regional laboratory.

21.5.2 Second series: 15 cases

When the results of the first series were analysed, two main problems were obvious; the low collection rate of villus material (53%) and an even lower chromosome analysis rate.

Collection problems were somewhat improved by the use of a higher resolution ultrasound machine, i.e. the Toshiba Sonylayer portable scanner. Villus material was transported in Hamm F10 medium which contained colchicine and at the laboratory end, Queen Elizabeth Cytogenetic Laboratory perfected a modified version of Simoni's method of direct chromosome analysis.

Table 21.2 Second series: chorion villus sampling direct chromosome analysis

Weight	*Total samples*	*Valli present*	*Chromosome analysis*
<1 mg	3	zero	zero
1–5 mg	2	1	1
5–10 mg	3	2	2
>10 mg	7	6	6
Total	15	9 (60%)	9 (60%)

In this series the collection rate for villi had only slightly improved to 60% but the laboratory's ability to produce a chromosome analysis had improved to 100% of all samples with villi present.

From the laboratory point of view the main criteria was adequate villus material. When 10 mg of tissue was obtained, of which 35–50% by weight was villi, chromosome analysis was virtually assured: 5–10 mg will usually produce enough cells in metaphase for an accurate result: below 5 mg the number of cells on which analysis is possible often fell below the minimum number which was set at 20 cells per patient.

In both series described there were relatively low weights of tissue, the maximum obtained was 20 mg compared to Ward (1983) who relied on 20–45 mg of tissue for DNA extraction in his work on diagnosis of thalassaemia. This variation may be explained by the limit on the cases described here to two attempts only at obtaining villi and no immediate check of the tissue microscopically, which, while better from the laboratory point of view, may tempt the operator to persist in trying to obtain more tissue with a possible increase in the abortion rate. Fourteen of these 15 cases had normal chromosome counts and one was a Trisomy 21. This was confirmed on analysis of aborted material.

At this stage of the work the laboratory side was successful but collection was still the weak link. Further attempts at terminations were planned but word of the work leaked out and the first patient arrived demanding the test on an ongoing pregnancy. She had previously had two mid-trimester abortions for abnormalities and requested termination before 12 weeks unless the baby could be proved chromosomally normal.

21.6 CHORION VILLUS SAMPLING IN ONGOING PREGNANCIES

The start of the clinical series was by patient demand and was limited to those women who had previously had chromosomally abnormal babies. The Hospital Ethics Committee demanded that all patients sign a consent form and were counselled that the procedure was experimental and that the abortion rate was not known but the only large reported series, that of Brambati (1984), suggested a rate of 3.6% compared with that of amniocentesis which was 0.3%.

Patients were counselled and offered a choice of amniocentesis or chorion villus sampling. Those that elected CVS were asked to sign the consent form, after which an ultrasound scan were performed to confirm gestational age and viability of the pregnancy. A date was given for the test, usually the following week. On the day of the test the patients were instructed to arrive with a full bladder accompanied by someone who would take them home afterwards. No drugs were given and the sampling performed in theatre as already described. After the sampling the patients were returned to the ward for an hours' rest before being sent home with instructions to put their feet up for the rest of the day. Bleeding was common due to the vulsellum marks on the cervix. Weekly scans were done on all those who bled until there bleeding had ceased for two weeks.

Analysis of the chromosomes in the 76 successful attempts showed 70 to be normal and one to have a 45XX—13—14+t(13q:14q)+translocation. A blood chromosome analysis on both parents showed that the mother had a

Essex County Hospital, Colchester

Consent to Chorionic Sampling

I.................................of...................................

....

hereby consent to the procedure of chorionic sampling being performed upon me. I understand that this is a new technique and that only some 600 samplings have been performed worldwide. I understand that present information suggests a miscarriage rate from this procedure is about 3.5% as opposed to the miscarriage rate from amniocentesis which is 0.3%. I also understand that, if it proves impossible to get a result from this sample, then I may need an amniocentesis at a later date.

Signed..Date......................

I confirm that I have explained the above procedure to the patient as requested by the Hospital Ethics Committee.

Signed..Date.....................

Figure 21.1 Consent for chorion villus sampling.

Table 21.3 Ongoing pregnancy for villus sampling

Came to theatre for sampling	93	
Found to have non-viable pregnancy	8	(no sampling)
Fundal placenta 12 weeks	1	(no sampling)
Sampling attempted	84	

Table 21.4 Results of 84 sampling in ongoing pregnancies

Successful sampling:			
first attempt	70		
second attempt	6		
Failed 1st attempt: no further attempts		5	amniocentesis at 16 weeks
Failed 2nd attempt: no further attempts		3	amniocentesis at 16 weeks

Table 21.5 Outcome 84 attempted chorion villus sampling in ongoing pregnancy

Delivered	50
Aborted	5
Ongoing pregnancy	24
Terminations	5

Table 21.6 Chromosome results on 76 successful villus samplings

Normal chromosomes	70		
Abnormal chromosomes	6:	Balanced translocation	delivered
		Trisomy 21	TOP
		Trisomy 18	TOP
		Partial trisomy 5p	TOP
		Trisomy 5q	TOP
		Trisomy 5p	TOP

similar translocation, so that the advice was that the fetus should be normal and the pregnancy is still ongoing. Five other abnormal chromosome counts were found and terminations performed.

21.7 DISCUSSION

Even within such a small series as this certain problems have been highlighted in the use of CVS for chromosome analysis.

21.7.1 Counselling of the patient

Within the United Kingdom only some 40% of patients at risk from age-related 'mongolism' are screened; this varies from 22% in Strathclyde to 56% in the North East Thames Region. This variation is mainly due to delay in referral of the patient to hospital. With a problem like this at 16 weeks a much greater problem must occur with CVS when referral is necessary before 11 weeks. Colchester, because of its high uptake of (alpha-feto protein) screening at 16 weeks, manages to pick up 70% of the risk group from age-related 'mongolism' by 18 weeks but in spite of advertising about CVS to local general practitioners the incidence of booking before twelve weeks is still only 35%. Thus, counselling of patients pre-conceptually may be necessary if the majority at risk are going to present early enough for chorion villus sampling.

21.7.2 Miscarriage rate

The morbidity rate is primarily the miscarriage rate. The difficulty is calculating a true percentage. Natural wastage before 12 weeks may be as high as 10% but this is not actually known. Even in this small series eight patients' pregnancies became non-viable over a six-day period from the original scan to the day of the sampling, i.e. 8.6%. Following the CVS three patients aborted at 19 weeks, two following villus sampling, giving a rate of 6%. Heckt *et al.* (1984), obtained results from six centres covering a total of 240 pregnancies with an abortion rate of 12%. Brambati (1984) quotes a miscarriage rate of 3.6%. Even with these apparently high miscarriage rates many patients would be prepared to take the risk in order to obtain an earlier diagnosis. Considering the experience of amniocentesis, it is probable that the abortion rate is linked to the number of attempts at CVSs, hence our limitation to not more than two attempts on any one day.

The success of collecting villus samples in the ongoing pregnancy group was 85%, but of the eight failures, four occurred in the first eight cases with only one attempt being made suggesting that, as with amniocentesis, there is a learning curve which improves with experience.

21.7.3 Accuracy of results

In all the 49 termination cases and ten patients who have delivered the chromosome analysis was accurate. The chosen method, that of direct chromosome analysis, should make mistakes virtually impossible.

21.7.4 Patient acceptance

CVS in comparison with amniocentesis takes longer (about 10 minutes) and is slightly more uncomfortable, but the ten patients in this series who had previously had an amniocentesis said that the fear and anxiety they experienced before amniocentesis was much greater than that before CVS. Table 21.4 shows that only 70 patients had successful samplings on the first attempt. Fourteen failures occurred, the first four of these were left for amniocentesis but the fifth patient demanded a re-test as she feared a second mid-trimester termination. This was successful so that the remaining failures on first attempt were offered a second attempt one week later, none of which have so far aborted. Patient acceptance of the test, even with the rather off-putting counselling demanded by the Hospital Ethics Committee, was very high. So far, only three patients, when described the test, have opted for primary amniocentesis.

21.7.5 Cost

Any new test must be shown to be cost effective. From the laboratory side direct chromosome analysis of chorionic villi costs £30 per sample compared with £60 for amniocentesis because there is no culturing stage. Collection and transport cost depends on whether the sampling is done in the operating theatre or ultrasound department, the cost being £88.50 and £35.00 respectively compared to amniocentesis in the ultrasound department, which costs £29. There would therefore be no economic reason to advocate amniocentesis as opposed to CVS.

The series described has been relatively small but does show that chorion villus sampling is practicable with the limited facilities of a district general hospital provided the specimen can be transported to the laboratory within six hours. Patient acceptance and enthusiasm for this method of chromosome analysis has been high and primarily responsible for pushing the pace of the work in the series described which will probably mean that attempts at a controlled prospective trial of CVS verses amniocentesis will be impossible to organize.

REFERENCES

Brambati, B. (1984) Figures to April, 1984; 221 continuing pregnancies, 8 losses, 70 delivered, percentage loss 3.6% as given to L. Jackson for Medical Research Council Meeting, 4 July, 1984.

Hecht, F., Heckt, B. K. and Bixenman, H. A. (1984) Caution about chorionic villus sampling, in the first trimester. *New Engl. J. Med.*, **310**, 1388.

Report on Confidential Enquiries into Maternal Death in England and Wales, 1976–1978. (1982) HMSO, London.

Simoni, G., Brambati, B., Danesino, C., Rosella, F., Terzoli, G. L., Ferrari, M. and Fraccaro, M. (1983) Efficient direct chromome analysis and enzyme determinations from chorionic villi samples in the first trimester of pregnancy. *Hum. Genet.*, **63**, 349–57.

Ward, R. H. T., Modell, B., Petrov, *et al.* (1983) Method of sampling chorionic villi in first trimester of pregnancy under guidance of real time ultrasound. *Br. Med. J.*, **286**, 1542–4.

22

The economic efficiency of prenatal screening

—— *John B. Henderson* ——

22.1 THE ECONOMIC EFFICIENCY OF PRENATAL SCREENING

It is increasingly being recognized that in order to make the best use of available resources economic efficiency must be considered in deciding whether or not, and to what extent, particular health care services should be provided. Economic efficiency simply means (a) maximizing the health and welfare produced from any given health care budget; (b) minimizing the cost of providing any given health care service; and (c) maximizing the excess of benefit over cost – where cost is defined as the loss of those benefits that the resources consumed would have produced in their next best alternative use. Cost-effectiveness analysis is used to help attain objectives (a) and (b) and cost-benefit analysis to help attain objective (c) (Sugden and Williams, 1978; Drummond, 1980; Drummond and Mooney, 1982).

While the principles of economic efficiency are clearly defined, putting them into practice is by no means straightforward – especially in the context of prenatal screening (Chamberlain, 1984; Henderson, 1985). Problems arise at several levels. For example there are problems of lack of information because certain relevant aspects, such as many of the costs borne by families, have not yet been studied. There are other problems associated with the methodology, for example those of measuring qualitative aspects of screening. Then there are problems of value judgements, whose resolution is not the professional job of economists (or, for that matter, of doctors either) such as deciding the weights to be attached to particular ethical viewpoints. (For example, to what extent should the views of those opposed to abortion affect the options open to those who desire prenatal diagnosis and abortion of a fetus with chromosomal or genetic anomaly?) Nevertheless, various studies have tried to evaluate the economic efficiency of prenatal screening. Their implications for the efficiency of chorion villus sampling are examined below.

22.2 COST-BENEFIT ANALYSIS

Cost-benefit analysis attempts to show whether the benefits of a programme exceed its costs. In this case the question to be posed is whether or not to provide a prenatal diagnostic service, using chorion villus sampling (CVS), for chromosomal and genetic anomalies. The first stage in analysing the costs and benefits of such a service is to identify all its costs and benefits over and above those of doing nothing. Table 22.1 lists the costs and benefits that ideally should be included in the evaluation. These are classified into tangible and intangible – material resource effects, and psychological and other effects – and into direct and indirect – effects arising through diagnosis and possible termination of the index pregnancy, and effects arising through the parents' 'replacement' of a terminated pregnancy.

The direct tangible costs and benefits are the easiest to study. Down's syndrome is the commonest chromosomal/genetic anomaly (Galjaard, 1978) and there have been several cost-benefit analyses of screening, using amniocentesis, for this condition. These have concluded that the total direct tangible benefits exceed the total direct tangible costs: if women aged 40 and over are screened (Glass, 1975, in the United Kingdom); if women aged 35 and over are screened (Hagard and Carter, 1976, in the west of Scotland; and Mikkelsen *et al.*, 1978, Denmark: public expenditure effects only); if women aged 36 and over are screened (Passarge, 1978, Federal Republic of Germany); if women aged 32 and over are screened (Andreano and McCollum, 1983, United States); and if women aged 38 and over are screened (Gardent *et al.* 1984a and 1984b, France).

In terms of the evaluation of the direct tangible benefits of screening these studies are incomplete in that they have not estimated the benefits of diagnosing conditions other than Down's syndrome (except for Andreano and McCollum, 1983, who included the benefits of diagnosing spina bifida, which would not, however, be possible with CVS). Down's syndrome represents no more than 25% of detectable chromosomal anomalies at maternal age 35 (Ferguson-Smith and Yates, 1984), although this rises to 80% at maternal age 46. A more complete evaluation would attempt to include the costs and benefits of detecting these other chromosomal anomalies (also taking into account the fact that many of these would have led to spontaneous abortion in the absence of a screening programme).

Another of the direct tangible effects that could have been more thoroughly evaluated is the costs falling on the families. The time taken to attend for diagnosis has been included in some studies along with the associated cost in terms of loss of the work (paid or unpaid) that would have been performed

Table 22.1 Classification of costs and benefits of prenatal screening

	Costs	*Benefits*
Direct tangible	1.1 Organization of primary health care services to identify women at high risk and inform them about prenatal diagnosis at an early stage of pregnancy. 1.2 Health service costs of diagnostic procedure. 1.3 Laboratory analysis of sample. 1.4 Woman's diagnosis attendance travel costs and opportunity cost of time. 1.5 Possible repeated costs of 1.2–1.4. 1.6 Health service costs of terminating pregnancy. 1.7 Woman's abortion attendance travel costs and opportunity cost of time. 1.8 Counselling after abortion.	Positive test result and termination of pregnancy leading to avoided: 2.1 Health services expenditure. 2.2 Education services expenditure. 2.3 Other public services expenditure. 2.4 Lost maternal output through rearing child. 2.5 Family expenditure on child. 2.6 Child's lifetime consumption of other goods and services net of lifetime output produced.
Direct intangible	3.1 Anxiety aroused through being informed of high risk 3.2 Discomfort of diagnostic procedure. 3.3 Anxiety before test result received. 3.4 Distress after miscarriage thought to be caused by diagnostic procedure. 3.5 Possible fetal damage caused by diagnostic procedure. 3.6 Abortion of non-handicapped fetus owing to false positive test result. 3.7 Possible complications for woman. 3.8 False reassurance and possible harm to relationship with child owing to false negative test result.	4.1 Avoided distress to parents (and others) of having handicapped child owing to positive test result and termination of pregnancy. 4.2 Reassurance to parents owing to true negative test result.
Indirect tangible	Replacement conception leading to: 5.1 Possible costs as at 1.1–1.8 above. Replacement birth leading to: 5.2 Health services expenditure. 5.3 Education services expenditure. 5.4 Other public services expenditure. 5.5 Lost maternal output through rearing child. 5.6 Family expenditure on child. 5.7 Child's lifetime consumption of other goods and services. 5.8 If replacement child is handicapped, but not aborted, then costs as at 2.1–2.6 above.	Replacement birth leading to: 6.1 Lifetime output produced.
Indirect intangible	Replacement conception leading to: 7.1 Possible costs as at 3.2–3.8 above.	Replacement conception leading to: 8.1 Possible benefits as at 4.1–4.2 above. Replacement birth leading to: 8.2 Joy, happiness, etc. to parents.

during this time – a cost that may be large when aggregated over a large number of women. However, little is known about the impact that a handicapped child has on the mother's propensity to go out to work. Hagard, Carter and Milne (1976) assumed that 70% of those mothers who would otherwise have been in paid employment would be prevented from doing so because of a handicapped child, an assumption followed by Henderson (1982), and Andreano and McCollum (1983). Hard evidence is difficult to come by. Piachaud *et al.* (1981), using data from the 1974 General Household Survey, compared the labour force participation rates of mothers of handicapped children with those of the mothers of non-handicapped children and found little difference. Gath (1978), in a controlled prospective study of 30 families with a Down's syndrome child, found that the mothers of such children went out to work no less often than the mothers of the control children, although the families had only been followed for a couple of years, which may not have been long enough for differences to have emerged. However, Baldwin (1985), using data from a family expenditure survey administered to applicants to the Family Fund (Bradshaw and Lawton, 1985), found that mothers of handicapped children engaged in paid employment less often than the mothers of non-handicapped children, and that the difference increased with the age of the child. The cost of the mother's lost output through being unable to work because of a handicapped child has been a major part of the total cost in those studies that have included it. Further research on this could make a considerable improvement to the accuracy of cost-benefit comparisons of the resource effects of screening.

It is not yet clear whether the direct tangible costs to the health service of prenatal diagnosis using CVS will be greater or less than those of using amniocentesis. More work is likely to be involved on the part of the primary health care service to get women to come for diagnosis at an early enough stage for CVS. Many centres use a larger team for the CVS diagnostic procedure. More laboratory work could be involved if the chorion villus sample is cultured, but perhaps less if the sample is analysed directly. However, failure to obtain a diagnosis may be more frequent with direct analysis leading to more false negative results and thus more handicapped children.

The direct intangible costs and benefits have not been measured, although some studies have attempted to identify them, as in parts 3, 4, 7, and 8 of Table 22.1 (Chamberlain, 1978; Gath, 1978; Gibson, 1978; Donnai *et al.*, 1981; and Muir Gray, 1984). Clearly the intangible aspects could be crucial in determining the acceptability of CVS. It would be helpful if those ratings of the quality of life that have already been developed could be adapted to try to measure these qualitative aspects of prenatal screening (Torrance, 1986).

The indirect costs and benefits are those that arise from the parents' response to therapeutic abortion. If a prenatal screening programme is available, it seems likely that they will try to 'replace' a terminated pregnancy, whereas in the absence of a screening programme fertility rates may be lower, particularly among those who perceive themselves to be at high risk of producing handicapped children (Morris and Laurence, 1976; Modell *et al.*, 1980). Thus there may be children conceived and born in the presence of a screening programme who otherwise would not be. The replacement rate – i.e. family size with a screening programme over family size without – could be between 0% and 100% or even higher than 100%, but since it has not been studied directly it is not known with any accuracy. Hagard and Carter (1976) attempted to include the effects of replacement, but did not allow for the delay of replacement (which becomes relevant when discounting future costs and benefits to their present values), the greater life expectancy of the non-handicapped replacement children, or the possibility of replacement rates higher than 100%. Replacement has been shown to have a potentially large impact on the total tangible costs and benefits of prenatal screening (Henderson, 1982) and deserves further study.

There have been cost-benefit analyses of prenatal screening for conditions other than Down's syndrome. Attanasio *et al.* (1980) examined the costs and benefits of screening for thalassaemia major, on Sardinia, for women at high risk and concluded that the direct tangible benefits exceeded the direct tangible costs. Nelson *et al.* (1978) and Dagenais *et al.* (1985) examined the costs and benefits of screening for Tay–Sachs disease, in Houston and Quebec respectively, for women at high risk and concluded that the direct tangible benefits exceeded the direct tangible costs.

The general conclusion that emerges from these studies is that screening offered to high risk groups is likely to produce a net saving in direct resource consumption. However, this is not the same as showing that the sum of the benefits exceeds the sum of the costs. To do so would mean including in addition the indirect and intangible aspects.

22.3 COST-EFFECTIVENESS ANALYSIS

Cost-effectiveness analysis attempts to show which of two or more options produces the greatest benefits from a given budget, or which provides a given level of output at least cost. One obvious alternative to CVS is amniocentesis and there are currently underway randomized controlled trials to determine their comparative effectiveness and safety (Modell, 1985). Conclusions on the cost-effectiveness of CVS as compared with amniocentesis will have to await their outcome. However trials also present appropriate opportunities to evaluate the efficiency of techniques such as CVS before, rather than after, they become established health service procedures (Mugford *et al.*, 1985).

There are several options that could be evaluated in a cost-effectiveness analysis of CVS versus amniocentesis, including the alternatives of direct analysis of chorion villus samples and/or analysis of cultured samples, and of different sizes of sampling procedure team. The sensitivity and specificity of the techniques could have important impacts on the costs. For example, if one detected only half as many anomalies as the other then even if the procedure costs were the same the cost per case detected by the former would be twice that of the latter. If one produced more false negative results than the other then it would also lead to more handicapped children being born and thus would have higher total costs. The earlier abortion allowed by CVS screening could well be less expensive to the health service (Catford and Fowkes, 1979) but whether this will be important to the total costs will depend on its frequency as well as its magnitude.

The most important difference between the two techniques might be the difference in intangible costs to the women. They may have strong preferences for the earlier diagnosis, the quicker results and the safer and much less unpleasant abortion that are possible with CVS. Ideally these preferences should be measured.

22.4 THE FUTURE

New technical developments will continue to arise which will require evaluation. It is likely that there will soon be available gene probes that will allow the accurate prenatal diagnosis of such conditions as Duchenne muscular dystrophy, Huntington's chorea, X-linked mental retardation and other gene defects. Economic evaluations would help to show whether offering screening for these conditions would yield positive net benefits. Once the high risk groups have been identified and counselled it is likely that the tangible benefits of offering prenatal diagnosis will exceed the costs, but comprehensive identification and effective counselling may have high resource costs. A general screen for several different conditions, if it became feasible, might reduce the costs (both tangible and intangible) per case detected and make it worthwhile offering prenatal diagnosis more widely.

Another development may be improvements in the comprehensiveness of the evaluations, particularly if the adoption of measures of 'quality adjusted life years' (QALYs) can be more widely promoted. Bush *et al.* (1973, New York State) measured the benefits of neonatal diagnosis of phenylketonuria in terms of QALYs gained. Prenatal diagnosis at present does not enable the QALYs of the fetus to be improved (although gene therapy for anomalies is a possibility at some future date). However it would now be appropriate to measure the benefits to the parents in terms of QALYs gained (Torrance, 1986).

22.5 CONCLUSIONS

Economic appraisal attempts to measure and compare the gains and losses to society arising from the provision of various programmes. Clearly this can be both relevant and helpful for devising effective health care policy, and is essential if the best uses are to be made of scarce resources for health care. Further research is needed to produce evidence to demonstrate that the intangible benefits of prenatal diagnosis are greater than the intangible costs, that the indirect benefits are greater than the indirect costs, and that CVS is more cost-effective than amniocentesis. However, if screening using CVS is offered to high risk groups – older women for the risk of chromosomal anomalies, and those who are known to have, or are likely to have, carrier status for gene defects – then the studies that have been undertaken to date seem to indicate that the direct tangible benefits would probably outweigh the direct tangible costs.

REFERENCES

Andreano, R. L. and McCollum, D. W. (1983) A Benefit-Cost Analysis of Amniocentesis. *Soc. Biol.*, 30(4), 347–73.

Attanasio, E., Galanello, R. and Rossi-Mori, A. (1980) Analisi Costi-Benefici di un Intervento Preventivo per la Talassemia. Estratto dal volume *La Prevenzione Delle Malattie Microcitemiche*, VI Congresso Internazionale dell'Associazione Nazionale per la lotta contro le microcitemie in Italia (Roma, 17–19 Aprile 1980).

Baldwin, S. (1985) *The Costs of Caring: Families with Disabled Children*, Routledge and Kegan Paul, London.

Bradshaw, J. and Lawton, D. (1985) 75,000 Severely Disabled Children. *Devel. Med. Child Neurol.*, 27, 25–32.

Bush, J. W., Chen, M. M. and Patrick, D. L. (1973) Health Status Index in Cost Effectiveness: Analysis of PKU Program. In *Health Status Indexes* (ed. R. L. Berg), Hospital Research and Education Trust, Chicago, pp. 172–94.

Catford, J. C. and Fowkes, F. G. R. (1979) Economic Benefits of Day Care Abortion. *Community Medicine*, 1, 115–22.

Chamberlain, J. (1978) Human Benefits and Costs of a National Screening Programme for Neural-Tube Defects. *Lancet*, ii, 1293–6.

Chamberlain, J. (1984) Which Prescriptive Screening Programmes are Worthwhile? *J. Epidem. Comm. Health*, 38, 270–7.

Dagenais, D. L., Courville, L. and Dagenais, M. G. (1985) A Cost-Benefit Analysis of the Quebec Network of Genetic Medicine. *Soc. Sci. Med.*, 20(6), 601–7.

Donnai, P., Charles, N. and Harris, R. (1981) Attitudes of Patients after 'Genetic' Termination of Pregnancy. *Brit. Med. J.*, 282, 621–2.

Drummond, M. F. (1980) *Principles of Economic Appraisal in Health Care*, Oxford University Press, Oxford.

Drummond, M. F. and Mooney, G. H. (1982) Essentials of Health Economics: V – Assessing the Costs and Benefits of Treatment Alternatives. *Brit. Med. J.*, 285, 1561–3.

Ferguson-Smith, M. A. and Yates, J. R. W. (1984) Maternal Age Specific Rates for

Chromosome Aberrations and Factors Influencing Them. Report of a Collaborative Study on 52,965 Amniocenteses. *Prenatal Diagnosis*, **4**, 5–44.

Galjaard, H. (1978) Early Diagnosis and Prevention of Genetic Disease: Molecules and the Obstetrician. In *Towards the Prevention of Fetal Malformation* (ed. J. B. Scrimgeour), Edinburgh University Press.

Gardent, H., Goujard, J., Fardeau, M. and Crost, M. (1984a) Analyse economique de la diffusion d'une innovation medicale: l'exemple du diagnostic prenatal par amniocentese precoce. 1re partie: les fondements epidemiologiques, medicaux et socio-economiques. La diffusion d'une innovation diagnostique. *Rev. Epidem. et Sante Publ.*, **32**, 88–96.

Gardent, H., Fardeau, M., Lanoe, J-L. and Kerleau, M. (1984b) Analyse economique de la diffusion d'une innovation medicale: l'exemple du diagnostic prenatal par amniocentese precoce. 2e partie: l'aide a la decision en Sante publique pour la diffusion optimale d'une innovation. *Rev. Epidem. et Sante Publ.*, **32**, 97–106.

Gath, A. (1978) *Down's Syndrome and the Family: the Early Years*, Academic Press, London.

Gibson, D. (1978) *Down's Syndrome: the Psychology of Mongolism*, Cambridge University Press.

Glass, N. (1975) Economic Aspects of the Prevention of Down's Syndrome (Mongolism). In *Systems Aspects of Health Planning* (eds N. T. J. Bailey and M. Thompson), North-Holland, Amsterdam.

Hagard, S. and Carter, F. A. (1976) Preventing the Birth of Infants with Down's Syndrome: A Cost-Benefit Analysis. *Brit. Med. J.*, i, 753–6.

Hagard, S., Carter, F. A. and Milne, R. G. (1976) Screening for Spina Bifida Cystica: A Cost-Benefit Analysis. *Brit. J. Prev. Soc. Med.*, 30, 40–53.

Henderson, J. B. (1982) An Economic Appraisal of the Benefits of Screening for Open Spina Bifida. *Soc. Sci. Med.*, **16**, 545–60.

Henderson, J. B. (1985) Appraisal of Screening Programmes. In *Health Economics Bulletin* (4), HERU, University of Aberdeen, Aberdeen.

Mikkelsen, M., Nielsen, G. and Rasmussen, E. (1978) Cost-Effectiveness of Antenatal Screening for Chromosome Abnormalities. In *Towards the Prevention of Fetal Malformation* (ed. J. B. Scrimgeour) Edinburgh University Press.

Modell, B. (1985) Chorionic Villus Sampling: Evaluating Safety and Efficacy. *Lancet*, i, 737–40.

Modell, B., Ward, R. H. T. and Fairweather, D. V. I. (1980) Effect of Introducing Antenatal Diagnosis on Reproductive Behaviour of Families at Risk of Thalassaemia Major. *Brit. Med. J.*, **280**, 1347–50.

Morris, J. and Laurence, K. M. (1976) The Effectiveness of Genetic Counselling for Neural-Tube Malformations. *Devel. Med. Child Neurol.*, **18** (Suppl. 37), 157–63.

Mugford, M., Drummond, M. F., Henderson, J. and Mooney, G. H. (1985) Chorionic Villus Sampling. *Lancet*, ii, 384–5.

Muir Gray, J. A. (1984) Needs of the Community. In *Antenatal and Neonatal Screening* (ed. N. J. Wald), Oxford University Press.

Nelson, W. B., Swint, J. M. and Caskey, C. T. (1978) An Economic Evaluation of a Genetic Screening Program for Tay–Sachs Disease. *Am. J. Hum. Genet.*, 30, 160–6.

Passarge, E. (1978) Screening Populations for Genetic Disease. In *Towards the Prevention of Fetal Malformation* (ed. J. B. Scrimgeour), Edinburgh University Press.

Piachaud, D., Bradshaw, J. and Weale, J. (1981) The Income Effect of a Disabled Child. *J. Epidem. Comm. Health*, **35**, 123–7.

Sugden, R. and Williams, A. (1978) *The Principles of Practical Cost-Benefit Analysis*. Oxford University Press.

Torrance, G. (1986) Measurement of Health State Utilities for Economic Appraisal. *J. Health Economics*, 5, 1–30.

Section IV

CHROMOSOMES AND DNA ANALYSIS

23

Prenatal karyotyping: amniotic fluid cells or chorion villus samples?

—— *Christine Gosden* ——

23.1 INTRODUCTION

If prenatal diagnosis is to have any impact in reducing the births of children who have major handicaps due to chromosome disorders, then effective methods for the detection of cytogenetic abnormalities in the fetus must be developed which are acceptable to the pregnant population. Such methods must detect clinically significant chromosome disorders with a high degree of efficiency, reliability and accuracy and distinguish these disorders from those abnormalities which have no significance for the fetus.

The experience of prenatal karyotyping to date has been disappointing. Only a small proportion of the pregnant population is recognized as being at risk for chromosome abnormalities such as Down's syndrome and even among those groups recognized as being at risk, such as older mothers, the uptake rates have been very low. The advent of new sampling methods such as chorion villus sampling (CVS) and other new techniques for fetal assessment may have much greater advantages and be much more acceptable for those currently eligible for prenatal testing and pave the way towards effective cytogenetic screening.

There are, however, a number of reasons for concern about chorion villus sampling. The risk of miscarriage is one of the principal issues, as it may ultimately affect the choice of procedure for any woman requesting prenatal diagnosis. Obviously one of the major aims of a randomized trial of chorionic villus sampling is to attempt to estimate the increased risk of miscarriage due to the method. There are a very large number of possible reasons for a miscarriage occurring (Lauritson, 1976). The geneticist, must undertake investigations to probe into possible causes. At what gestation did the miscarriage occur, and how is evidence of the developmental, genetic and cytogenetic anomalies of the fetus and placenta best studied? Even a superficial investigation in each case would increase the workload associated with CVS quite substantially.

It is known that the frequency of chromosome abnormalities is very high at conception, but it falls throughout pregnancy because of loss through spontaneous abortion of chromosomally abnormal embryos and fetuses. This means that there will be substantially more chromosomally abnormal fetuses in the first trimester than in the second, particularly for older mothers, and the types of abnormality pose different problems for first-trimester diagnosis.

The spectre of diagnostic error always looms large in prenatal diagnosis. Fears that prenatal karyotyping from CVS is less sensitive and less specific than that from amniocentesis and amniotic fluid (AF) cell culture, have been expressed (Feeny *et al.*, 1985). The major concerns are not just those of maternal contamination and mosaicism in culture, but also other factors which might influence diagnostic accuracy. It has been suggested (Kalousek and Dill, 1983) that certain types of chromosome mosaicism might be confined to the placenta, and this would clearly compromise diagnostic accuracy in CVS where only trophoblast is being sampled.

The risk of maternal or fetal infection due to the sampling procedure is of great concern because of the possible complications for the mother and her fetus. The presence of potentially pathogenic micro-organisms may also compromise the laboratory part of the diagnosis, particularly if the villi have to be cultured, both because of the risk of culture loss through contamination or *in vitro* changes induced by high antibiotic concentrations in the culture medium. For CVS, antibiotic concentrations tend to be higher and include more exotic agents than are used in AF cell culture (where the risk of infection is less).

The range of cytogenetic and genetic conditions for which prenatal diagnosis can be carried out is increasing very rapidly. For example, fragile X-linked mental retardation and certain chromosome instability syndromes can now be detected prenatally, but only using specialized culture techniques and conditions. With a widening of the range of conditions amenable to prenatal diagnosis, it is crucial to compare those which are at present only possible after later second-trimester sampling with those which can be carried out in the first trimester.

The potential advantages for the patient for first-trimester diagnosis either in providing reassurance that certain abnormalities can be excluded, or of offering earlier termination if this is necessary, are obvious. What is rather less clear are the potential problems, pitfalls and restrictions of first trimester karyotyping when compared with that in the second trimester. The purpose of this paper is to try and examine these issues in more detail.

23.2 ORIGINS OF CELLS AND CELL TYPES

Any diagnostic system will have advantages and drawbacks according to the material upon which the investigations are carried out. Both amniotic fluid cells and chorionic villi are unusual tissues for study if the desire is to gain information about the fetus. Amniotic fluid cells might be considered effete fetal cells discarded by the fetus into liquor which will eventually be lost. Chorionic villus cells come from extra-embryonic cells which are of a cell lineage which diverged from the fetus proper very early in embryonic development (probably at or before the 64 cell stage). Extra placentae villi are destined to degenerate once the implantation site and placenta are established or, for placental villi, these will form the placenta programmed to last only the short duration of the pregnancy.

Both these tissues may seem relatively unprepossessing as predictors of the future human being, but their major advantages are in the relatively non-invasive procedures for the fetus by which they can be obtained.

23.2.1 Amniotic fluid (AF) cells

Uncultured amniotic fluid cells are usually classified according to the epithelia from which they originate – fetal periderm or epidermis, amnion, trophoblast and mucosae of respiratory, digestive and urogenital tracts. When sampling is carried out in a normal pregnancy, then only those cell surfaces which are in contact and can exfoliate cells into the amniotic fluid will be represented in the amniotic fluid cell population. If, however, the fetus has a structural abnormality, then other cells may be contributed into the amniotic fluid. For example, neural tube defect cells in anencephaly and spina bifida, peritoneal cells in exomphalos and gastroschisis and trophoblastic cells from the placenta if the integrity of the amnion is compromised (Gosden, 1983).

In the second trimester, only a small proportion of the total cells (usually less than 20%) are viable. Since cells in the uncultured amniotic fluid are very rarely dividing, these cells cannot be used for karyotyping. It is thus necessary to grow AF cells in culture in order to obtain mitotic figures for cytogenetic studies.

Those cells which proliferate in AF cell culture represent only a very few original cells from the relatively small proportion of viable cells in the original sample. Three major cultured cell types have been described (although this classification is by no means universally accepted, see Gosden, 1983). About 70% of cells are described as 'amniotic fluid cells' (AF cells). These are probably derived from fetal membrane and trophoblast as, in addition to their characteristic morphology, they synthesize hormone chorionic gonadotrophin (HCG) and have type IV-like procollagen. The second most predominant cell type (20%) is the epithelioid cell (EC). These are squames, probably derived from fetal skin and bladder. They form desmosomal complexes, but do not produce HCG. The third and rarest cell type (10%) the 'fibroblastic cell' (FC) has the greatest cloning efficiency and these cells may be derived from fibrous connective tissue and dermal fibroblasts.

23.2.2 Chorionic villus cells

Much less is known about different cell types in chorionic villi than is known about amniotic fluid (AF) cells and, in particular, knowledge about properties of cultured chorionic villus cells is very limited. Although the basic structure of the villous stems and their branches at both light microscope and EM level is well characterized, the origin of the mitotic cells for both direct chromosome preparations and cultured villus preparations is rather contentious. Unfortunately, using current preparation methods for metaphase spreads, chromosomes can only be seen if the cell membrane and cytoplasm are destroyed, which effectively limits the information about the cell types from which the dividing cells were derived. Although it is known that cells in the chorionic villi produce human chorionic gonadotrophin (HCG), human placental lactogen (HPL), various progestogens and other substances and that a number of specialized cell types are present, such as macrophages, fibroblasts, Hofbauer cells, endothelial cells lining the blood vessels and collagen producing cells, associations between morphological type, origin and function are not well characterized.

The basic structure of a chorionic villus stem is of a central mesenchymal core in which the ground matrix is predominantly of collagen fibres containing a number of morphologically different cell types. The core is surrounded by a basement membrane resting upon which is a single layer of trophoblastic (Langhans) cells. The outermost layer is of syncytiotrophoblast, consisting of pyknotic nuclei, vacuoles, fat droplets, vesicles and inclusions and this has irregular microvilli on the external surface. The syncytiotrophoblastic layer consists only of free nuclei without individual cell walls, so these do not divide. It is thus clear that *in vitro* culture of cells from chorionic villi will only yield possible growth of cells from the cytotrophoblast and mesenchyme. The relative growth and proliferative properties of the different cells types are not yet well understood.

23.3 METHODS AND SPECIALIZED CYTOGENETIC TECHNIQUES

The range of genetic and cytogenetic conditions for which prenatal diagnosis can now be carried out is increasing rapidly. Among these conditions are the fragile X syndrome, chromosome instability syndromes, such as Fanconi's anaemia, Bloom's syndrome and Cockayne's syndrome and small chromosomal deletions associated with major genetic conditions such as aniridia-Wilms' tumour, Prader–Willi syndrome and retinoblastoma. Can the same range of conditions be encompassed by CVS as for AF cell culture? In addition to asking about those diagnostic tests which can be applied in the first or second trimesters it is also important to question whether prenatal diagnosis for conditions such as these should only be applied where there is relevant family history. For example, the fragile X syndrome which leads to mental handicap in males, may have a frequency as high as 1.8 per 1000 new-born males and where 40% of cases may be the result of new mutations (Sherman *et al.*, 1984). In such cases, a large number of affected infants will be born to women with no previous history. It then becomes important to debate whether the frequency and severity of the conditions involved, and the cost effectiveness, would merit screening programmes.

23.3.1 Direct or cultured preparations

Methods for chromosome preparations from chorion have already been covered in this volume. Direct preparations have tremendous advantages in that results can be given to the patient relatively quickly after sampling and the time, effort and dangers of culture infection and failure are reduced. However, at present, detailed cytogenetic studies prove more difficult on direct preparations than after culture. Fragile X analysis on direct preparations has been described by Brambati *et al.* (1985), but Tomerrup *et al.* (1985) found it necessary not only to culture villi but also to add methotrexate as a folate antagonist.

For detailed high resolution banding studies, cell synchronization is necessary. In amniotic fluid cells, the mixed cell populations have different cell cycle times and are relatively refractory to such techniques. For chorionic villus cells where maternal contamination and increasing polyploidy with time in culture can be major problems, synchronization, exposure to special compounds or other techniques tend to be much more difficult than those for AF cells.

23.3.2 Fragile X

The fragile X syndrome is an X-linked genetic condition in which mental handicap is associated with a fragile site at the distal end of the long arm of the X chromosome at Xq28, and is second only to Down's syndrome in its contribution to genetic mental handicap. Affected males have the fragile X in 2–50% of their cells and obligate carrier females in a lower proportion of cells. There is a danger of false negative results which is probably greater for CVS than AF cells, and thus for more definitive diagnosis it is felt that fetal blood sampling may be carried out in those pregnancies where there is a male fetus at risk for fragile X (Webb *et al.*, 1983). At present chorion presents more problems than AF cell culture because recognition of fragile X by cytogenetic analysis demands cell culture in the presence of low folate medium or with a folate antagonist in order to achieve satisfactory expression of the fragile X. There are two drawbacks of this culture method. First, the mitotic index is greatly reduced so that obtaining sufficient mitoses for analysis is difficult. Secondly, although this requirement for more cells can be achieved by growing the cells for longer, the problem of CV cells becoming polyploid (tetraploid or octoploid) during this time also increases. Will fragile X analysis from CVS soon enable it to be used as a general screening method for the fragile X syndrome as well as being useful in families at risk? The fragile X syndrome may soon be amenable to prenatal diagnosis using recombinant DNA analysis and this would influence the way in which diagnosis was undertaken.

23.4 PROBLEMS AND PITFALLS

23.4.1 Maternal cell contamination

Maternal cell contamination has always been considered a serious potential source of error in prenatal diagnosis. For amniotic fluid cell cultures, the European figures (Thirkelsen, 1979) from 40,000 cases in 61 laboratories showed that a mixture of male and female cells was seen in 0.229% of all cases, and a misdiagnosis resulting from the growth of maternal cells alone occurred in a further 0.085% of all cases. The combined US data from 6,520 cases (Simpson *et al.*, 1976; Golbus *et al.*, 1979; Crandall *et al.*, 1980; Benn *et al.*, 1983) gives a figure for mixed male and female cells in 0.123% of cases and misdiagnosis due to maternal cell contamination of 0.23%. Since recognition is of mixed male/female cell populations, these figures must be doubled to allow for those cases of maternal contamination which would not have been detected because the fetus was female.

Are the estimates for maternal cell contamination in CVS likely to be different from those of AF cells? It might be argued that for direct preparations the level of maternal contamination would be comparatively low although there are no estimates for this yet. However, when karyotyping of CVS occurs after cell culture, the dangers are much greater. The sampling of chorionic villi gives fetal tissue which is embedded in the maternal decidua and bathed in maternal blood cells. Even with excellent sampling and separation of the villi, there is a much higher risk of maternal tissue being co-cultured with the fetal maternal cells than for AF cells. Furthermore, our recent observations (Gosden and Davidson, 1985), show that in the vast majority of cases with cultured cells, maternal decidual cells in culture grow at least twice as fast as chorionic villus cells; this results in progressively greater maternal contamination with time in culture. Both maternal and fetal cells show increasing polyploidy (from initial diploidy through tetraploidy to octoploidy), as time in culture increases. There are a number of ways of either trying to prevent or of testing for maternal cell contamination, all of them labour intensive. For those laboratories where relatively large numbers of amniotic fluid samples have maternal contamination in the absence of heavy blood contamination, discarding the first 1–2 ml of fluid obtained may be beneficial. Where samples are heavily blood-stained, a Kleihauer test may help identify those samples with maximum risk (e.g. those containing > 75 million maternal red blood count in each millilitre of fluid). For CVS samples, careful sorting of the tissue under a dissecting microscope to remove any contaminating decidua and washing to remove maternal blood cells, will help minimize problems. Ultimately, comparison of maternal and fetal markers (for example, by comparison of fluorescence heteromorphisms between mother and fetus) is the definitive test.

23.4.2 Trisomies 2, 16 and 20

We must question why Trisomy 2 and Trisomy 20 (and mosaicism for these lines) are commonly encountered in amniotic fluid cell cultures (but not in the fetus itself). This is usually described as pseudomosaicism. It has been suggested that these cell lines are derived from trophoblastic lines (perhaps from AF cells) and so it is important to study the cell types from which these trisomies emanate. The major problem with pseudomosaicism in CVS samples (which obviously consists of pure trophoblastic tissue) seems to involve Trisomy 16. It has been known for some time that Trisomy 16 is the most common abnormality among first-trimester spontaneous abortions (Hassold and Chiu, 1985; Kajii *et al.*, 1980), but karyotyping was usually performed on extra-embryonic membranes and seldom, if ever, upon the embryo or fetus, so the significance and dilemmas of seeing Trisomy 16 where diagnosis was being undertaken in an ongoing pregnancy in CVS were not at first apparent. Given that Trisomy 16 was common in first-trimester abortions, when Trisomy 16 karyotypes were initially encountered in a viable pregnancy after CVS it was assumed that this was an abnormal pregnancy destined to abort. However, careful karyotyping after termination of these pregnancies showed that although cells from extra-embryonic membranes and trophoblast might have a Trisomy 16 karyotype, those of the fetus itself were normal.

It now appears that Trisomy 16 may be found after CVS both in direct preparations and cultures from chorion, but where there is a viable fetus, the fetus itself will probably have a normal karyotype and the Trisomy 16 will be restricted to extra-embryonic membranes and trophoblast.

Thus, if Trisomy 16 is found after CVS in a viable pregnancy it would seem prudent to assume that the fetus is probably chromosomally normal. A number of approaches are possible. Careful surveillance of the pregnancy and ultrasound monitoring should be considered and if the patient aborts spontaneously then detailed karyotyping on all available different tissues in the products of conception might prove helpful. Fetal karyotyping of a different cell population, for example, amniocentesis at 16–17 weeks gestation might be of reassurance.

The problems of encountering Trisomy 16 may, however, have wider implications than simply providing a false positive cytogenetic result from either direct or cultured villus preparations. The presence of Trisomy 16 might create other diagnostic problems. For example, the α-like globin genes are clustered on the short arm of chromosome 16 (Weatherall and Clegg, 1981). For many genetic studies it is important to try and identify the origin of the extra chromosome and from which cell type it was derived. It is tempting to speculate that Trisomy 16 in placenta and membrane might convey a special advantage to certain cells, for example, by giving three copies of a gene involved in the synthesis of a placental hormone. As the trophoblast is destined only to survive for the duration of the pregnancy, then the advantages for synthesis are obvious and the karyotypic abnormality would be self-limiting.

23.4.3 Mosaicism

The problem of mosaicism occurring in prenatal diagnosis should be taken seriously. The consequences of failing to distinguish true mosaicism in the fetus (with the risks of a child surviving with serious handicap) from pseudomosaicism (where there are no serious clinical consequences and might lead to a termination of a potentially normal fetus) are considerable.

Mosaicism has always been a problem in amniotic fluid cell culture and although the proportions of cultures in which it is detected, and the types of abnormality vary quite widely from one laboratory to another, everyone recognizes the potential hazards. The recent suggestion that the risks of mosaicism in CVS are probably greater than those for AF cells because mosaicism is confined to the placenta (Kalousek and Dill, 1983) is thus very disconcerting.

The scientific background of frequency of chromosomal abnormalities in the first trimester has been derived largely from spontaneous abortion surveys. Unfortunately, not only does wide variation exist between the findings of different groups, but recent studies of viable pregnancies examined after chorionic villus sampling demonstrate that certain trisomies, particularly Trisomy 16, but also Trisomies 2 and 20, may be restricted only to the placental villi and extra-embryonic membranes while the fetus itself has a normal karyotype, a fact not well-recognized before. This thus poses questions about the significance of certain trisomies in spontaneous abortuses karyotyped exclusively from villi and membranes.

For mosaicism in first trimester abortuses, Niikawa *et al.*, 1977 found only one mosaic abortus (46XX/47XX+22) in 447 karyotyped abortuses, a frequency of 0.2%. The authors concluded that this abortus probably started as a 47XX+22 zygote resulting from a maternal non-disjunction but then lost the extra chromosome 22 in one cell line and became mosaic. This conclusion is supported by Richards (1969), who estimated that 80% of children with mosaic Down's syndrome actually started as trisomic zygotes. In contrast with the figure of 0.2% from Niikawa, Warburton *et al.* (1978) gave data showing that nearly 10% (10 of 103) of the autosomal trisomies in their abortion survey were trisomy/normal mosaics in a total of 592 karyotyped specimens. However, eight had Trisomy 2, one had Trisomy 3, 43 had Trisomy 16 and five had Trisomy 20. These are all trisomies which have recently been demonstrated to be restricted to the villi and membranes alone while the fetus usually has a normal karyotype. If these are excluded from the calculations (and, of course the validity of this is questionable) then the calculation on the basis of this exclusion gives only 46 trisomies in a total of 592 karyotyped abortuses, of which two were mosaics (0.3%). In surviving children, the most frequently encountered mosaicism is that for Trisomy 21 (Down's syndrome), where the overall frequency appears to be less than 1%. Other forms of mosaicism, such as marker chromosome mosaicism, are also seen at similar levels, but clearly we do not yet know what effects chromosomal mosaicism for the various karyotypic abnormalities has in influencing prenatal lethality.

When CVS is undertaken, current results suggest that bacterial infection of the uterine cavity may perhaps be associated with complications later in pregnancy such as pre-term labour or fetal death rather than acute intra-uterine infection. High rates of positive cultures for cervical swabs (Garden *et al.*, 1985; Brambati *et al.*, 1985) show that attempts to cleanse the vagina and cervix have only limited efficacy. In addition to the risks from infection to mother and fetus, two other major concerns arise from this. The first is that little is currently known of the teratogenic or other potentially harmful effects on fetus or mother for the different routes of first-trimester administration of the variety of agents active against the micro-organisms found in the female genital tract. The second is that the effects of these antimicrobials *in vivo* or *in vitro* are, as yet unquantified. Perhaps these would have little effect on changes of the tissue in culture, such as those leading to chromosomal mosaicism. However, as pseudomosaicism is now known to lead to significant problems in CVS karyotyping, it becomes crucial to examine any factors which might influence such problems.

23.5 WHICH CHROMOSOME ABNORMALITIES ARE CLINICALLY SIGNIFICANT?

Some 5–7% of all recognized pregnancies are estimated to have a chromosome aberration at six weeks gestation but with loss due to spontaneous abortion, this figure falls to 1–1.5% in the second trimester, the exact proportion depending largely on the maternal age distribution of the population (Gustavii, 1984). Only 0.6% of live births have chromosome abnormalities but 5% of stillbirths have major chromosomal anomalies (Angell *et al.*, 1984).

As chorion villus sampling is carried out at an earlier stage in gestation than amniocentesis, karyotypically abnormal conceptuses which would have spontaneously aborted before 16 weeks are discovered. These swell the numbers of chromosomally abnormal pregnancies at first trimester CVS compared with AF cell culture. This expectation of a higher proportion of abnormalities in the first trimester, combined with relatively limited knowledge of the true frequencies of abnormalities in the viable fetus in first trimester, may tend to obscure critical questioning of whether the abnormality predicts the possibility of severe handicap in the fetus. The risks of diagnostic error and methodological problems may also be greater.

For many major chromosome disorders the associated malformation syndromes are well characterized. However, for some anomalies such as *de novo* translocations, rearrangements or supernumerary markers there are few data available and the information about early pregnancy is very limited. Furthermore, for abnormalities such as mosaicism it is difficult to evaluate the extent of true mosaicism in the fetus for example, or fetal brain cells from the limited information gained from chorionic villi, AF cell culture or even fetal blood cells.

23.5.1 Trisomies

Although trisomies are the most commonly identified chromosome abnormalities in man (at least 4% of all clinically recognized pregnancies are trisomic), the dangers of identifying a pure trisomy in prenatal diagnosis which is entirely artefactual (giving a false positive result) does exist. There is thought to be a greater risk for first trimester CVS rather than AF cell culture because in the former all cells are derived from trophoblast which has a greater tendency to pseudotrisomy. Furthermore, in the first trimester, there is a greater expectation that the conceptus might be chromosomally abnormal (with more unusual trisomies than those for chromosomes 8, 9, 10, 13, 18 and 21 seen in the second trimester) which might influence the assumption that abnormalities (which are not real) are of significance. At present, there is little background information about false positive rates for trisomy in CVS because spontaneous abortion data was often restricted to karyotypes of membrane and villi only with no information on a fetus. CVS is only carried out in viable pregnancies and comparison of karyotypes between the villi and the fetus itself have proved instructive in highlighting those abnormalities restricted to extra-embryonic tissue.

23.5.2 Mosaicism

The dangers of mosaicism in culture have already been discussed and the most significant point in comparing CVS with AF cell culture is that the risk of pseudmosaicism in CVS appears greater than that for AF cell culture. If, however, further sampling suggests that true mosaicism is present then the dilemmas of the prognosis for the fetus begin. The mixture of different cell lines (usually two but sometimes more) means that the phenotype may be extremely variable although it is usually less severe than non-mosaic cases. Studies of children with mosaic Down's syndrome have shown that the situation is very complex (Taylor, 1970). The proportion of normal and trisomic cells varies from tissue to tissue and the two (or more) cell types are often not in equilibrium, so that there are changes with time. In some babies there is selection of normal cells while in others the trisomic cell line increases.

The extent to which mosaicism in culture might influence diagnostic accuracy in the first trimester compared with that in second trimester sampling has yet to be examined in a large series. More importantly, strategies for investigating the significance of mosaicism when it is discovered must be developed.

A number of different forms of mosaicism may be encountered in prenatal diagnosis. As each of these seems to be associated with different risks and problems we will examine each group in turn. A major prerequisite for all studies is that when mosaicism is discovered the basic analysis is extended to a much larger number of cells, and if the *in situ* method is used, as many different colonies (clones) as possible should be karyotyped.

(a) Sex chromosome mosaicism

It is important to distinguish XX/XY mosaicism (or more complex forms of sex chromosome mosaicism) which might indicate possible intersexuality, from that which results from maternal contamination. Where a 45X cell line is present it is important to remember that this may occur by simple chromosomal loss in a trophoblastic line as well or it may suggest that mosaicism for Turner's syndrome might be present.

Exclusion of maternal contamination, careful testing of parental markers and the possibility of further sampling, for example amniocentesis following

CVS or fetal blood sampling to resolve problems encountered from amniocentesis, should be considered.

(b) Mosaicism for a normal cell line and Trisomy 2, 16 or 20

The difficulties involved with Trisomies 2, 16 and 20 (mentioned earlier) should alert all those undertaking prenatal diagnosis to the possible dangers here.

(c) Mosaicism for a normal cell line and a trisomy other than 2, 16 or 20

These cases pose a number of problems. A careful analysis of the literature shows that the vast majority (at least 80%) are due to culture artefact and probably have no significance for the pregnancy (Gosden, 1984; Gosden *et al.*, 1985). The possible association of the trisomy in question with a recognizable clinical syndrome (for example, Trisomy 13, or Trisomy 21), is of no help whatsoever in trying to assess whether this is true or pseudomosaicism, and it is important to realize the fallaciousness of such an association. In all cases of mosaicism, the arguments against carrying out a repeat of the same sampling procedure (either CVS or amniocentesis) is that the same abnormal result may be found in the repeat sample but still may not indicate true mosaicism. If, however, two different results are obtained there is no predictive factor to indicate which one is correct!

Studying parental markers might be of help, but it may be misleading. Again, the possibility of further sampling to give access to a different tissue is most important. Of these cases, 20% might well have severe phenotypic effects due to trisomic mosaicism. None the less, on statistical grounds there is less than a one in five chance of the mosaicism being real, with a > 80% chance of pseudomosaicism.

(d) Mosaicism involving structural chromosomal aberrations

A number of cases have been studied involving complex but unique rearrangements. In some cases the fetus may have mosaicism involving two or more different abnormal cell lines. There is, at present, insufficient data to be able to quantitate the risks in such cases but the information available suggests the risks for the fetus are relatively high and such mosaicism should be regarded as having potential clinical significance. Again, in order to gain more information further sampling should be considered.

(e) Mosaicism for a normal cell line and a supernumerary marker chromosome

As with the structural chromosomal aberrations above, mosaics for supernumerary chromosomes in AF cell culture which have had further testing by fetal blood sampling, have frequently shown confirmation of the abnormality in the blood cell line (Gosden *et al.*, 1985). Since the possession of a *de novo* supernumerary marker chromosome, even in mosaic form, is frequently associated with moderate to severe mental handicap (Buckton *et al.*, 1985), then it is important to assess the risks for the fetus. This varies according to the size, type, and origin of the marker and proportion of cells in which it is found.

Most of the information about mosaicism in culture is at present derived from second trimester amniocentesis surveys. The extent to which mosaicism is present in first trimester samples and differences between direct chromosome preparations and cultured villous preparations are factors which may well influence the way in which prenatal karyotyping is done in the future.

23.5.3 Sex chromosome abnormalities

The discovery of a sex chromosome abnormality in prenatal diagnosis poses a number of dilemmas. Decisions should be based upon information about individuals with sex chromosome anomalies but preferably that from unbiased sources such as longitudinal follow-up studies of children originally ascertained in new-born surveys.

23.5.4 Triploidy and tetraploidy

It is important to recognize that there are a number of different forms of polyploidy, some with clinical significance, others simply as culture artefacts. Triploidy is relatively common in first trimester pregnancy (some 2–3% of all human conceptions are thought to be triploid) and it rarely occurs as a culture artefact, but less so in the second trimester because of the lethality for triploid conceptuses. If triploidy is diagnosed later in pregnancy it is usually associated with severe fetal abnormalities such as cardiac and renal malformation, omphalocele, hydrocephalus and hydatidiform degeneration of the placenta. Abnormal ultrasound scan in these cases should suggest the probability of fetal anomaly. Triploidy may be present in pure or mosaic form.

Tetraploidy provides a more complex problem because it usually arises from endoreduplication in culture. Pure tetraploidy in the fetus appears to be lethal early in gestation. Diploid/tetraploid mosaicism is rather more common because it leads to greater fetal survival than pure triploidy, but must be distinguished from tetraploidy arising as a culture artefact. For fetal blood cultures it is possible to identify those cells undergoing a second round of replication *in vitro* by using bromodeoxyuridine (BUdR) labelling to distinguish first from second divisions. Failure to do this can lead to false assumptions that diploid/tetraploid mosaicism is real, whereas in fact it is one of the most common culture artefacts.

23.5.5 *De novo* rearrangements

The difficulties in trying to predict risks when a *de novo* rearrangement is found are considerable. In many cases the arrangements are apparently balanced, but it is impossible to discern at the gross light microscope level whether small deletions or gene mutations have arisen as a result of the breakage and reunion. The principal risk, derived from studies of individuals with *de novo* rearrangements, is generally considered to be that of mental handicap, but many cases involve unique break-points, and thus the literature provides very little help in these cases which would guide decisions for the parents. There is thus a need to make an overall assessment of risk. For apparently balanced *de novo* translocations the general risk is about one in six to one in nine of moderate to severe mental handicap, whereas for *de novo* supernumerary markers the risks vary according to the size, structure and origin (Buckton *et al.*, 1985).

The disadvantage of first trimester karyotyping is that it is usually more difficult to obtain sufficiently long 'stretched' chromosomes to undertake the detailed cytogenetic studies. These are essential for the identification of the chromosomes involved and the evaluation of risks. However, the advantages of CVS are that early sampling allows more time for detailed studies to be carried out, further sampling if necessary, and more time for the parents to consider the risks and reach a decision. Detailed ultrasound scanning to try to detect anomalies is unlikely to be of help, as even the more severely mentally handicapped individuals with *de novo* rearrangements are usually phenotypically normal.

23.6 DISCUSSION

A number of new approaches to identifying potentially abnormal fetuses have recently been developed. Some of these are at present applicable only in second trimester pregnancy, but may be important in identifying pregnancies in those women who would not otherwise be recognized as being at risk. Two examples of these are the use of low maternal serum alpha-feto protein (AFP) levels to identify an increased risk of Down's syndrome (Cuckle *et al.*, 1984), and detailed ultrasonography to identify major structural abnormalities in the fetus which have been found to be associated with a 25% risk of chromosome abnormality (Gosden *et al.*, 1985). Obviously both of these can only be applied in second trimester.

Perhaps the advantages of using first trimester diagnosis are that it can be used for those patients in which it is currently applicable and where the risks are acceptable, together with the possibility of carrying out prenatal karyotyping during the second trimester in those women who present with problems or indications later in pregnancy. This combined approach would enable more fetuses with chromosome abnormalities to be identified.

The thoughts and efforts of those who undertake fetal karyotyping must encompass not only those aspects of the sampling procedures which determine the amount, quantity, possible contamination and problems inherent in each method, but also how to respond to the challenge of recognizing as many as possible of those pregnancies in which the fetus has a significant chromosome abnormality.

REFERENCES

Angell, R. R., Sandison, A. and Bain, A. D. (1984) Chromosome variation in perinatal mortality: a survey of 500 cases. *J. Med. Genet.*, **21**, 39–44.

Benn, P. A., Schonhant, A. G. and Hsu, L. Y. F. (1983) A high incidence of maternal cell contamination of amniotic fluid cell cultures. *Am. J. Med. Genet.*, **14**, 361–5.

Brambati, B., Simoni, G., Danesino, C., Oldrini, A., Ferrazzi, E., Romitti, L., Terzoli, G., Rossella, F., Ferrari, M. and Fraccaro, M. (1985) First trimester fetal diagnosis of genetic disorders: clinical evaluation of 250 cases. *J. Med. Genet.*, **22**, 92–9.

Buckton, K. E., Spowart, G., Newton, M. S. and Frans, H. J. (1985) Forty-four probands with an additional 'marker' chromosome. *Hum. Genet.* **69**, 353–70.

Crandall, B. F., Lebherz, T. B., Rubenstein, L., Robinson, R. D., Sample, W. F., Sarti, D. and Howard, J. (1980) Chromosome findings in 2,500 second trimester amniocentesis. *Am. J. Med. Genet.*, **5**, 345–56.

Cuckle, H. S., Wald, N. J. and Lindenbaum, R. H. (1984) Maternal serum alpha fetoprotein measurement: a screening test for Down Syndrome. *Lancet*, i, 926–9.

Feeny, D., Fuller, P. J., Milner, R., Mottide, P. T., Tomkins, D. J. and Torrance, G. W. (1985) Chorionic villus sampling. *Lancet*, i, 1269–70.

Garden, A. S., Reid, G. and Benzie, R. J. (1985) Chorionic villus sampling. *Lancet*, i, 1270.

Golbus, M. S., Loughman, W. D., Epstein, C. J., Halbasch, G., Stevens, J. D. and Hall, B. D. (1979) Prenatal genetic diagnosis in 3,000 amniocentesis. *New Engl. J. Med.*, **300**, 157–63.

Gosden, C. M. (1983) Amniotic fluid cell types and culture. *Br. Med. Bull.*, **39**, 348–54.

Gosden, C. M. (1984) Diagnostic problems in chromosome analysis. In *Prenatal Diagnosis*: Proceedings of the 11th study group of the Royal College of Obstetricians and Gynaecologists (ed. C. H. Rodeck and K. H. Nicolaides), London. pp. 65–84.

Gosden, C. M. and Davidson, Z. (1985) Manuscript in preparation.

Gosden, C. M., Rodeck, C. H., Nicolaides, K. H., Campbell, S., Eason, P. and Sharp,

J. C. (1985) Fetal blood chromosome analysis: some new indications for fetal karyotyping. *Br. J. Obstet. Gynaecol.*, **92**, 915–20.

Gustavii, B. (1984) Chorionic biopsy and miscarriage in the first trimester. *Lancet*, i, 562.

Hassold, T. and Chiu, D. (1985) Maternal age-specific rates of numerical chromosome abnormalities with special reference to trisomy. *Hum. Genet.*, 70, 11–17.

Kajii, T., Ferrier, A., Niikawa, N., Takahara, H., Ohama, K. and Avirachan, S. (1980) Anatomic and chromosome anomalies in 630 spontaneous abortuses. *Hum. Genet.*, 55, 87–98.

Kalousek, D. K. and Dill, F. J. (1983) Chromosome mosaicism confined to the placenta in human conceptions. *Science*, **221**, 665–7.

Lauritsen, J. G. (1976) Aetiology of spontaneous abortion. *Acta Obstet. Gynecol.*, Supplement, 52, 4–29.

Niikawa, N., Merotto, E. and Kajii, T. (1977) Origin of acrocentric trisomies in spontaneous abortuses. *Hum. Genet.*, 40, 73–8.

Richards, B. W. (1969) Mosaic mongolism. *J. Ment. Defic. Res.*, **13**, 66–83.

Sherman, S. L., Morton, N. E., Jacobs, P. A. and Turner, G. (1984) The marker (X) syndrome: a cytogenetic and genetic analysis. *Ann. Hum. Genet.*, **48**, 21–37.

Simpson, N. E., Dallaire, L., Miller, J. R., Siminovitch, L., Hamerton, J. L., Miller, J. and McKeen, C. (1976) Prenatal diagnosis of genetic disease in Canada: Report of a collaborative study. *Can. Med. Assoc. J.*, **115**, 739–46.

Taylor, A. I. (1970) Further observations of cell selection *in vivo* in normal-G trisomic mosaics. *Nature* 227, 163–4.

Thirkelsen, A. J. (1979) Cell culture and cell technique. In *Prenatal Diagnosis* (eds J. D. Murken, S. Stengel-Rutkowski, E. Schwinger), Proceedings of 3rd European Conference on Prenatal Diagnosis of Genetic Disorders, Ferdinand Publishers, Stuttgart, pp. 258–70.

Tomerrup, N., Sondergaard, F., Tonneson, T., Kristensen, M., Arveiler, B. and Schinzel, A. (1985) First trimester prenatal diagnosis of a male fetus with Fragile X. *Lancet*, i, 870.

Warburton, Yu, C-Y, Kline, J. and Stein, Z. (1978) Mosaic autosomal trisomy in cultures from spontaneous abortions. *Am. J. Hum. Genet.*, 30, 609–17.

Watanabe, M., Ito, T., Yamamoto, M. and Watanabe, G. (1978) Origin of mitotic cells in the chorionic villi in direct chromosome analysis. *Hum. Genet.*, **44**, 191–3.

Weatherall, D. J. (1983) *The new genetics and clinical practice.* Nuffield Provincial Hospital Trust, Oxford.

Weatherall, D. J. and Clegg, J. B. (1981) *The thalassemia syndromes.* 3rd edn, Blackwells Scientific Publications, Oxford.

Webb, T., Gosden, C. M., Rodeck, C. H., Hamill, M. A. and Eason, P. J. (1983) Prenatal diagnosis of X-linked mental retardation with fragile (X) using fetoscopy and fetal blood sampling. *Prenat. Diag.*, 3, 131–9.

24

Chorionic villi and direct chromosome preparation

—— D. E. Heaton and B. H. Czepulkowski ——

24.1 INTRODUCTION

The presence of spontaneous mitoses in chorionic villi was first noted in the cytotrophoblast layer, and it was later demonstrated that these were confined to the Langhans cells (Boyd and Hamilton, 1966; Hamilton, 1972; Wynn, 1975; Pritchard and MacDonald, 1976; Watanabe *et al.*, 1978). In 1971, Moe claimed to have demonstrated mitotic activity in the syncytiotrophoblast, particularly in the syncytial sprouts, and in the syncytial bridges. The mitoses were, however, infrequent.

Spontaneous divisions were first utilized for the chromosome analysis of induced abortions (Yamamoto *et al.*, 1975, 1982), and preparations were made using a modification of the technique originally described for obtaining chromosomes from membranes and tail tips of embryonic and new-born mice (Evans *et al.*, 1972). During this time the possibility of using trophoblast material for prenatal diagnosis of genetic disorders had been suggested, although preliminary work was concentrated on the use of long-term tissue cultures for cytogenetic analysis (Hahnemann *et al.*, 1974; Niazi *et al.*, 1981). A different approach was, however, employed by a Chinese group from the Tietung Hospital of Anshan Iron and Steel Company, who, in 1975, achieved a 93.9% success rate of fetal sex prediction by direct analysis of X-chromatin of aspirated chorionic villi.

In 1983, Simoni *et al.* published an adaptation of the Evans technique which they applied to chorionic villus samples aspirated from first trimester pregnancies immediately prior to therapeutic termination. The procedure was used in 20 cases and karyotyping was successful in all of them. The successful application of the direct method to a total of 250 diagnostic cases was subsequently reported by this group (Simoni *et al.*, 1984a; Brambati *et al.*, 1985).

Although the many advantages of a method for obtaining chromosome preparations from chorionic villus material without the need for long-term tissue culture are evident, these must be weighed against the information which can be reliably obtained in this way. This in turn depends on the quality and quantity of the metaphase spreads obtained when compared to the results which are possible from long-term tissue cultures (Czepulkowski *et al.*, 1986).

This chapter will discuss the following aspects of the direct method:

1. The techniques available.
2. Reliability of the technique and quality of metaphase spreads obtained.
3. Accuracy of result.
4. Future developments.
5. The place of the direct technique in routine first trimester diagnosis.

24.2 THE METHODS

The original Evans technique (Evans *et al.*, 1972) for the preparation of chromosomes from the membranes or tail tips of embryonic or new-born mice involved five stages:

1. a colcemid treatment;
2. a hypotonic treatment using sodium citrate;
3. fixation in 3:1 ethanol:acetic acid;
4. exposure to 60% aqueous acetic acid;
5. preparation of slides treated on a hotplate.

The first three steps are standard treatments in the preparation of most human tissues for chromosome analysis. The exposure to 60% aqueous acetic acid had the effect of releasing cells from the membranes. Slides could not be prepared by conventional drying methods since evaporation of the 60% aqueous acetic acid was not sufficiently rapid to allow adequate spreading of the metaphases. A more extreme treatment was therefore necessary. For this purpose, Evans applied a dropping and withdrawing technique using a Pasteur pipette, together with slides heated on a hotplate. This caused the cells to attach to the slide at the retreating edge of the fluid, those in mitosis being left as chromosome spreads. An alternative method of spreading was to apply the cell suspension to the heated slide and blow from a rubber bulb or to tilt the slide from side to side.

Yamamoto *et al.* (1975) omitted the colcemid treatment, but otherwise used essentially the same technique. Spreads were stained with Giemsa in most cases, but Q-banding was used for the analysis of abnormal karyotypes and for sex determination.

The technique of Simoni *et al.* (1983, 1984a, personal communication) is as follows:

1. Wash villi in Hanks' solution and place in a petri dish containing 3 ml RPMI without serum.
2. Add colcemid to a final concentration of 0.04 μg/ml and leave for 1 hour.
3. Remove medium completely with a pasteur pipette and replace with 3 ml 1% sodium citrate for 10 min.
4. Remove citrate completely and add 3 ml 3:1 methanol:acetic acid fixative. Leave for 10 min. Repeat this twice more.
5. Remove fixative thoroughly and gather villous pieces together in crease of petri dish. Add a few drops (0.5 ml approx.) 60% acetic acid solution.
6. Leave tipped for 5–10 min and observe dissociation of cells under phase contrast.
7. Make slides by placing a large drop of cell suspension at one end of a cleaned slide placed on a hotplate at 40°C and by pulling the drop up and down the slide with the bent tip of a pasteur pipette until the acid has almost evaporated. Any surplus drops can then be sucked back into the pipette. It is important that the bent pipette tip does not touch the slide during this process but that it is suspended just above the surface holding the drop by surface tension. Slides can also be prepared using a specially developed machine (GI-RO 3283) multi-slide machine, Ma-re, Milan, Italy).

Villi can be incubated for 12–24 hours in complete medium with 20% fetal calf serum in a 5% CO_2 atmosphere at 37°C. The above procedure is then followed.

Modifications of the Evans technique have been described by Burgoyne (1983) and Ferguson-Smith *et al.* (1984). Burgoyne's modification avoids the laborious slidemaking procedure necessary for Simoni's technique by introducing a further fixative wash after the acetic acid treatment. Both techniques involve essentially the same steps as Simoni's method, but the treatments are carried out in centrifuge tubes instead of petri dishes so that reagents can be removed at each stage after centrifugation. Chang medium is used instead of RPMI for the initial colcemid treatment.

An entirely different approach to direct chromosome preparation from chorionic villi was described in 1983 by Ford and Jahnke. These workers used collagenase to dissociate the cells of the cytotrophoblast layer before hypotonic and fixative treatments thus avoiding the use of acetic acid. Slides could then be made by conventional methods. The method is as follows:

1. Mince villous material with a scalpel for 0.5 min.
2. Transfer to a centrifuge tube containing 1 mg/ml collagenase type V (Sigma) in Hams F10 and colchicine 1 μg/ml.
3. Incubate for 1 hour at 37°C
4. Rinse in Dulbecco's phosphate buffer (pH 6.8) and then suspend in 75 mmol/l KCl at 37°C for 20 min.

5. Fix in 3:1 methanol:acetic acid.
6. Make slides preferably after overnight storage at 4°C.

More recently, Blakemore *et al.* (1984) developed a technique which allows both direct preparations and long-term cultures to be made simultaneously from a single villus sample. The method is as follows:

1. Place cleaned villi into 2 ml trypsin-EDTA solution (1X) with 20 μg/ml DNase 1.
2. Mince villi with fine scissors and gently stir in the solution for 5 min at 37°C with a Teflon coated magnetic stirring bar.
3. Aspirate the cell suspension carefully leaving the tissue pieces behind.
4. Place the suspension into 3 ml MEM with 20% FBS and 0.07 μg/ml Colcemid at room temperature.
5. The process of stirring for 5 min and aspirating the cell suspension is repeated twice more. Each cell suspension is added in turn to the colcemid solution.
6. The remaining tissue fragments are rinsed and suspended in MEM with 10% FBS for establishing cultures.
7. Direct harvest is performed on the cell suspension by first exposing it to 0.075 M KCl for 20 min, and fixing in two successive 15 min exposures to 3:1 methanol:acetic acid. At each stage the pellet should be re-suspended gently to avoid cell loss.
8. Cell suspension is blown onto cold wet slides which are then rapidly transferred to a 60°C hotplate for 90 seconds.
9. Tissue fragments are placed in flasks or on to coverslips in MEM with 20% FBS for long-term cultures.

24.3 RELIABILITY AND QUALITY OF RESULTS

24.3.1 Mitotic index

Watanabe *et al.* (1978) obtained an average of approximately 4.4 mitoses per 500 cells in his samples when examining only Langhans cells. No mitoses were observed in syncytium or stromal cells.

Simoni *et al.* (1983) obtained 15–131 mitoses from 5 mg or more of villous material in all of the 20 cases to which they applied the direct technique. In a series of 250 diagnostic cases, this group successfully karyotyped 247 cases out of the 248 in which fetal material was obtained (Brambati *et al.*, 1985). The sample size ranged from 5 mg to 100 mg in these cases, and it is evident from the 1983 report that the majority of the first 100 cases involved sample sizes of 20 mg or more (75 out of 96 cases).

Ford and Jahnke (1983) obtained from 50 to over 400 metaphase spreads per 40 mg sample, and successful karyotypes were obtained in all cases. Both

Simoni (1984a) and Burgoyne (1983) have found that the mitotic index can be increased by incubating villous aspirates for 12–48 hours in complete medium at 37°C before applying the appropriate harvesting procedures. In contrast Ferguson-Smith *et al.* (1984) found that the 24-hour 'direct' treatment produced a very low success rate. The experience in the St. Mary's laboratory has also been that the mitotic index is lowered after prolonged incubation.

Although the mitotic index and success rates obtained by the above groups are encouraging, in practice many laboratories who have applied these techniques to their own diagnostic cases have not been able to obtain consistently satisfactory results by the direct method.

There are two possible reasons for variability in mitotic index:

1. Quantity and quality of villous sample.
2. The interval between sampling and receipt of specimen by laboratory.

The quantity and quality of villous material available for the technique will vary with the experience of the obstetrician who is sampling. It is important for the ongoing pregnancy that disturbance to the sac is minimal, but further data correlating sample size with fetal loss is necessary to establish how much tissue can be safely removed. Burgoyne, and Ford and Jahnke developed their techniques on material obtained after termination of pregnancy and could, therefore, use large samples. Most of Simoni's results were also obtained from large samples, although this group maintain that the mitotic index is not necessarily correlated with sample size (Simoni *et al.*, 1986).

The interval between sampling and receipt of the sample by the laboratory is likely to be the most important factor influencing the number of mitoses recovered by the direct technique. Samples may have to be transported considerable distances, with some laboratories receiving them the day after sampling if this has been done late in the day. It is likely that the temperature will have a considerable effect during this time, and rough handling of the sample during transportation will almost certainly result in some loss of the syncytial 'sprouts' which represent the most mitotically active regions of the chorionic villus. It is, perhaps, significant that the diagnostic samples described by Simoni were obtained from a clinic in the same building as the laboratory, and could thus be attended to immediately.

Blakemore *et al.* (1984) drew attention to this point stating that they were able to begin the direct preparations within 20 minutes of sampling and that this maximized the number of recovered metaphase spreads. Ford and Jahnke (1983) collected their abortus specimens into medium containing 1μg/ml colchicine, and processed them 30 minutes to two hours after collection. Satisfactory preparations were obtained but shorter chromosomes resulted from the longer colchicine exposures. At least one United Kingdom laboratory uses this approach in their routine treatment of diagnostic samples which are taken at a hospital 30 miles away and then transported to the laboratory by train (Palmer, personal communication). Results from the direct preparations of these samples appear to be adequate. This is, however, a somewhat risky procedure since delays of more than a few hours are possible within such a system, and there may be little chance of salvaging the sample with a long-term culture if exposure to colchicine has been excessive.

24.3.2 Quality of mitoses and banding resolution

Evans (1972) in his original paper noted that chromosome spreads tended to be distorted and incomplete, and that the quality of fixation and sharpness of staining were not as satisfactory as in the conventional air-dried preparations. He could, however, use at least five selected spreads to establish the karyotype with confidence, although the preparations were not banded. These observations have also been true of many preparations made with Simoni's direct technique, and several ways of minimizing the problems have been suggested. The tendency for direct spreads to be incomplete can be overcome to some extent by placing villi suspended in 3:1 methanol:acetic acid fixative into a deep freeze (−20°C) for 24 hours before preparations are made (Gregson and Seabright, 1984). This treatment also improves the chromosome morphology. Simoni observed that the number of broken mitoses was lower in preparations made after 12–24 hour incubation in complete medium at 37°C.

A major criticism of Simoni's direct method is that chromosome morphology may be poor, and that Giemsa banding resolution achieved routinely from other cultured material, including amniocytes, cannot be consistently obtained from direct spreads (Brambati *et al.*, 1983; Sachs *et al.*, 1983; Mackenzie *et al.*, 1983; Gregson and Seabright, 1983; Ford and Jahnke, 1983; Blakemore *et al.*, 1984; Heaton *et al.*, 1984; Gosden, 1984). Figure 24.1 illustrates a G-banded metaphase spread obtained from a chorionic villus aspirate by the direct technique of Simoni (1983).

The preparations do seem to be suitable for routine Q-banding, and many laboratories, particularly those in Europe, are using this as an acceptable alternative. In addition, Sachs *et al.* (1983) reported the detection of complex chromosome rearrangement using Reverse Heat Acridine orange banding (RHA). Many laboratories, however, find the dependence on fluorescent banding techniques unacceptable, and have attempted to improve G-banding quality on the direct preparations. Certainly the most consistent results have been produced by the techniques which avoid the acetic acid treatment by the use of enzymes to dissociate the cells of the cytotrophoblast (Ford and Jahnke, 1983; Blakemore *et al.* 1984). Gregson and Seabright (1983) were able to obtain improved G-banding on preparations made from villi incubated overnight in Chang medium, and processed by the Simoni tech-

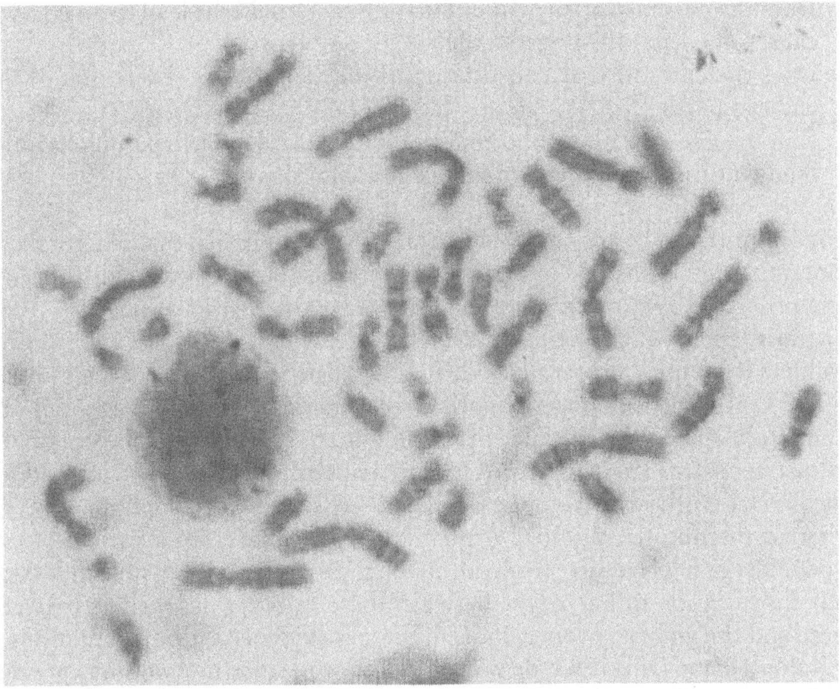

Figure 24.1 G-banded metaphase spread obtained from chorionic villus aspirate (Simoni, 1983).

nique. Slides were first stained conventionally with Leishman or Giemsa stain and then decolourized with 3:1 methanol:acetic acid fixative. G-banding was then carried out, and the process monitored under phase contrast microscopy. The monitoring process allowed optimum banding to be achieved for each slide. Ferguson-Smith *et al.* (1984) described a banding technique involving hydration and dehydration treatment prior to trypsin banding. This was successful when used in conjunction with their modified direct method.

Simoni *et al.* (1984a) demonstrated the suitability of the direct preparations for C-banding, and for sister chromatid exchange (SCE) studies, using Bromodeoxyuridine (BudR).

24.4 ACCURACY OF RESULTS

There are three questions that must be answered when considering the accuracy and reliability of karyotypes obtained from chorionic villus samples both by the direct method and from cultures (see Chapter 23).

1. Does the presence of any contaminating maternal cells lead to an equivocal result?
2. Does the chromosome constitution of the trophoblast reflect that of the embryo paper?
3. Can the chromosome abnormalities which can be detected on amniotic fluid cultures be detected on villous preparations?

A recent report by Blakemore *et al.* (1985) has suggested that maternal cell contamination is possible in direct preparations of undissected villi although Simoni *et al.* (1986) cite only 2 known cases of this in a series of 1000 diagnostic samples. Both these authors conclude that this is not a significant problem if samples are carefully cleaned by experienced staff.

The karyotypes obtained by both direct and culture techniques should be compared, since the cell types are representative of different layers of the villous structure. The majority of spontaneous mitoses which are utilized for the direct method arise from the Langhans' cells of the cytotrophoblast layer, whereas the mitoses obtained from culture originate from a variety of cell types most of which derive from the mesenchyme core. It is possible that there may be variation in karyotype between these cell types as well as between these and the embryo proper. Indeed, there is evidence for both situations.

Kalousek and Dill (1983) demonstrated chromosome mosaicism expressed exclusively in placental chorionic cells which was not detected in cells derived from the embryo proper. Brambati *et al.* (1985) reported two diagnostic cases from their series of 250, in which such a discrepancy was found. A Trisomy 3 mosaicism, and a Trisomy 16 detected by the direct technique were not confirmed after termination on fetal fibroblasts. Similar discrepancies have been reported by Simoni (1985) which have occurred in other Italian centres. Since cultures were not set up from the initial villus samples a comparison cannot be made of karyotypes of the different cell types. This is, perhaps, regrettable since discrepancies between results obtained from direct preparations and corresponding cultures have been demonstrated by Jackson (personal communication) (Table 24.1). Five of Jackson's cases involved mosaicism which was detected on direct preparation but not on cultured material.

More recently three cases of false-negative findings on chorion villus sampling have been reported. Two of these cases involved 46,XY/47,XXY mosaicism where the direct preparations revealed only normal cells whereas the mosaicism was detected on long term cultures and subsequently confirmed on the fetus (Eichenbaum *et al.* (1986), Linton and Lilford (1986)). The other case, reported by Martin *et al.* (1986) involved a fetus with trisomy 18 which was not detected on direct preparations which gave only normal cells. We know of a similar case which has occurred in London (Kearney, personal communication).

The third question can be answered by comparing the quality of banding

Table 24.1 Discrepancies found at CVS (Jackson, personal communication)

Direct	*Culture*	*Amniocentesis*	*Fetal tissue*	*Pregnancy outcome*
48XXY+A	46XY	—	46XY (chorion)	IUFD 1 week
46XX/ 47XX+13	46XX	46XX	—	continuing
46XX/ 47XXX	46XX	—	46XY (chorion)	terminated
46XX/ 47XXX	46XX	46XX	—	delivered
46XX/ 47XX+ Marker	46XX	—	—	continuing
46XX/ 45X	46XX	—	—	continuing
47XX+20	47XX+20	46XX/ 47XX+20	—	pending
92XXYY	46XY	—	—	continuing

obtained from villous preparations with that from cultured amniocytes. It has been suggested that the direct preparations are only suitable for the detection of trisomies and major rearrangements, while it is necessary to culture villi to find more subtle abnormalities (Heaton *et al.*, 1984). Of the 250 cases reported by Brambati *et al.* (1985), an abnormal chromosome constitution was found in 21, of which 16 were aneuploid, three were Robertsonian translocations, one had an inversion in the X chromosome, and one had a balanced insertion inherited from the father. Mackenzie *et al.* (1983) reported an unbalanced translocation, involving chromosomes 4 and 18, detected on direct villous preparations, though this had already been identified in the balanced form in the father. The most convincing example of detection of subtle abnormality is that reported by Sachs *et al.* (1983) where complex structural rearrangements on four chromosomes were involved. Although the double translocation had already been characterized in both the female carrier and her mother, at least one of the derivative chromosomes would have required banding of good resolution to be identified. The unbalanced translocation was detected by RHA banding on direct villous preparations.

There are no accounts in the literature of subtle rearrangements detected on direct villus preparations alone, without abnormality in the family having been previously characterized. It can be argued, however, that there are no reports in the literature of chromosomal abnormality detected in a fetus delivered after chorionic villus sampling which was not found by direct analysis.

The situation regarding the necessity or otherwise for culture for the detection of fragile X is unclear at present. Simoni (1984b) at the Rapallo symposium reported the detection of fragile X in villi incubated for 48 hours in TC 199. Two out of 140 mitoses had the fragile X, and on subsequent analysis of the maternal lymphocytes 3/300 were found to be fragile X positive. Tommerup *et al.* (1985) reported a fragile X which they detected in long-term tissue culture, both untreated and treated with methotrexate, but not in the direct or 24 hour direct preparations.

24.5 FUTURE DEVELOPMENTS

Since the direct method of chromosome preparation from chorionic villi depends on the presence of spontaneous mitoses, it would seem logical to assume that they can be synchronized in some way. Such improvements have been made on the preparation of chromosome spreads from bone marrows using methotrexate or FudR (Webber *et al.*, 1983). FudR (Fluorodeoxy-uridine) is an anti-metabolite which acts at a specific binding site in the biosynthesis of thymine derivatives, leading to a block in the DNA production. Adding FudR thus has the effect of blocking DNA synthesis and hence inhibiting cell division. This block can then be released by exposure to thymidine which then enables the cell division to progress. Since cell division will now be synchronized, a short colcemid treatment is sufficient after which preparations can be made by the method of Simoni (1983). It is important to collect villi in a thymidine-depleted medium such as RPMI since the FudR will be ineffective in the presence of thymidine. The following method has been applied to 13 cases to date, and an improvement in chromosome morphology has been noted in these cases (Czepulkowski, 1984).

1. Clean sample and place in RPMI (complete) overnight at 37°C.
2. Add FudR (final conc. 0.1 μg/ml) and uridine (final conc. 4 μg/ml) for 2 hours.
3. Add thymidine (final conc. 10 uM) for 1–2 hours.
4. Add colcemid (0.04 μg/ml) for 30 min.
5. Proceed according to method of Simoni *et al.* 1983.

Yu *et al.*, (1986) have recently reported encouraging results from the use of a cold 'holding' period between incubations at 37°C which they believe may introduce some degree of synchronization.

24.6 THE PLACE OF THE DIRECT TECHNIQUE IN ROUTINE FIRST-TRIMESTER DIAGNOSIS

The direct approach to chromosome preparation from chorionic villus samples has several important advantages over long-term tissue culture. It is possible to obtain a result within a few hours of sampling, although in practice better results may be obtained over a period of up to 2–5 days. The presence of maternal cells in a sample does not influence the result in the way that it may in a culture, and the presence of contaminating micro-organisms does not jeopardize the chance of obtaining a result. The system is cheaper to operate than one which requires tissue culture since it is possible to do without sophisticated incubators or sterile facilities. For this reason it is well suited to use in developing countries which may be lacking in facilities. Medium consumption is also comparatively less. Of these advantages, the time factor is probably the most important since the concept of first-trimester diagnosis was introduced to minimize the period of anxiety experienced during pregnancy by couples at risk for genetic abnormality, and to enable earlier, and consequently less traumatically, termination of pregnancy where necessary. Certainly the direct method can mean the difference between an early or late termination in cases where sampling has taken place at 12 weeks gestation or more.

There are, however, several serious disadvantages of this technique which would suggest that to rely solely on this approach for diagnosis without supporting cultures would be unwise. Although most laboratories are able to obtain mitoses from the majority of their direct villous preparations, the number of mitoses suitable for analysis, both banded and unbanded, can be variable to the extent that it can sometimes be difficult to establish even a chromosome count with confidence. The QFQ banding favoured by Simoni *et al.* is not in routine use in the majority of United Kingdom laboratories, and the quality of G-banding obtained from direct preparations does not satisfy the rigorous standards of those laboratories that routinely G-band their amniotic fluid preparations. Cultured preparations, on the other hand, provide G-banded chromosomes comparable to those obtained from other tissues. The effect of delay between sampling and receipt of the sample by the laboratory is a serious drawback both from the point of view of quality of results, and also from that of inconvenience since direct preparations must be made immediately. Indeed, for laboratories with limited personnel the direct treatments represent a greater burden than culturing since timing of treatments is more rigid. A culture, however, can be set up at any time after receipt of the sample (or even the next day), in 10–20 minutes. The actual time spent preparing villous samples both by direct methods or culture is probably about the same.

The major advantage of using cultured villous material is that there is a potentially unlimited supply of cells available for examination should difficulties arise during analysis, e.g. in the case of suspected mosaicism. The sample is exhausted once direct preparations have been made, and if a problem is encountered further slides cannot be prepared.

Brambati *et al.* (1985) suggested that additional investigations in the second trimester should be offered when a mosaic or rare type of autosomal trisomy normally associated with non-viable pregnancies is found in the trophoblast. In the light of evidence showing that discrepancies can occur between the results obtained by the direct method and by culture, it would appear to be insufficient to give counselling solely on the basis of the direct method. It is possible that unnecessary termination of some pregnancies may be avoided if further information, which can be obtained from a culture, is available at the time of decision within the first trimester. It therefore seems evident that, at present, it is advisable to prepare both direct and cultured preparations from diagnostic chorionic villus samples for the maximum information to be obtained.

ACKNOWLEDGEMENTS

Our thanks are due to Dr Laird G. Jackson, Jefferson Medical College, Philadelphia, for granting us permission to cite his unpublished data, and to Dr D. V. Coleman for her critical review of the manuscript. Figure 24.1 was supplied by Lyndal Kearney, Harris Birthright Centre, King's College Hospital, London.

REFERENCES

Blakemore, K. J., Watson, M. S., Samuelson, J., Breg, W. R. and Mahoney, M. J. (1984) A method of processing first-trimester chorionic villous biopsies for cytogenetic analysis. *Am. J. Hum. Genet.*, **36**, 1386–93.

Blakemore, K. J., Samuelson, J., Breg, W. R. and Mahoney, M. J. (1985) Maternal metaphoses on direct chromosome preparation of the first trimester decidua. *Hum. Genet.* **69**, 380.

Boyd, T. P. and Hamilton, W. J. (1966) Placental Septa. *Z. Zellf.*, **69**, 613–34.

Brambati, B., Oldrini, A., Simoni, G., Terzoli, G. L., Romitti, L., Rossella, F. and Ferrari, M. (1983) First trimester fetal karyotyping in twin pregnancy. *J. Med. Genet.*, **20**, 58–60.

Brambati, B., Simoni, G., Danesino, C., Oldrini, A., Ferrazzi, E., Romitti, L., Terzoli, G., Rossella, F., Ferrari, M. and Fraccaro, M. (1985) First trimester fetal diagnosis of genetic disorders: clinical evaluation of 250 cases. *J. Med. Genet.*, **22**, 92–9.

Burgoyne, P. (1983) Direct chromosome preparations from chorionic villi. *Prenat. Diag. Group Newsletter*, **7**, 3–4.

Czepulkowski, B., Heaton, D. E. and Coleman, D. V. (1984) Recent developments in the preparation of villous samples for cytogenetic studies: use of FudR to improve banding of chromosomes prepared directly from chorionic villi. *Prenat. Diag. Group Newsletter*, **8**, 18.

Czepulkowski, B. H., Heaton, D. E., Kearney, L. and Coleman, D. V. (1986) Chorionic villus culture for first trimester diagnosis of chromosome defects: evaluation by two London centres. *Prenat. Diag.* **6**, 271–86.

Eichenbaum, S. Z., Krumine, E. J., Fortune, D. W. and Duke, J. (1986) False-negative finding on chorionic villus sampling. *Lancet*, **ii**, 391.

Evans, E. P., Burtenshaw, M. D. and Ford, C. E. (1972) Chromosomes of Mouse

Embryos and Newborn Young: Preparations from Membranes and Tail Tips. *Stain Technol.*, **47**, 229–34.

Ferguson-Smith, M. E., Frew, C., Gilmore, D. H., Chatfield, W. R. and Ferguson-Smith, M. A. (1984) Chromosome Studies from Chorionic Villi: Glasgow Results. *Prenat. Diag. Group Newsletter*, **8**, 13–15.

Ford, J. H. and Jahnke, A. B. (1983) Handling Chorionic Villi for Direct Chromosome Studies. *Lancet*, **ii**, 1491–2.

Gosden, C. M. (1984) Problems of first trimester prenatal diagnosis. *Prenat. Diag. Group Newsletter*, **8**, 19–20.

Gregson, N. M. and Seabright, M. (1983) Handling chorionic villi for direct chromosome studies. *Lancet*, **ii**, 1491.

Hahnemann, N. (1974) Early Prenatal Diagnosis: a study of biopsy techniques and cell culturing for extraembryonic membranes. *Clin. Genet.*, **6**, 296–306.

Hamilton, W. J. (1972) *Human Embryology*, London, Macmillan.

Heaton, D. E., Czepulkowski, B. H., Horwell, D. H. and Coleman, D. V. (1984) Chromosome analysis of first trimester chorionic villus biopsies prepared by a maceration technique. *Prenat. Diag.*, **4**, 279–87.

Kalousek, D. K. and Dill, F. J. (1983) Chromosomal mosaicism confined to the placenta in human conceptions. *Science*, **221**, 665–7.

Linton, G. and Lilford, R. J. (1986) False-negative finding on chorionic villus sampling. *Lancet*, **ii**, 630.

MacKenzie, I. Z., Lindenbaum, R. H., Patel, C., Clarke, G., Crocker, M. and Jonasson, J. A. (1983) Prenatal diagnosis of an unbalanced chromosome translocation identified by direct karyotyping of chorion biopsy. *Lancet*, **ii**, 1426–7.

Martin, A. O., Elias, S., Rosinsky, B., Bombard, A. T. and Simpson, J. L. (1986) False-negative finding on chorionic villus sampling. *Lancet*, **ii**, 391–2.

Moe, N. (1971) Mitotic activity in the syncytiotrophoblast of the human chorionic villi. *Am. J. Obstet. Gynec.*, **110**, 431.

Niazi, M., Coleman, D. V. and Loeffler, F. E. (1981) Trophoblast sampling in early pregnancy. Culture of rapidly dividing cells from Immature Placental Villi. *Br. J. Obstet. Gynaecol.*, **88**, 1081–5.

Pritchard, J. A. and Macdonald, P. C. (1976) The placenta and fetal membranes. In *Williams' Obstetrics*. Appleton-Century-Crofts, New York. 101–143.

Sachs, E. S., Van Hemel, J. O., Galjaard, H., Nirmeijer, M. F. and Jahoda, M. G. (1983) First trimester chromosomal analysis of complex structural rearrangements with RHA banding on chorionic villi. *Lancet*, **ii**, 1426.

Simoni, G., Brambati, B., Danesino, C., Rossella, F., Terzoli, G. L., Ferrari, M. and Fraccaro, M. (1983) Efficient Direct Chromosome Analysis and Enzyme Determinations from Chorionic Villi samples in the First Trimester of Pregnancy. *Hum. Genet.*, **63**, 349–57.

Simoni, G., Brambati, B., Danestino, C., Rossella, F., Terzoli, G. L., Ferrari, M. and Fraccaro, M. (1984a) Diagnostic application of first trimester trophoblast sampling in 100 pregnancies. *Hum. Genet.*, **66**, 252–9.

Simoni, G. (1984b) The Cytogenetics of First Trimester Fetal Diagnosis. International Symposium on First Trimester Fetal Diagnosis, Rapallo.

Simoni, G., Gimella, G., Cuoco, C., Terzoli, G. L., Rossella, F., Romitti, L., Dalprà, L., Nocera, G., Tibiletti, M. G., Tenti, P. and Fraccaro, M. (1985) Discordance between prenatal cytogenetic diagnosis after chorionic villi sampling and chromosomal constitution of the fetus. In *First Trimester Fetal Diagnosis* (eds M. Fraccaro, G. Simoni and B. Brambati) Springer-Verlag, Berlin.

Simoni, G., Rossella, F. and Fraccaro, M. (1986) Maternal metaphases on direct preparation from chorionic villi and in cultures of villi cells. *Hum. Genet.* 72, 104.

Tietung Hospital of Anshan Iron and Steel Company, Anshan. (1975) Fetal sex prediction by sex chromatin of chorionic villus cells during early pregnancy. *Chin. Med. J.*, 1, 117–26.

Tommerup, N., Sondergaard, F., Tonnesen, T., Kristensen, M., Arveiler, B. and Schinzel, A. (1985) First trimester prenatal diagnosis of a male fetus with fragile X. *Lancet*, i, 870.

Watanabe, M., Ito, T., Yamamoto, M. and Watanabe, G. (1978) Origin of mitotic cells of the chorionic villi in direct chromosome analysis. *Hum. Genet.*, 44, 191–3.

Webber, L. M. and Garson, M. (1983) Fluorodeoxyuridine synchronisation of bone marrow cultures. *Cancer Genet. Cytogenet.*, 8, 123–32.

Wynn, R. M. (1975) Placental ultrastructure. In *Human Placentation* (eds I. A. Brosens, G. Dixon and W. B. Robertson), Exerpta Medica, Amsterdam.

Yamamoto, M., Fujimori, R., Ito, T., Kamimura, K. and Watanabe, G. (1975) Chromosome studies in 500 induced abortions. *Humangenetik*, 29, 9–14.

Yamamoto, M., Ito, T., Watanabe, M. and Watanabe, G. (1982) Causes of Chromosome Anomalies suggested by Cytogenetic Epidemiology of Induced Abortions. *Hum. Genet.*, 60, 360–4.

Yu, M-T., Yu, C-Y., Yu, C-X., Maidman, J. and Warburton, D. (1986) Improved methods of direct and cultured chromosome preparations from chorionic villous samples. *Am. J. Hum. Genet.* 38, 576–81.

25

Cytoculture of chorionic tissue

D. V. Coleman, D. E. Heaton,
B. H. Czepulkowski and A. S. Tyms

25.1 INTRODUCTION

25.1.1 Early studies on trophoblast culture

The earliest investigations into the culture of human placental cells began during the 1920s. Early culture methods depended on the use of plasma clots to attach tissue explants to the floor of the culture vessels after which they were flooded with medium (Jones *et al.*, 1943; Stewart *et al.*, 1947). Although cell growth was obtained in this way, a variety of cell types were evident. This led to conflicting results from different groups who were using this technique to study cell function. Stewart *et al.* (1947) cultured trophoblast material derived from placentae obtained from therapeutic abortions and from placentae obtained at delivery. Cultures from early pregnancies (5–7 weeks) showed a profuse growth of what Stewart describes as Langhan's cells, which were seen to have a characteristic clear halo around the nucleus. Fibroblasts were also obtained in early cultures. Cultures from later pregnancies (3–9 months) tended to be composed of fewer 'Langhans cells' but more fibroblasts, with the latter cell type completely outgrowing trophoblast cells in term placentae.

Thiede (1960) described an alternative method for growing trophoblast material *in vitro* which avoided the use of explants. This enabled him to limit the number of cell types obtained to three, which he then attempted to match with cells seen in tissue sections. The technique he employed consisted of a trypsinization treatment, followed by filtration through a gauze mesh, resulting in a cell suspension which could then be inoculated into culture vessels. This was applied to trophoblast material derived from placentae obtained from therapeutic abortions performed at 9–14 weeks.

Several groups at this time attempted to obtain karyotypes from cultured trophoblast material with varying degrees of success, including Carr (1963), and Hall and Källén (1964) who used placentae obtained from term pregnancies shortly after delivery. In 1965, however, Valenti reported successful karyotyping of trophoblast tissue using a modification of the technique described by Thiede (1960) which he applied to tissue obtained from therapeutic abortions performed at early gestations. Valenti was able to demonstrate the removal of most of the cytotrophoblast and syncytiotrophoblast layers of the villus by enzyme and filtration treatments, leaving behind the exposed mesenchyme cores which could then be cultured.

25.2 CULTURE OF ASPIRATED CHORIONIC VILLUS SAMPLES

25.2.1 Culture of chorionic villus aspirates for chromosome studies

In 1968 the first attempt to culture aspirated chorionic villus samples was reported by Hahnemann, who obtained villi from first-trimester pregnancies by transvaginal sampling using a modified hysteroscope (Hahnemann and Mohr, 1968, 1969). Sixty-two samples were obtained and prepared for examination using a dissecting microscope. Histological studies confirmed that chorionic villi were present in 51 of these samples, although decidua was also noted in 36%. Culture was largely unsuccessful and karyotypes were obtained in only 12 of 34 cultures (35%).

Several years later, Hahnemann reported the results of a further series of 35 samples in which culture had been more successful (Hahnemann, 1974). Cultures were set up from 22 samples which were thought to contain villi or amniotic membrane only, and all but two were karyotyped (91%). Hahnemann pooled the results of his studies (Hahnemann, 1968, 1969, 1974) and found that 30 karyotypes were normal, and four were abnormal. Karyotypes were identified from those obtained from the corresponding fetus, in the 24 normal cases where this was compared. There was an even sex distribution (16 males: 18 females). Two trisomies were detected and mosaicism was noted in two cultures; one karyotype was recorded as 46XX/47XX+G and the other as 46XX/47XX+C, although the latter was derived from culture of amniotic membrane. Confirmation by analysis of fetal parts were not attempted in these two cases nor were banding studies done.

In 1973, Kullander and Sandahl reported the successful culture of placental samples obtained under transcervical endoscopic vision from first trimester pregnancies. Thirty-nine samples were cultured and karyotypes obtained from 20 (57%). A normal male karyotype was obtained in 12 cases and a normal female karyotype in seven. In one case, two fragments of tissue were taken. The karyotype obtained from one fragment was 46XX, and from the other, 46XY. Tissue culture from the corresponding fetus revealed a normal male karyotype. In the remaining cases a correlation was noted between the karyotype obtained from the cultured cells and the sex of the aborted fetus.

25.2.2 Exfoliated trophoblast in the endocervical canal

An alternative source of trophoblast material, avoiding direct sampling from the gestation sac, was investigated in 1971, when Shettles demonstrated the presence of exfoliated trophoblast in aspirated endocervical tissue. The endocervical specimens were stained with quinacrine and Y bodies were found in some of them. Both Shettles (1971) and Warren *et al.* (1972) reported the successful use of this material for Y body sex determination from aspirated endocervical tissue obtained at all stages of pregnancy.

Rhine *et al.* (1977) postulated that if the fetal cells in the endocervical canal were viable, they could perhaps be cultured for first trimester diagnosis of chromosome defects and inborn errors. This group developed the antenatal cell extractor (ACE) for the purposes of obtaining endocervical tissue, and they were able to obtain samples from 66 pregnancies. At first the success of culturing was poor, since only six of 32 samples grew and none could be karyotyped. A further 21 samples yielded growth in 18 cases (86%) but karyotypes in only five. Cells from these five cultures could be distinguished from maternal cells on the basis of chromosome polymorphisms. Twelve of the last 13 samples grew sufficiently well to provide karyotypes. Since all karyotypes were female, Q-band polymorphisms were compared between cultured preparations and maternal cells. Differences were found in nine cases, but in one case no differences were observed and in two there appeared to be a mixture.

In a further study Rhine and Milunsky (1979) reported growth of 37 out of 53 endocervical samples (70%) of which 26 were confirmed as being of fetal origin when compared with cultures of fetal tissues. The quality of metaphase spreads obtained was, however, frequently poor.

Encouraged by the results of Rhine *et al.*, Goldberg *et al.* (1980) undertook a pilot study of 30 cases to replicate their work. Goldberg and his colleagues concentrated on the 12 cases in which fetal tissue was male, since they considered interpretation of polymorphisms to be somewhat subjective. Of these 12 cases, karyotypes were obtained in nine, all of which were female. This clearly demonstrated the maternal origin of the ACE cultured cells in each informative case, and these workers were of the opinion that their results cast serious doubt upon the validity of the findings of Rhine *et al.* who had obtained only female karyotypes.

25.2.3 Recent studies on trophoblast culture for chromosome analysis

Coleman (1982) reported similar findings to those of Goldberg (1980) based on a series of 12 samples obtained by blind transcervical aspiration from pregnancies of 8–12 weeks gestation immediately prior to termination. A portion of each aspirate was retained for histological studies, while the remainder was briefly trypsinized, and cultured. Histological sections revealed the presence of both chorionic villi and decidua in all 12 samples. Karyotypes were obtained from 11 of the 12 cultures, and in each case this was 46XX. Karyotypes from the corresponding fetuses were available in eight cases, three of which were 46XY. Tissue types of cells cultured from two of the aspirates with a corresponding fetal karyotype 46XX were identical to those of the maternal lymphocytes. The origin of the cultured cells in the remaining six cases could not be established. It was therefore clear that at least five of the 11 cultures were of maternal origin.

Niazi (1982) undertook an investigation of the reasons for maternal overgrowth of fetal cells in transcervical aspirates. She approached this by thoroughly washing placental tissue with PBS solution, and then dissecting the villi from the membranes. A fragment of tissue was retained for histological examination, while remaining fragments were cultured using plasma clots to adhere the tissue to the surface of a flask. Histological sections showed that the tissues were composed of intact chorionic villi only, with no evidence of maternal tissue. Five of eight cultures yielded karyotypes of which two were 46XY and three were 46XX. Cell growth was, however, very slow, and karyotypes were only obtained after 8–10 weeks in culture. Niazi postulated that the low growth potential of the immature placental villi accounted for their overgrowth by maternal cells.

Several authors had already noted that cells from the mesenchyme stroma tended to grow more rapidly, and survive longer in culture, than those from the outer trophoblast layers. This led Niazi to investigate the possibility of accelerating cell growth of transcervical aspirates by removing these outer layers. By using a trypsinization treatment followed by filtration through a wire mesh gauze, Niazi was able to collect tissue composed entirely of mesenchyme cores which was trapped on the gauze. The filtrate contained a mixture of cytotrophoblast strips, red blood cells and single cells of unknown origin. These components could be separated on a density gradient, and the cytotrophoblast strips recovered from the base. Syncytiotrophoblast was destroyed by the treatment.

Mesenchyme cells were found to grow rapidly in culture, whereas cytotrophoblast cells grew very slowly. The trypsinization/filtration technique was applied to transcervical aspirates, and the mesenchyme tissue was cultured. Five cultures were tissue-typed and compared with maternal lymphocytes. In each case the fetal origin of the cells was demonstrated.

Chromosome preparations were made from 17 cultures. Normal female karyotypes were obtained in six cases of which four were confirmed by comparison with fetal fibroblasts. Normal male karyotypes were obtained in six cases, and two abnormal karyotypes were detected, 47XX+21 and 69XXY. Cultures were karyotyped in 20 days (mean).

Further studies were undertaken to evaluate the accuracy of this culture method when applied to samples obtained by blind transcervical aspiration. In 25 cases, tissue was aspirated using a 16-gauge Medicut cannula attached to a 20 ml syringe. Eleven of the samples contained chorionic villi, together with other tissues in some cases. Five of the samples were cultured, of which two failed due to fungal infection. A normal male karyotype was obtained from two of the successful cultures, and a normal female karyotype from the third, which correlated with the karyotype obtained from fetal cells (Niazi, 1982). A further series of nine cultures successfully yielded karyotypes within 18 days, of which five were male and four were female. The karyotypes of the mesenchymal cells were identical to those of the corresponding fetuses (Niazi *et al.*, 1981).

Simoni *et al.* (1983) adapted Niazi's method for *in situ* culture of villi on coverslips. They applied this modification to 32 villous specimens, and obtained growth in all of them. Karyotypes were obtained in 30 cases, 11 of which were male, and 14 female. Maternal cell contamination was detected in five samples where a male karyotype was subsequently detected from fetal control cultures. In one case, where the fetus was female, four of 11 cultured cells were found to be of maternal origin, while the remaining seven cells had identical polymorphisms as those of the control culture. After the fifteenth sample, however, no evidence of maternal cell contamination was found and this improvement was attributed to more accurate selection of the villi with increasing experience. This group were able to obtain karyotypes in 8–16 days if RPMI supplemented with 20% FCS (fetal calf serum) was used as the culture medium, but this could be reduced to 4–7 days when cells were grown in Chang medium (Chang *et al.*, 1982).

Schwab *et al.* (1984) also used a medium which, like Chang medium, was supplemented with hormones and growth factors. By seeding petri dishes with a cell suspension dissociated from chorionic villi with trypsin and collagenase treatments, this group obtained cell growth suitable for chromosome analysis in 4–8 days.

Martinez *et al.* (1983) investigated several parameters to determine optimal conditions for culturing trophoblast cells and an assessment of the suitability of these cells for fetal chromosome studies. Material derived from term placentae was minced into 1 mm^2 pieces, and treated with trypsin/EDTA. Supernatant was removed several times during the enzyme treatment, after which the fractions were centrifuged. After an erythrocyte lysis treatment, trophoblast cells were inoculated into flasks. Factors such as cell density, oxygen concentration, medium volume, medium changes and glucose concentration in the medium were analysed, and optimum conditions for culture were defined. Despite these results, the authors still noted an extremely slow pace of cell replication which was barely sufficient to provide enough metaphases for karyotyping. Maternal cell contamination was demonstrated in five of eight placentae from male fetuses. In addition, Down's syndrome. It is possible that this group's poor success with trophoblast culture was due to their use of material obtained from term placentae, since it is clear from earlier work such as that of Stewart *et al.* (1947) that growth potential decreases with increasing gestational age. Indeed, the most successful of these earlier workers were those who used material from early gestations (Thiede, 1960; Valenti, 1965), in contrast to those who used term placentae (Carr, 1964; Hall and Källén, 1964).

Despite the promising results obtained by Niazi *et al.* (1981) and Simoni *et al.* (1983) using the trypsinization/filtration approach to chorionic villus culture, it was clear that, in practice, the procedure was time-consuming and needed to be simplified for routine use. Simoni *et al.* (1983) turned their attention to the development of a method for obtaining metaphase spreads directly from spontaneous mitoses in the cytotrophoblast, which had the potential advantages of speed, and freedom from the problem of maternal cell contamination.

The group at St Mary's Hospital, London, continued their investigations into long-term tissue culture of trophoblast. Niazi *et al.* (1981) had shown that rapid cell growth from chorionic villi could only be achieved if the mesenchyme core was exposed, and this had been accomplished by the use of enzyme treatments. With this in mind, Heaton *et al.* (1984) postulated that the mesenchyme core could be exposed without the need for trypsinization, by simply mincing the villi with a blade. This idea represented a return to the 'explant' approach originally employed in early studies, but differed from these techniques in two ways. First, the tissue was minced beyond the 1 mm^2 fragment stage described by other authors; indeed, it was 'macerated' to a mushy consistency achieved only by repeated cutting with a scalpel blade. Secondly, by spreading the pieces across the surface of a flask, and subsequently inverting it for 24 hours, or 'sandwiching' between two coverslips, the need for plasma clots for tissue adherence was eliminated. Numerous tiny villous fragments could be generated by this method, many of which were composed of mesenchyme core, or which exposed mesenchymatous material along at least part of the fragment surface.

This technique was applied to 50 chorionic villus samples aspirated by blind aspiration. Growth was obtained in 39 (78%) cases of which 18 had a normal male karyotype, and 21 had a normal female karyotype. Karyotypes from fetal fibroblasts were available in 11 of the cases where villous cells had a female karyotype, and of these, eight were 46XX and two were 46XY. Karyotypes were obtained in 16 days (mean). Most of the samples which failed to grow were either degenerating villi probably aspirated from the chorion laeve, or were too small (less than 1 mg). Maternal cell contamination was demonstrated in at least two cases, but these were among the first to be examined, and as experience of handling villous material increased, so did the accuracy of the results.

The effects of this 'learning curve' were substantiated by the results obtained from a further series of 125 experimental cultures established from chorionic villus samples aspirated under ultrasound guidance (Czepulkowski *et al.*, 1986). Karyotypes were obtained from 121 (97%) of the samples, of which 66 (55%) were normal male, 51 (42%) were normal female, and four (3%) had an abnormal chromosome constitution. Of the cultures with a female karyotype, 32 (56%) were confirmed as fetal by comparison with fetal fibroblasts. An overall success rate of 97% was achieved in this series, and 84% of the cultures were confirmed as being of fetal origin. In no case was there evidence of maternal cell contamination. Karyotypes were obtained in 18 days (mean), although this was reduced to 11 days (mean) when cells were cultured in Chang medium.

At this point the culture method of Heaton *et al.* (1984) was applied to diagnostic cases both at St Mary's Hospital, London, and King's College Hospital, London, and combined data from the first 100 cases were reported (Czepulkowski *et al.*, 1986). Karyotypes from 97 of the 100 samples were obtained within two weeks, of which 47 (48%) were normal male, 39 (40%) were normal female, and 11 (11%) had an abnormal chromosome constitution. Of the 39 samples with a female karyotype, 28 were confirmed as being of fetal origin by comparison with cultures from fetal or maternal tissues, or with direct preparations. Thus, to date of publication, the accuracy of 87% of the successful cultures was demonstrated. The remaining results have since been verified.

Gustavii *et al.* (1984) also used an explant technique to culture trophoblast tissue, but this group used a Flaskette chamber attached to a microscope slide, instead of flasks or dishes. Minced villous fragments were distributed on to the floor of the chamber, which could be removed when colonies of actively dividing cells were observed. Harvest techniques could then be applied directly to the cell colonies on the slides. Villi were sampled by the 'direct vision' technique (Kullander and Sandahl, 1973; Gustavii, 1983) which enabled selection of placental villi, recognizable by an abundance of blood vessels and 'buds', which were free from contaminating maternal tissues.

The early problems associated with chorionic villus culture, namely poor growth potential, and maternal cell contamination, have now been overcome to the extent that the procedure is suitable for the routine diagnosis of chromosome defects. The relative merits of culture and direct techniques are fully discussed in the chapter dealing with direct chromosome preparation from chorionic villi.

25.3 CHORIONIC VILLUS CULTURE TECHNIQUE

25.3.1 The Maceration Technique (modified from Heaton *et al.*, 1984)

(a) Media

Wash medium: 100 ml basic medium (e.g. MEM, TC199)
5 ml heparin without preservatives (5000 units)
20 ml fetal calf serum
3 ml penicillin/streptomycin (5000 units/ml)
2 ml kanamycin (100×) (10 000 μg/ml)
1.5 ml mycostatin (100 000 units)

Culture media: Chang medium (Hana Biologicals inc., Berkeley, California) supplemented with *L*-glutamine and antibiotics, and reconstituted as recommended by the manufacturer.
Hams Nutrient Mixture F10 as normally used for routine culture of amniotic fluid.

(b) Preliminary treatment of specimens

1. Prepare six-well multi-dishes (Nunc) with 2 ml wash medium in each.
2. Collect samples directly into wash medium. This is best achieved by taking 5 ml medium into the syringe before sampling so that the aspirate is sucked through the cannula and straight into medium. This is then expelled into the well.
3. If the sample is bloodstained it may be necessary to remove solid material from the well and place it into an adjacent well. Villous material is recognizable from its white, frond-like appearance and will be apparent with the naked eye. Examination with a microscope or light box may be useful for assessment.

(c) Culture of the specimen

1. Wash the specimen in wash medium as many times as necessary, until villous material can be clearly identified. Remove all other tissue by teasing off with a 1 ml syringe (without needle) or Pasteur pipette. It is important to remove all material with a loose amorphous appearance.
2. Place pure villous pieces in a small plastic petri dish and add two to three drops of Chang medium from 0.2 ml held in a 1 ml syringe.
3. Macerate to a very fine consistency (less than 0.5 mm^2) by repeatedly cutting with a size 22 scalpel blade.

4. Suspend the fragments in the remainder of the 0.2 ml Chang medium. Mix thoroughly and draw suspension into syringe.
5. Inoculate into flasks or on to coverslips as follows:

(d)(i) Flask cultures

Distribute macerate evenly on to the surface of a 25 cm^2 tissue culture flask and invert. Add 5 ml Chang medium so that it is not in contact with adhering tissue fragments. Incubate overnight and reinvert so that medium now bathes adherent fragments.

(d)(ii) Coverslip cultures

Four-well multi-dishes (Nunc) are prepared with cleaned, and sterilized glass coverslips diameter 13 mm. One drop of macerate from the 1 ml syringe is placed on to the coverslip in each of the four wells. Another coverslip is placed on top, thus sandwiching the tissue fragments. 0.75 ml Chang medium is added to each.

(e) Maintenance of cultures

All cultures are incubated at 37°C. If they are to be grown in an 'open' system, an atmosphere of 5% CO_2 and 97% humidity is used. Cultures can, however, be grown in a closed system if a final concentration of 200 mM HEPES buffer is added to the culture media.

Once satisfactory growth has been established, Hams F10 can be substituted for Chang medium, and the cultures can be maintained in this. Trypsinization, and *in situ* methods of cell harvest can be applied to cultures as for amniotic fluid cultures.

Fig. 25.1 illustrates a G-banded metaphase spread obtained from an *in situ* harvested chorionic villus culture.

25.4 CELL TYPES PRESENT IN CHORIONIC VILLUS CULTURES

Many authors have described, and attempted to identify, the cell types obtained from placental cultures by morphology, enzyme histochemistry, and hormone synthesis. This work has been extensively reviewed by Loke (1983) to which the reader is referred for a more detailed account than is possible within the scope of this chapter.

Three cell types have been recognized in cultures from term placentae and from earlier villous material. These are as follows:

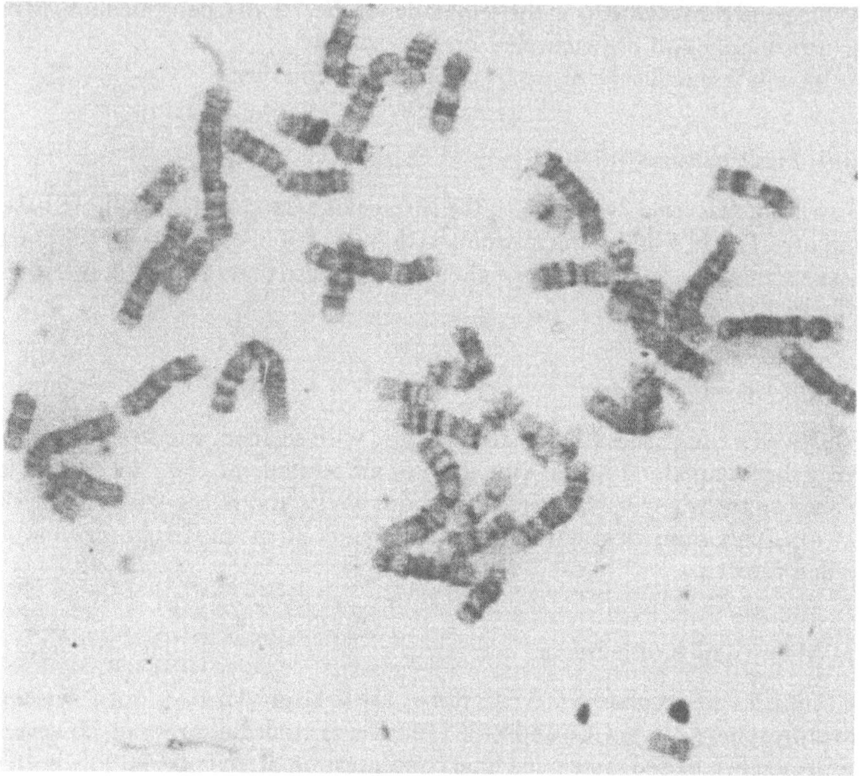

Figure 25.1 G-banded metaphase spread obtained from *in situ* harvested chorionic villus culture.

1. spindle-shaped cells
2. small round or polygonal cells
3. large multi-nucleated cells

The spindle-shaped cells tend to predominate in most cultures, and some authors have described these as fibroblastic (Niazi *et al.*, 1981; Loke, 1983; Heaton *et al.*, 1984). It is likely that only a few of these cells are fibroblastic, the majority being derived from the mesenchyme stroma, since they show a content of enzymes very similar to that of the villous stromal cells in the intact placenta (Fox and Kharkongor, 1970b). Niazi *et al.* (1981) obtained this cell type only in cultures from mesenchyme core tissue which had been stripped of the trophoblast layers, and they were not associated with secretion of human chorionic gonadotrophin (HCG).

The small round, or polygonal cells have been shown to be cytotrophoblastic in origin, and have been described as 'epithelioid' (Thiede,

1960; Thiede and Rudolph, 1961). This cell type has been shown to produce HCG (Loke and Borland, 1970). Niazi *et al.* (1981) obtained these cells from cultures of cytotrophoblast strips which had been removed from the chorionic villi. They did not proliferate, however, and rapidly died out. Stewart *et al.* (1947) described these cells as Langhans cells.

The large, multi-nucleated cells were also seen in cultures from cytotrophoblast strips (Niazi *et al.*, 1981), but these also disintegrated after a few days. Fox and Kharkongor (1970) noted that the histochemical reactions of these cells were very similar to those of the syncytiotrophoblast of the intact placental villi.

The behaviour of the cell types varied as the cultures progressed, and depended also on whether the culture had been established from explants or by enzyme dissociation. Up to four additional cell types have been described by various authors (Loke, 1983; von Koskull, 1985). One of these, a large ovoid cell described by Fox and Kharkongor (1970a), was thought by these authors to be Hofbauer cells since the enzyme histochemistry is suggestive of this. Another cell type, prominent in cultures from basal plate villi containing abundant cytotrophoblast cell columns, are of a large, irregular shape and form colonies with a 'crazy-paving' morphology (Loke, 1983; Lueck and Aladjem, 1980). Loke suggests that these may be derived from maternal decidual cells of the basal plate. Heaton *et al.* (1984) demonstrated the presence of this cell type, which they described as 'convoluted cells', in cultures of chorionic villi obtained by blind transcervical aspiration. Polyploid karyotypes were obtained from this cell type, but this always corresponded to the fetal sex, thus showing that these cells are not of maternal origin.

The nature and origins of the various cell types present in chorionic villus cultures is of particular importance for the study of cell function and diagnosis of inborn errors of metabolism. The cytogeneticist, however, can make use of any cell type providing it is capable of rapid cell division, and accurately reflects the fetal karyotype. The spindle-shaped cells are the most suitable for chromosome studies. It is, however, difficult to distinguish these from fibroblasts which may be maternal in origin, so a culture cannot be identified as fetal, maternal or a mixture on the basis of morphology alone.

A further application of chorionic villus culture has been suggested by the work of Tyms *et al.* (in press) involving the use of trophoblast cells for the study of virus replication.

25.5 TROPHOBLAST CELLS AND VIRUS REPLICATION

The use of cell culture systems for the isolation and growth of viruses is valuable for diagnosis and research but probably provides an artificial environment when compared with virus growth *in vitro*. In the case of viruses that cause human disease, the conditions of growth *in vitro* are often totally alien with respect to the host species and cell type. In addition, it is not clear how representative the fraction of virus that freely replicates in cell culture relates to the virus that actually causes disease. Analysis of the specific characteristics of cells used in medical research, coupled with a better understanding of cell growth *in vitro* has led to the availability of novel cell culture for the study of virus infections. This is illustrated by the work of Tyms *et al.* (in press) which involves the isolation and growth of human cytomegalovirus (CMV) in human trophoblast cells derived from first trimester chorionic villus samples (Plates I and II). CMV is a member of the herpes virus family, and is an important cause of morbidity and mortality in neonates and in patients who are immuno-suppressed (Tyms, 1982; Betts, 1982).

This virus is highly species specific and grows well *in vitro* only in cells of fibroblastic origin, whereas in the whole animal the virus is known generally to infect epithelial cells. Tyms *et al.* (in press) have demonstrated that clinical isolates of CMV replicate far more efficiently in cells cultured from chorionic villi than in fibroblast cells. The placental cells have been shown to express markers which characterize them as cells of trophoblastic origin.

The transplacental passage of virus is considered to be the major route for infection of the fetus with CMV. The efficiency of transmission of the virus to the fetus during primary infection in the mother is between 20% and 50%. One reason for this relatively inefficient transmission may well relate to variation in the pathogenicity of the virus strain involved or to the genetic disposition of fetus and placenta, which can be considered as a partial allograft. The novel interaction between human CMV and the natural environment of the early placental cells should provide important information in the study of congenital infections due to this virus.

25.6 FUTURE DEVELOPMENTS

The development of chorionic villus culture for diagnostic purposes is concerned primarily with eliminating the risk of maternal cell contamination, and reducing the time taken for a result to be obtained. Preliminary studies on the use of monoclonal antibodies for selective elimination of maternal cells have been initiated at St Mary's Hospital, London. The most significant advance has, however, been the application of the 'Pipette method', developed by Claussen (1980) for the early harvesting of amniotic fluid cells, to chorionic villus cultures. This harvesting method enables the first mitotic cells appearing in the culture to be utilized, while the remainder of the culture can be maintained if necessary.

The 'sandwich' coverslip cultures described by Heaton *et al.* (1984) are separated after 4–5 days, and treated with colcemid on the following day.

Plate I

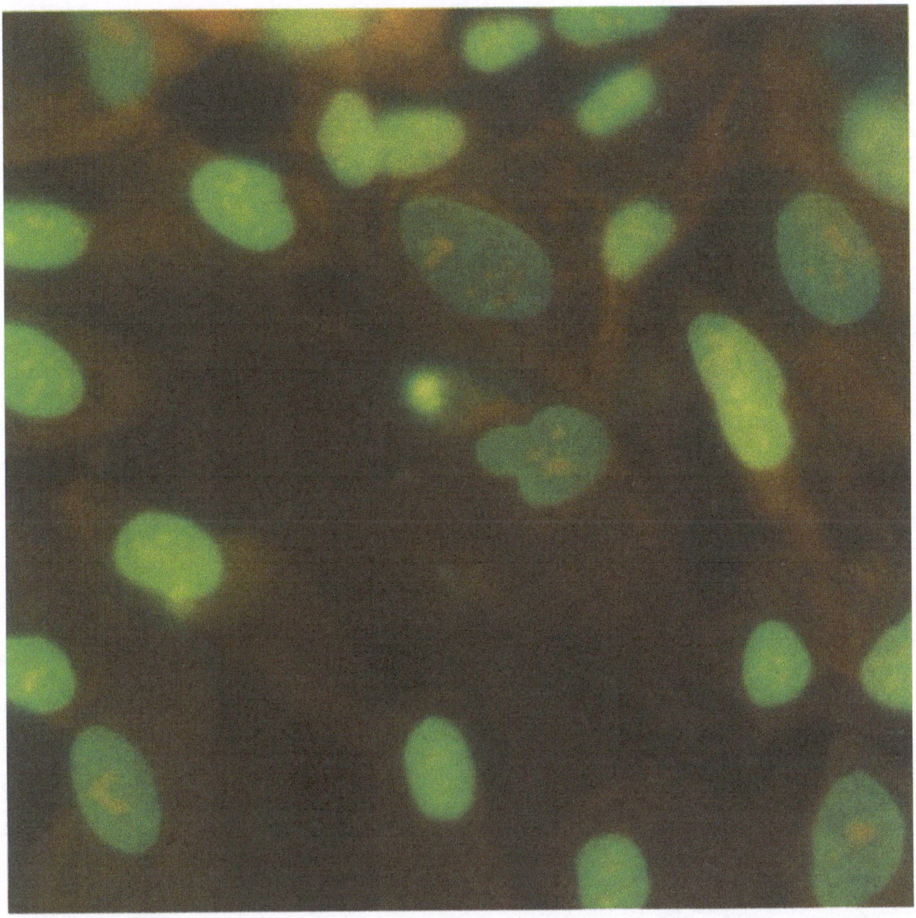

Plates I and II Cells obtained from chorion villus sampling material by the method of Heaton *et al.* (1984) were expanded in cell culture. Monolayers of cells were either sham-infected (*Plate I*) or infected with a low-passage clinical isolate of human cytomegalovirus and incubated at 37°C for five days (*Plate II*). The intra-nuclear and intra-cytoplasmic sites containing viral DNA in the infected cells were resolved as apple-green inclusions by acridine orange staining.

Plate II

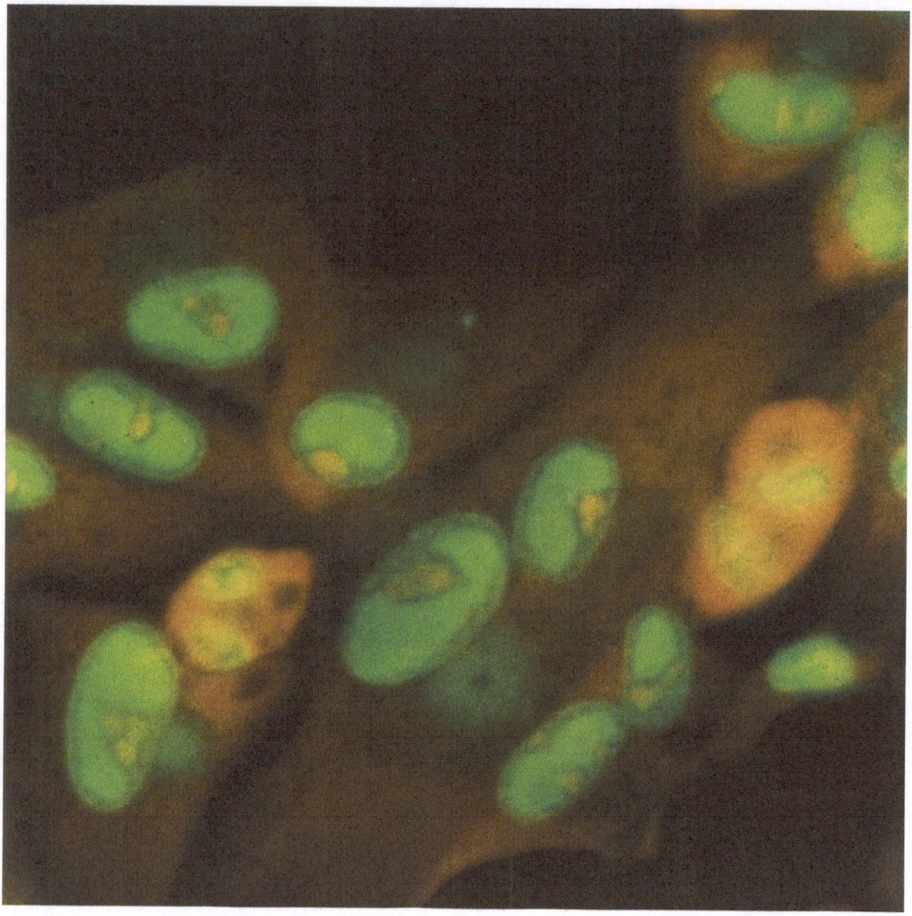

The coverslips can then be placed cell side upwards into a petri dish which is placed on a X63 invertoscope. An attenuated Pasteur pipette of tip bore size 20–60 μm, held in a simple micromanipulator, is positioned over the cell colonies and guided towards those in mitosis. Gentle suction is applied via a tube attached to the pipette and mitotic cells are individually detached and taken into the pipette. They are then expelled into hypotonic KCl solution and once more drawn into the pipette. The cells are then fixed by drawing a small volume of 3:1 methanol/acetic acid into the pipette. Drops of cell suspension are then expelled onto cleaned, wet slides, and routine staining and banding techniques can be applied.

A preliminary series of eight chorionic villus cultures harvested in this way were all karyotyped in seven days, some 3–4 days earlier than is usual with conventional harvesting procedures (Claussen *et al.*, 1986).

25.7 THE PLACE OF CHORIONIC VILLUS CULTURE IN PRENATAL DIAGNOSIS

Cells cultured from chorionic villi are suitable for the prenatal diagnosis of all chromosome defects, many inborn errors of metabolism, and DNA hybridization studies. The latter uses are considered in other chapters, and will not be repeated here.

When considering the use of chorionic villus culture for cytogenetic studies, it is necessary to evaluate the reliability of the technique, and the accuracy of the results obtained when compared with the standards expected from amniotic fluid culture. Furthermore, this technique must be assessed in relation to the direct methods of preparing fresh trophoblast material for karyotyping, which are examined in Chapter 24.

REFERENCES

Betts, R. F. (1982) CMV-induced disease in transplant patients. *Prog. Med. Virol.*, **28**, 44–64.

Carr, M. C. (1964) Human term placental villi in explant tissue culture. *Am. J. Obstet. Gynecol.*, **88**, 584–91.

Chang, H. C., Jones, O. W. and Masui, H. (1982) Human amniotic cells grown in a hormone supplemented medium. *Proc. Natl. Acad. Sci. USA.*, **79**, 4795–9.

Claussen, U. (1980) The Pipette Method: A new rapid technique for chromosome analysis in prenatal diagnosis. *Hum. Genet.*, **54**, 277–8.

Claussen, U., Heaton, D. E. and Coleman, D. V. (1986) Rapid karyotyping of chorionic villus cultures by a single cell harvest technique. *J. Med. Genet.*, **23**, 79.

Coleman, D. V. (1982) Endocervical lavage in early pregnancy. *Am. J. Obstet. Gynecol.*, **142**, 118–19.

Czepulkowski, B. H., Heaton, D. E., Kearney, L. U., Rodeck, C. H. and Coleman, D. V. (1986) Chorionic villus culture for first trimester diagnosis of chromosome defects: Evaluation by two London centres. *Prenat. Diag.*, **6**, 271–86.

Fox, H. and Kharkongor, F. N. (1970a) Morphology and enzyme histochemistry of cell derived from placental villi in tissue culture. *J. Path.*, **101**, 267–76.

Fox, H. and Kharkongor, F. N. (1970b) Immunofluorescent localisation of chorionic gonadotrophin in the placenta and in tissue cultures of human trophoblast. *J. Path.*, **101**, 277–81.

Goldberg, M. F., Chen, A. T. L., Ahn, Y. W. and Reidy, J. A. (1980) First-trimester fetal chromosome diagnosis using endocervical lavage: A negative evaluation. *Am. J. Obstet. Gynecol.*, **138**, 436–40.

Gustavii, B. (1983) First-trimester chromosomal analysis of chorionic villi obtained by direct vision technique. *Lancet*, **ii**, 507–8.

Gustavii, B., Chester, M. A., Edvall, H., Iosif, S., Kristoffersson, U., Lofberg, L., Mineur, A. and Mitelman, F. (1984) First-trimester diagnosis on chorionic villi obtained by direct vision technique. *Hum. Genet.*, **65**, 373–6.

Hahnemann, N. and Mohr, J. (1968) Genetic diagnosis in the embryo by means of biopsy from extraembryonic membranes. *Bull. Europ. Soc. Hum. Genet.*, **2**, 23–9.

Hahnemann, N. and Mohr, J. (1969) Antenatal fetal diagnosis in genetic disease. *Bull. Europ. Soc. Hum. Genet.*, **3**, 47–54.

Hahnemann, N. (1972) Possibility of culturing foetal cells at early stages of pregnancy. *Clin. Genet.*, **3**, 286–93.

Hahnemann, N. (1974) Early prenatal diagnosis; A study of biopsy techniques and cell culturing from extraembyronic membranes. *Clin. Genet.*, **6**, 294–306.

Hall, B. and Kallen, B. (1964) Chromosome studies in abortuses and stillborn infants. *Lancet*, **ii**, 110.

Heaton, D. E., Czepulkowski, B. H., Horwell, D. H. and Coleman, D. V. (1984) Chromosome analysis of first trimester chorionic villus biopsies prepared by a maceration technique. *Prenat. Diag.*, **4**, 279–87.

Jones, G. E. S., Gey, G. O. and Gey, M. K. (1943) Hormone production by placental cells maintained in continuous culture. *Bull. Johns Hopkins Hosp.*, **72**, 26.

Kullander, S. and Sandahl, B. (1973) Fetal chromosome analysis after transcervical placental biopsies during early pregnancy. *Acta Obstet. Gynec. Scand.*, **52**, 355–9.

Loke, Y. W. (1983) Human Trophoblast in culture. In *Biology of Trophoblast* (eds Loke and Whyte), Elsevier Science Publishers BV,

Loke, Y. W. and Borland, R. (1970) Immunofluorescent localization of Chorionic Gonadotrophin in monolayer cultures of human trophoblast cells. *Nature*, **228**, 561–2.

Lueck, J. and Aladjem, M. D. (1980) Time-lapse study of normal human trophoblast *in vitro*. *Am. J. Obstet. Gynecol.*, **138**, 288–92.

Martinez, F., Cheung, S. W., Crane, J. P. and Arias, F. (1983) Use of trophoblast cells in tissue culture for fetal chromosomal studies. *Am. J. Obstet. Gynecol.*, **147**, 542–7.

Niazi, M., Coleman, D. V. and Loeffler, F. E. (1981) Trophoblast sampling in early pregnancy. Culture of rapidly dividing cells from immature placental villi. *Brit. J. Obstet. Gynaecol.*, **88**, 1081–5.

Niazi, M. (1982) PhD Thesis. University of London, London.

Rhine, S. A., Palmer, C. G. and Thompson, T. F. (1977) A simple alternative to amniocentesis for first trimester prenatal diagnosis. *Birth Defects*, **13**, 231.

Rhine, S. A. and Milunsky, A. (1979) Utilisation of trophoblast for early prenatal diagnosis. In *Genetic Disorders and the Fetus* (ed. A. Milunsky), Plenum Press. New York, p. 527.

Schwab, M. E., Muller, C. H. and Schmid-Tannwald, I. (1984) Fast and reliable culture method for cells from 8–10 week trophoblast tissue. *Lancet*, **i**, 1082.

Shettles, L. B. (1971) Use of Y chromosome in prenatal sex determination. *Nature*, **230**, 52.

Simoni, G., Brambati, B., Danesino, C., Rossella, F., Terzoli, G. L., Ferrari, M. and Fraccaro, M. (1983) Efficient direct chromosome analysis and enzyme determination from chorionic villi samples in the first trimester of pregnancy. *Hum. Genet.*, **66**, 252–9.

Stewart, H. L., Sano, M. E. and Montgomery, T. L. (1947) Hormone secretion by human placenta grown in tissue culture. *J. Clin. Endocrinol. Metab.*, **8**, 175–88.

Thiede, H. (1960 Studies of the human trophoblast in tissue culture. *Am. J. Obstet. Gynecol.*, **79**, 636–47.

Thiede, H. and Rudolph, J. H. (1961) A method for obtaining monolayer cultures of human fetal cells from term placentas. *Proc. Soc. Exp. Biol. Med.*, **107**, 565–9.

Tyms, A. S. (1982) Human cytomegalovirus infection of the fetus and neonate. *Med. Lab. Sci.*, **39**, 275–86.

Tyms, A. S., Davis, J. M., Clarke, J. R., Coleman, D. V. and Heaton, D. E. (in press) The growth of human cytomegalovirus in trophoblast cells from first trimester chorionic villus biopsies.

Valenti, C. (1965) Chromosomal study of trophoblastic tissue. *Am. J. Obstet. Gynecol.*, **92**, 211–20.

Von Koskull, H. Ämmälä, P., Aula, P. and Virtanen I. (1985) Cytoskeletal and lectin marker for cells cultured from chorionic villi and decidua. In *First Trimester Fetal Diagnosis* (eds M. Fraccaro, G. Simoni and B. Brambati) Springer-Verlag, Berlin.

Warren, R., Sanchez, L., Hammond, D. and McLeod, A. (1972) Prenatal sex determination from exfoliated cells found in cervical mucosa. *Am. J. Hum. Genet.*, **24**, 29a.

26

Recombinant DNA technology and prenatal diagnosis

Stephen R. Barnes

26.1 INTRODUCTION

The ability to detect genetic lesions at the DNA level has improved both the speed and precision of prenatal diagnosis. Conventional assays, based on the protein products of defective genes, frequently depend upon quantitative differences between normal and affected individuals. Furthermore, they require the gene in question to be active in the tissue used for sampling – a condition that is not always fulfilled. Since virtually all human cell types contain a full complement of DNA, the structure of any gene may be determined with confidence using DNA from any tissue. The purpose of this chapter is to introduce the principles and methodology that are used in prenatal diagnosis at the DNA level. Specifically, we will consider the types of mutation that may be distinguished, and the particular techniques best suited to each type. Provided that a suitable cloned sequence of DNA is available, it should be possible to make a qualitative distinction between alleles at a locus responsible for a given inherited condition.

26.2 BASIC PRINCIPLES

The problem of distinguishing two genes that differ by a single base pair – a normal and a mutant allele – is not minor. Its solution has two components:

1. the detection of the particular sequence of DNA among the rest of the genome – the human genome contains 3×10^9 base pairs (bp) of DNA, so that a single gene of 3000 bp (3 kbp) makes up only one millionth of the total DNA present;

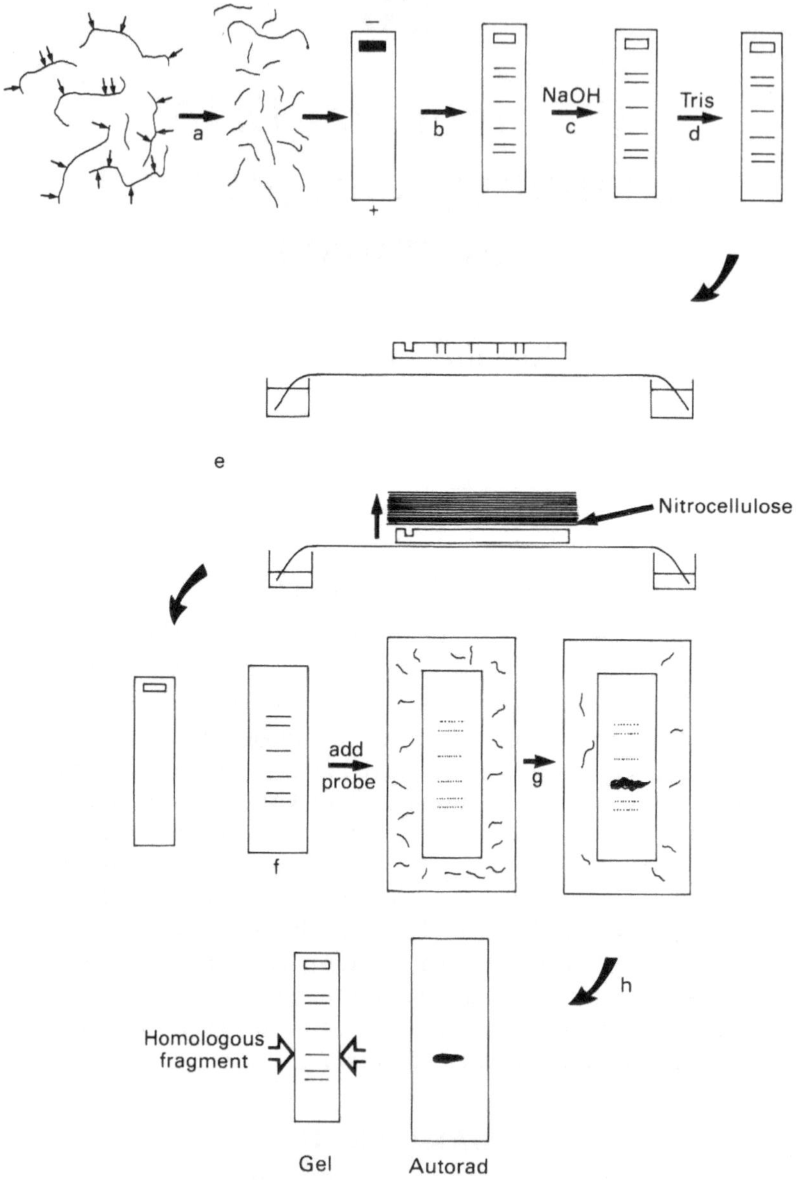

Figure 26.1 *The Southern 'blot' technique.* Purified DNA is digested with the appropriate restriction enzyme(s) (a), and the fragments resolved using agarose gel electrophoresis (b). DNA may be visualized by UV fluorescence in the presence of ethidium bromide at this point. The DNA is rendered single-stranded by alkaline denaturation (c), neutralized (d), and transferred to a nitrocellulose or nylon membrane by the flow of transfer buffer, drawn upwards by a blotting pad (e). The DNA bands retain their relative position and are baked onto the membrane (f). The

2. the detection of the difference in base sequence between the normal and mutant alleles.

Thus the problem is not dissimilar from that of finding the proverbial needle in its haystack.

The first part of the problem (that of identifying the gene of interest) may be solved provided that we have a purified copy of the particular sequence that we seek. This will normally be in the form of a recombinant molecule: the gene will have been isolated by molecular cloning, usually in bacterial cells. Pieces of DNA that are homologous in sequence to our cloned fragment may be identified using the specificity of complementary base pairing in double-stranded DNA. The cloned sequence will be able to form a stable duplex (or *hybridize*) only with its homologous region in the DNA under analysis; by radio-labelling the purified sequence (chemical labelling is also possible, see below) we have a 'probe' that may be used to identify such regions within any sample of DNA.

The second part of the problem (determining the structure of the gene in the bulk DNA preparation) may be tackled in various ways, depending upon the difference between mutant and normal genes. In general, however, these rely upon the combined use of DNA probes, restriction endonucleases, and gel electrophoresis. Bacterial *restriction endonucleases* recognize specific DNA sequences (usually four or six base pairs in length), and cleave within that site. Any particular region of the DNA will contain these sequences at defined sites, and will therefore be cleaved in a predictable way to yield DNA fragments of defined sizes. The fragments that result from restriction enzyme digestion may be resolved according to molecular weight by electrophoresis in agarose gels, and the particular fragments that are homologous to a specific cloned probe may be identified by DNA:DNA hybridization. The separated fragments are denatured in the gel, and transferred to a membrane filter (made of nitrocellulose or nylon) where they retain the pattern of separation achieved in the gel during electrophoresis. This procedure, known as Southern blotting (Southern, 1975) is illustrated in Fig. 26.1. The immobilized DNA is now available for hybridization to a suitable labelled probe sequence; any probe that binds non-specifically may be removed using carefully controlled salt/temperature combinations for the rinses, and the bands of DNA within the gel that are homologous to the probe may be visualized by autoradiography of the filter. Thus, using this approach, it is possible to determine the number and size of DNA fragments that correspond to the probe of interest.

---

membrane is now incubated in a solution of labelled, single-stranded probe DNA, which forms stable hybrid duplices only with complementary sequences bound to the filter (g). The position(s) of hybridization may be visualized by autoradiography (h).

26.3 DETECTION OF SPECIFIC TYPES OF MUTATION

26.3.1 Changes that lead to different sizes of restriction fragments

Where individuals have regions of the chromosome that differ in their pattern of restriction sites, digestion with the enzymes concerned will clearly result in fragments of differing lengths; they are said to display restriction fragment length polymorphism, or RFLP. RFLPs are the simplest class of changes that may be used to distinguish normal from mutant genes. They may be considered simply as another form of allelic variation, scored at the level of the DNA, visualized as a difference in hybridization pattern to restriction enzyme-digested DNA. Their usefulness in prenatal screening depends upon the position of the polymorphic restriction site in relation to the mutation that is of prime interest; four cases will be considered briefly, to illustrate the application of this technique, and to highlight its advantages and limitations.

(a) The mutation itself leads to the introduction or loss of a restriction site

When the change in DNA sequence that leads to the mutation under analysis happens to lie within a restriction enzyme recognition site, the change in sequence will result in the *loss* of that site; the enzyme will no longer cut at that point, and the DNA fragment(s) homologous to the probe will change in size and/or number, the nature of the change being dependent upon the position of the restriction site change relative to the region of homology with the labelled probe. A similar type of change in restriction fragments will be seen in cases where the primary lesion in the DNA leads to the *generation* of a new site. These possibilities are illustrated in Fig. 26.2(a).

This type of change is rare. Since only a limited number of sequences form sites for restriction endonucleases, only those mutations that lie within such sites (actual or potential) can give rise to such changes. Where they do occur, however, they are extremely useful – the change that is being scored in the analysis is precisely the difference responsible for the inherited condition.

(b) Insertions and deletions

In cases where the mutation is caused by the insertion or deletion of genetic material, the fragment(s) homologous to the probe will change size; the change may be detected by blot hybridization (Fig. 26.2(b)).

(c) Changes in restriction sites linked to the mutation

Most mutations do not lead directly to changes in the restriction pattern of the affected region of the DNA. The human genome is not monomorphic,

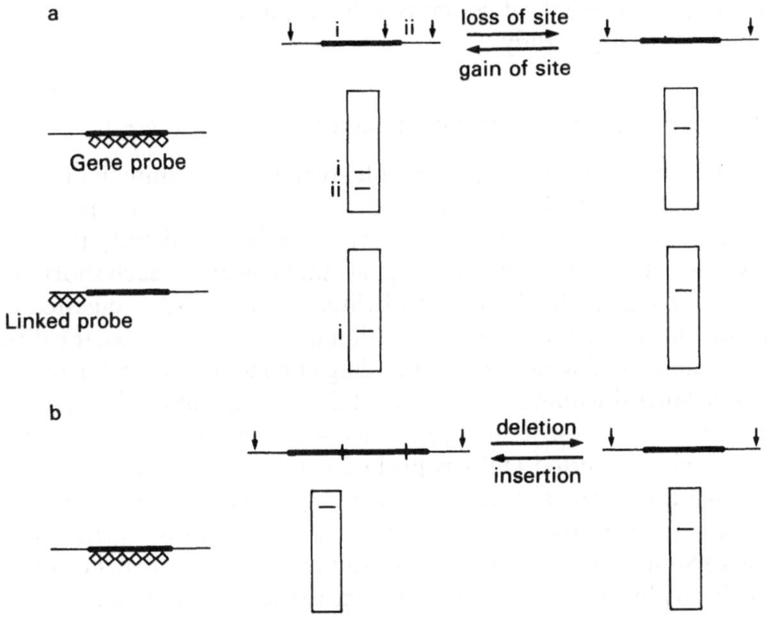

Figure 26.2 *RFLP caused by the mutation under diagnosis.* (a) If mutation introduces or removes a restriction site. Depending upon the nature of the probe used (homologous to ◇◇◇, in figure), either the number or molecular weight of hybridizing fragments will change. (b) Effect of an insertion or deletion on the size of restriction fragments.

however, and most individuals differ at a large number of nucleotides, many of which lead to changes in restriction enzyme cutting sites (leading to RFLPs). Provided that such a site is linked tightly to the mutant gene in question, it may be possible to use this RFLP as a marker for the mutant allele. For this approach to be useful it is necessary to establish, for the family under study, that the linked site is indeed polymorphic, and to find out whether the presence or the absence of this polymorphic site is linked to the mutant allele in question.

It is clearly possible to use more than one linked polymorphism to distinguish between chromosomal regions carrying mutant and normal genes. Since the diagnosis is making use of linkage, rather than detecting the lesion itself, the degree of confidence that may be placed in the diagnosis will depend upon the number of sites used and their spatial relationships with the gene itself.

The use of linked RFLPs is perhaps the most generally applicable of approaches, since it does not require any specific information about the nature of the DNA lesion responsible for the disease in question; all that is needed is a DNA probe that originates from a chromosomal site linked to the affected region, which itself contains polymorphisms that are segregating in the population under study.

(d) The use of repetitive sequences linked to genes of interest

The recent discovery of hypervariable regions in mammalian genomes (Jeffreys *et al.*, 1985a,b) has raised the possibility of using the repeated sequences responsible for this variability as probes to identify the variable regions themselves. The number of repeats that constitute each short tandem block varies considerably between individuals. If the DNA is digested with a restriction enzyme that does not cut within the repeated region, the differing size of the array will lead to corresponding changes in particular restriction fragments. Since the human genome contains several hundred such blocks, a similar number of restriction fragments – all variable in size – may be visualized when digested DNA is probed with a cloned repeat (Fig. 26.3).

Although these arrays of repeats are highly variable, they are likely to be sufficiently stable for use in pedigree analysis over one or two generations. By analysis of Southern blot patterns using this probe it may, then, be possible to identify individual bands that show linkage to the condition under diagnosis; the variability over a longer time-scale means that in all but consanguineous unions there will be extensive differences between parental genomes, rendering such analyses feasible.

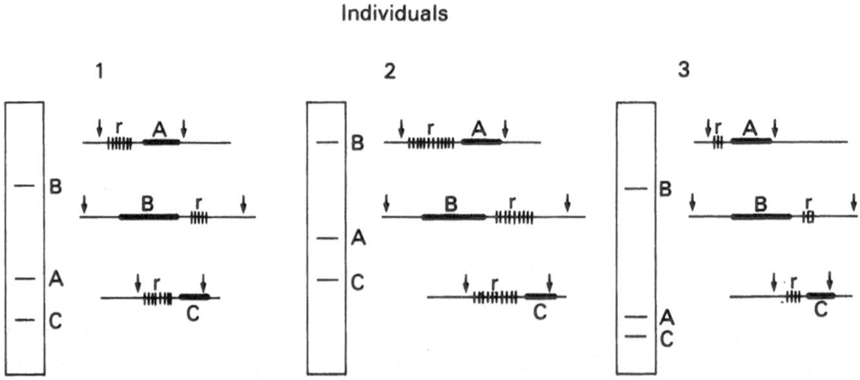

Figure 26.3 *Use of linked hypervariable regions for diagnosis.* Hypervariable regions have recently been shown to be due to variation in the number of copies of short repeated units (r) at a particular site. The effect of this is that, for a particular site, unrelated individuals will have different sized restriction fragments, shown schematically for three genes in each of three individuals. For simplicity, only one copy of each gene is shown.

If, by chance, one such region is closely-linked to the gene of interest, then one of the bands of hybridization to a labelled r probe will segregate with the mutant allele in the family under study.

26.3.2 Changes that do not lead to an alteration of restriction pattern

The approaches already described rely upon changes in the *size* of observable DNA fragments that are homologous to a given probe. A second way is to manipulate experimental conditions such that the probe will hybridize to one, and not the other, of the genes that are to be distinguished. By altering the 'stringency' under which the hybridization is performed, and provided that the probe sequence is sufficiently short, a difference of only one base pair between the probe and the DNA under test may be enough to reduce the stability of the duplex formed by a significant amount. Two methods have been developed that make use of this phenomenon, and are described below.

(a) The use of synthetic oligonucleotide probes

In those cases where the change in DNA sequence responsible for a particular mutation has been determined, it may be possible to devise a short oligonucleotide of DNA that will hybridize preferentially to either the normal or the mutant sequence. Under carefully chosen conditions a probe of, say, seventeen nucleotides will only form stable hybrids when perfectly matched; a single mispaired base will reduce duplex stability to the point where hybridization will not be seen (Fig. 26.4).

Although this method may only be applied in cases where the molecular nature of the mutation has been determined, the speed with which DNA may be sequenced and oligonucleotides synthesized mean that new mutations may

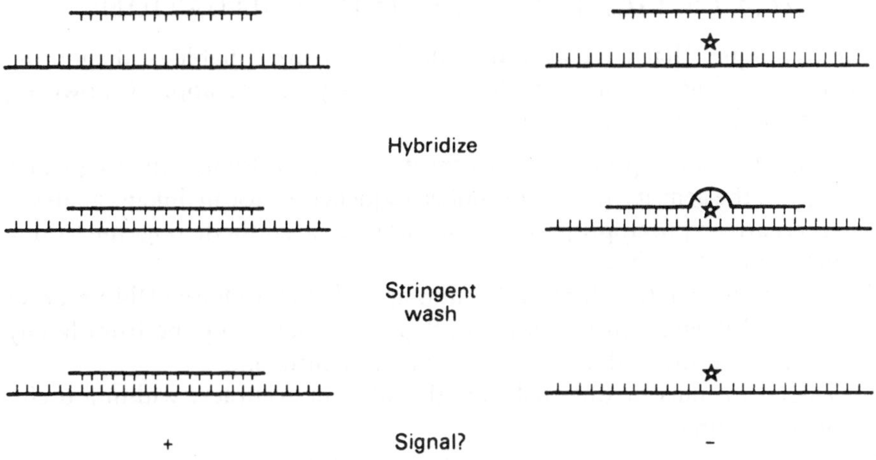

Figure 26.4 *Use of specific oligonucleotide probes to detect single nucleotide changes.* The single base pair difference between the normal and mutant alleles (*) reduces the stability of the duplex formed with the labelled synthetic oligonucleotide (right); in this case, only the normal allele (left) will form a stable hybrid.

be characterized fairly rapidly. The relative expense of this method, however, will probably mean that oligonucleotide probing will only be of real practical use for common conditions of a relatively uniform cause.

(b) The detection of *any* mutation in a defined DNA sequence

A method has been described by which any mutation affecting a defined region of DNA may be detected (Myers *et al.*, 1985). The DNA under analysis is digested and allowed to hybridize with a labelled copy of the normal gene of interest. The hybrid DNA is then electophoresed through a gel that contains a gradient of denaturant. The point at which a hybrid duplex is denatured depends upon the degree of mismatch with the probe sequence, and migration through the gel effectively stops as soon as denaturation occurs. Mutant genes will therefore lead to bands at positions in the gel that differ from the normal bands (Fig. 26.5).

Although this method provides no information about the precise nature of a mutant allele, it is none the less a means of screening any defined sequence of DNA for alterations in nucleotide sequence. A positive result from such an analysis must, of course, be treated with great caution: mutations identified by this method would not necessarily lead to any functional defect in the gene product. It is clearly important to establish the relationship between a 'mutant' band identified in this way, and the inherited defect for which the screening is being carried out. Family studies may, therefore, be needed.

26.4 APPLICATION TO CLINICAL SITUATIONS

The techniques that have been described above are capable of diagnosing most types of genetic abnormality. Before they can be applied, however, certain conditions must be met:

1. A suitable cloned probe sequence must be available for use; this might be a copy of the gene itself, or some linked sequence for use in linkage analysis. Alternatively, in appropriate circumstances, a synthetic oligonucleotide probe may be suitable.
2. The linkage relationships of the mutant allele to the chosen DNA marker site (RFLP, etc.) must be known; this may entail sampling from family members in order that linkage may be established.
3. The result must be obtainable, with sufficient accuracy, within a useful period of time.

Of these preconditions, the first is the most likely to be limiting at present; few probes have yet been identified as being useful in this type of diagnosis, and it is by no means a simple task to isolate more. In general, probes for linkage analysis have been identified by screening a large number of cloned

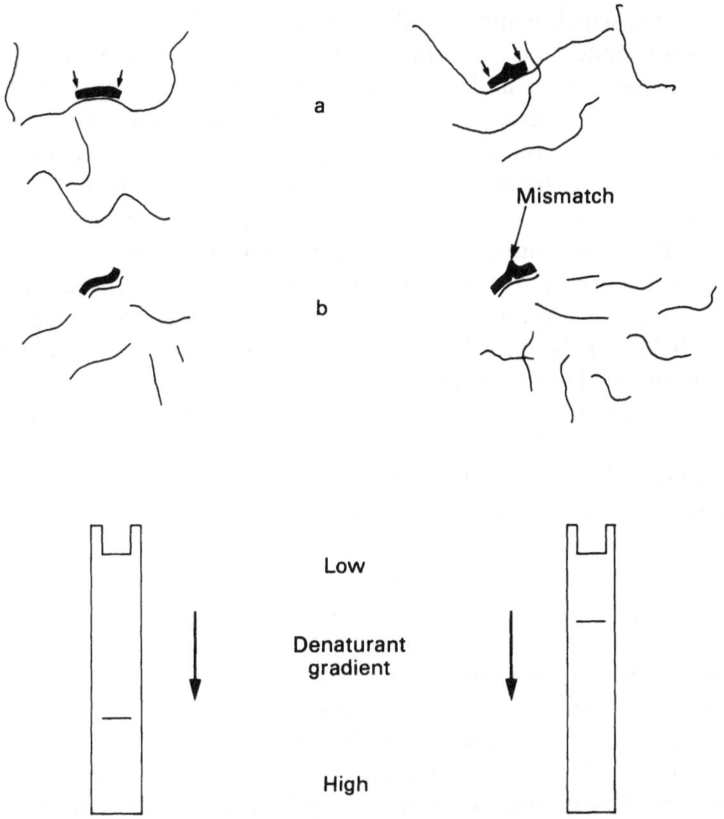

Figure 26.5 *Detection of any change in DNA sequence by using denaturant-gradient gels.* The probe is hybridized to the DNA under test (a), and the hybrid digested with restriction endonculease (b). The point at which the DNA stops in the gel is determined by the concentration of denaturant needed to render it single-stranded; thus a hybrid with mismatched base-pairs (right) will stop before a perfectly matched duplex (left).

unique sequences to find one that is both polymorphic in the population and segregates with the disease of interest. Techniques of chromosome sorting (to purify DNA from one particular chromosome) and chromosome micro-dissection and micro-cloning (for the isolation of DNA from one particular chromosomal location) may well prove to be useful ways of isolating probes that will show linkage to defined chromosomal sites (of use when the chromosomal position of a particular deleterious gene is known). The difficulty of isolating suitable probes may mean that, for many rare conditions, these techniques may prove impractical on purely economic grounds.

The time taken for a diagnosis will vary considerably; clearly, when family studies are required, the whole process may take many weeks to complete. A second factor, which is more easily controlled, is the speed of detection of hybridization bands, etc. Commonly, DNA probes are labelled with ^{32}P-containing precursors, and detection relies upon autoradiography. This presents several problems: detection may often take many days, and since radioactive decay is continuing during the autoradiographic exposure, if a first exposure proves inadequate, then subsequent ones will take even longer. This latter factor is aggravated by ^{32}P's short half-life of 14 days. The short half-life of the radioisotope presents the additional factor that probes must be used soon after preparation; for conditions where diagnoses are comparatively rare (less than once per week, for example), this means that a freshly-labelled probe must be produced each time, thereby increasing both delay and financial costs. Many of these considerations may be overcome by the use of chemical and/or immunochemical detection systems: DNA probes may be labelled using biotin-tagged precursors, and molecules that hybridize may be detected using standard histochemical or immunological methods. Detection may be carried out immediately hybridization has been completed, eliminating the need for time-consuming autoradiography; furthermore, the labelled molecules are stable for many months, suiting them to occasional use. The only possible drawback of biotinylated probes is the slight reduction in sensitivity reported by some workers, but this should be overcome in the near future, as detection systems are improved.

While all of the procedures outlined above are, in theory, straightforward, the technical expertise required for their successful application to clinical cases is considerable. The isolation of DNA, its digestion with restriction enzymes and Southern blot analysis may be carried out with only a few months' training by a competent biochemical technician; other methods would usually require considerably more experience, both in the execution and in the interpretation of results. This type of diagnosis would thus probably be best concentrated in regional centres, unless a particular local population carried sufficiently high frequencies of a condition that local screening programmes for that condition alone would be worthwhile. In general, however, the frequency with which diagnosis of any particular condition is attempted will be low; each will require a different approach for diagnosis – some will simply use RFLP, others oligonucleotide probes, etc. – and it therefore seems desirable to concentrate resources for the diagnosis of each condition in a limited number of centres. Each centre must have the services of molecular biologists and genetic counsellors, experienced in the inheritance and molecular biology of its specialist range of inherited conditions.

Molecular biology has provided the tools needed for its application to the prenatal diagnosis of inherited disease; it is now the turn of health agencies to widen the range of conditions to which this form of screening may be applied, and to establish facilities to make such diagnosis more widely available.

REFERENCES

Jeffreys, A. J. Wilson, V., and Thein, S. L. (1985a) Hypervariable 'minisatellite' regions in human DNA. *Nature*, **314**, 67–73.

Jeffreys, A. J., Wilson, V. and Thein, S. L. (1985b) Individual-specific 'fingerprints' of human DNA. *Nature*, **316**, 76–9.

Myers, R. M., Lumelsky, N., Lerman, L. S. and Maniatis, T. (1985) Detection of single base substitutions in total genomic DNA. *Nature*, **313**, 495–8.

Southern, E. M. (1975) Detection of specific sequences among DNA fragments separated by gel electrophoresis. *J. Mol. Biol.*, **98**, 503–17.

27

Genetic engineering and detection of haemoglobinopathies

J. M. Old

27.1 INTRODUCTION

The haemoglobinopathies are a diverse group of inherited recessive disorders which form the commonest single gene disorder in the world population. A World Health Organisation working party has estimated recently that there are over 200 000 000 carriers for the haemoglobinopathies and that between 200 000 and 300 000 severely affected homozygotes or compound heterozygotes are born each year. Clinically, the most important of these conditions are the α- and β-thalassaemias, sickle-cell anaemia and its variants, and the compound heterozygous state for haemoglobin E and β-thalassaemia (Weatherall and Clegg, 1981). Because there is no definitive treatment for these diseases, and because symptomatic management is expensive and unsatisfactory, their prevention has become a major public health goal for many countries, especially those with a high incidence of β-thalassaemia. The method of control adopted by these countries is to screen the population for carriers, identify pregnant women at risk of carrying a severely affected fetus, offer them the possibility of antenatal diagnosis and, if indicated, a therapeutic abortion.

Prenatal diagnosis of the haemoglobinopathies was first achieved in 1974 by the estimation of the relative rates of globin chain synthesis in a fetal blood sample following the development of fetal blood sampling. This approach, which directly quantifies the product of the mutant globin gene, has been adopted by most countries with a haemoglobinopathy control programme and has been remarkably successful, with over 3000 cases being reported to date (Alter, 1984). It suffers from the disadvantage, however, that fetal blood sampling is not possible until about the 18th week of pregnancy which means a long wait for the mother and, if required, a relatively difficult therapeutic abortion. Such a late diagnosis is not acceptable to some at-risk ethnic groups. In addition, the fetal blood sampling procedure carries a 5% risk of fetal loss, therefore as soon as techniques for the detection of haemoglobinopathies by gene analysis were developed, several centres started using fetal DNA from fetal cells obtained by the safer procedure of amniocentesis. However, amniocentesis is also a mid-trimester procedure and it is often difficult to obtain sufficient cells for DNA analysis without first growing them in culture for several weeks. Following development of procedures for chorion villus sampling, it has been shown to be possible to obtain sufficient fetal DNA between the 9th and 11th week of pregnancy for the diagnosis of the haemoglobinopathies by gene analysis (Old *et al.*, 1982).

27.2 THE DEVELOPMENT OF GENETIC ENGINEERING TECHNIQUES

The haemoglobinopathies are the first group of genetic disorders to be comprehensively studied by the techniques of molecular biology and recombinant DNA technology. This occurred because considerable information about the globin genes was already known from the study of the protein sequence of haemoglobins and the naturally occurring haemoglobin variants and, secondly, because reticulocytes are a good source of relatively pure globin mRNA. The discovery of the enzyme reverse transcriptase enabled DNA probes for hybridization studies to be made from a mRNA template and globin mRNA was quickly used to make DNA copies of the globin gene (cDNAs) which were used to study genomic DNA from patients with various haemoglobinopathies. These cDNA/DNA hybridization experiments led to the discovery that α-thalassaemia was due to a deletion of the α-globin genes and enabled the first prenatal diagnosis of a genetic disease to be made in 1976 by Kan *et al.*, who showed that a fetus with α-thalassaemia could be detected by the reduced hybridization of an α-cDNA probe to fetal DNA obtained from cultured amniotic fluid cells.

Although very useful, these globin cDNA probes were not very pure because they were always made from mRNA which coded for two or more different globin genes (for example, mRNA from normal reticulocytes contains approximately equal amounts of α and β-globin mRNA) and attempts to purify a single cDNA species were never 100% successful. However the development of recombinant DNA technology enabled pure cDNA probes to be prepared by genetically engineering the insertion of a globin cDNA molecule into a plasmid vector. Plasmids are naturally occurring small circular pieces of DNA in the cytoplasm of bacteria which replicate independently of the host bacterial DNA. A bacterium can be infected by only one plasmid (carrying the foreign cDNA insert) and therefore if the infected bacteria are spread out thinly enough on an agar plate, single bacterial cells will grow up into colonies in which every bacterial cell contains the same plasmid with the same cDNA insert. By this method pure α, β and γ-globin gene plasmid probes were isolated (Wilson *et al.*, 1978) which gave much cleaner hybridization signals in Southern blotting experiments than the old cDNA probes.

In 1970, the discovery of restriction endonucleases (enzymes which cut DNA at specific recognition sites) meant that DNA fragments of reproducible size could be produced from genomic DNA. Genomic DNA, however, is cleaved into hundreds of thousands of differently sized fragments, of which only a few contain globin gene sequences and the problem remained of how to identify these few globin gene fragments among all this DNA. This problem was solved in 1975 by Southern who introduced the technique of 'Southern' blotting. By this technique DNA is cleaved by a restriction endonuclease and the resulting fragments are separated according to their size by agarose gel electrophoresis. The gel is then soaked in alkali to make the DNA fragments single stranded so that they will subsequently hybridize with a complementary DNA probe. After neutralizing the gel, the DNA fragments are transferred by a blotting process onto a nitrocellulose filter laid over the top of the gel. The DNA fragments then become firmly bound to the filter in the same positions they had migrated to inside the agarose gel (the smaller fragments migrating further than larger ones). The filter-bound DNA fragments are then hybridized to a single-stranded radioactively labelled DNA probe containing sequences of a particular gene of interest. After washing off the unhybridized probe, the DNA fragments that have formed double-stranded hybrids with the radioactive probe can be identified by subjecting the filter to autoradiography.

The globin gene plasmid probes containing cDNA inserts were ideal for the Southern blotting technique and a great deal of information about the location of restriction enzyme sites in and around the globin genes was quickly obtained. Gene deletions responsible for α-thalassaemia, Hb Lepore thalassaemia, δβ-thalassaemia and hereditary persistence of fetal haemoglobin disorders were identified by this technique and the first introns were discovered by Southern blotting experiments using rabbit globin gene probes. However, the human β-globin like genes were too far apart from each other to be detected as a group by Southern blotting and very little information was obtained about the overall gene arrangement of the β-globin gene cluster.

This knowledge was gained by a development of genetic engineering techniques pioneered by Maniatis and his colleagues, who in 1978 reported the first successful construction of a human gene library (Lawn *et al.*, 1978). DNA sequences from the entire human genome were cloned by inserting random restriction fragments into a bacteriophage vector which could be grown up and stored. Overlapping restriction fragments covering the whole α- and β-globin gene clusters were isolated from this library and a complete map of each globin gene cluster obtained. Large amounts of pure genomic DNA fragments could be obtained by this technique, suitable for DNA sequencing by the methods developed by Sanger and by Maxam and Gilbert, with the result that the entire DNA sequence of the β-globin gene cluster (48 kb of continuous sequence) is now known. The cloned DNA fragments were also used to generate smaller genomic DNA fragments which were then inserted into plasmids to make genomic DNA plasmid probes which are more useful than cDNA plasmid probes because they can be made for any unique DNA sequence.

Once the normal sequence of the β-globin genes had been derived, cloning techniques were quickly applied to DNA from patients with various thalassaemias and the molecular defects of most types α- and β-thalassaemia have now been determined. At least 30 different specific β-thalassaemia mutations have been identified, most of which involve single base substitutions or small deletions or insertions within or just upstream of the β-globin gene (Orkin and Kazazian, 1984). These mutations all affect some aspect of gene function: either DNA transcription, RNA processing or mRNA translation, with the end result of either none or only very little amounts of β-globin being synthesized.

There are now several different approaches to the detection of these mutations for prenatal diagnosis by DNA analysis and the precise method chosen depends on what type of molecular defect is responsible. Table 27.1 summarizes the most important types of haemoglobinopathies together with their molecular defects and the main methods of their detection. These methods can be conveniently divided into those which detect the mutation directly and those which rely on the indirect method of linkage analysis using DNA polymorphisms.

27.3 DIRECT DETECTION OF THE HAEMOGLOBINOPATHIES

Gene deletions can be detected directly either by the absence of any hybridizing restriction fragments in a Southern blot analysis if the deletion encompasses the whole of the proble DNA sequence, or by the appearance of a characteristic abnormal fragment if only part of the complementary probe sequence is missing. α-Thalassaemia, Hb Lepore thalassaemia, δβ-thalassaemia, the deletion forms of hereditary persistence of fetal haemoglobin (HPFH) and the Indian β°-thalassaemia gene can all be detected in this way (Old, 1984).

There are three common types of gene deletions which in their homozygous

Table 27.1 The common types of haemoglobinopathies

Disorder	*Homozygous state*	*Molecular defect*	*DNA analysis*
α^+-thalassaemia	Low MCH and MCV	3.7 or 4.2 kb deletion removing one α-gene	α-probe – characteristic 10 kb Bam H1 fragments.
α°-thalassaemia	Hb Barts hydrops fetalis syndrome	Three types of large DNA deletions removing both α-genes.	1. α-probe – absence of normal bands in homozygote. 2. ζ-probe – characteristic 10.5 or 13.9 kb abnormal Bg1 II fragments.
β-thalassaemia:			
β°-	Thalassaemia major, Hb F 98%	One common gene deletion (Indian β°), remainder are point mutations or small deletions or insertions.	1. β-probe – characteristic 4.6 kb Bg1 II fragment for Indian β°. 2. Globin gene probes – linkage analysis using DNA polymorphisms (all types) 3. Oligonucleotide probe analysis (some types)
β^+-	Thalassaemia major, Hb F 70–95%		
β^+-	Thalassaemia Intermedia HB F 20–40%		
Hb S	Sickle-cell anaemia	Point mutation	β-probe – characteristic 1.3 kb Mst II fragment
Hb S/β-Thalassaemia	Variable sickle-cell anaemia	As above	Mst II + β-thalassaemia method
Hb S/Hb C	Moderate sickle-cell anaemia	Hb C – point mutation	Mst II + Hpa 1 polymorphism
Hb E/β-thalassaemia	β-thalassaemia major to intermedia	Hb E – point mutation	Linkage analysis only for Hb E

state, result in infants with haemoglobin Bart's hydrops fetalis syndrome (Higgs and Weatherall, 1983), for which prenatal diagnosis is desirable. All three deletions occur in the α-globin gene cluster removing all or most of both α-globin genes. Therefore the homozygous conditions for these three types of α°-thalassaemia can be detected by the absence of any normal α-globin gene fragment in a Southern blot analysis. However, the ς-gene is present in all three types and if a ς-probe is used characteristic abnormal bands can be detected as an alternative method of prenatal diagnosis.

In the case of β-thalassaemia, so far only one type has been found with a DNA deletion large enough to be detected by Southern blotting. This is a β°-thalassaemia mutation found only in Asian Indians and results from a 619 base pair deletion at the 3′ end of the β-globin gene, giving rise to a characteristic 4.6 kb Bgl II β-gene fragment instead of the normal 5.2 kb globin gene fragment. One of the first reported examples of a first trimester diagnosis of the haemoglobinopathies was for a couple at risk of having a fetus homozygous for the Indian β°-deletion type of thalassaemia (Old *et al.*, 1982).

All the other β-thalassaemia mutations cannot be detected directly by Southern blotting using plasmid probes unless the point mutation or small deletion/insertion of nucleotides occurs at the recognition site of a restriction endonuclease which generates easily detectable fragments at that particular locus. In practice, DNA fragments are only easily detected by the Southern blotting method if they are larger than 500 base pairs in size. Only six of the thirty or more β-thalassaemia mutations fall into this category (Orkin *et al.*, 1983) and only one is common, the β39 nonsense mutation which can be diagnosed by the enzyme Mae I (Thein *et al.*, 1985). Interestingly one of the six types is caused by a mutation in the same codon as the sickle cell mutation and can be detected directly by the same method.

The sickle cell mutation is a single base change of A to T in codon 6 of the β-globin gene and this mutation abolishes three different enzyme recognition sites present in the normal β^A-gene sequence. The first two to be discovered, Mn1 I and Dde I, produced DNA fragments which were too small to be detected easily by the Southern blotting method. This resulted in a very limited use of the direct method for prenatal diagnosis in preference to the previously established method of linkage analysis using the nearby Hpa I polymorphic site. However, the third restriction enzyme recognition site to be discovered at the mutation locus, Mst II, generated easily blottable fragments of 1.1 kb from β^A genes and 1.3 kb from β^S genes and this approach is now the standard method of prenatal diagnosis of sickle cell anaemia, although the sickle mutation has been shown to be directly detectable by yet another method, the oligonucleotide probe technique.

The main application of the oligonucleotide technique appears to be for the detection of β-thalassaemia. The approach relies on short, synthetic DNA probes (called oligonucleotides), tailor-made to detect single base changes in a DNA restriction fragment. Two probes are hybridized to Southern blots or dried gels, one probe complementary to the normal DNA sequence, the other to the DNA sequence containing the point mutation, and the presence of the mutant gene in a genomic DNA sample is determined by the presence or absence of hybridization of each of the probes. Studies have shown that only a few β-thalassaemia mutations are present in each population and therefore only a limited number of pairs of oligonucleotide probes are required to detect most of the β-thalassaemia mutations in a particular population. However, although this technique is extremely useful in theory, in practice it is more difficult and less sensitive than the standard method of Southern blotting and hybridization with plasmid probes and the application of this technique has so far been best suited for populations in which one β-thalassaemia gene accounts for the majority of cases of β-thalassaemia, such as the β39 nonsense mutation in Sardinia (Rosatelli *et al.*, 1985).

27.4 INDIRECT DETECTION OF THE HAEMOGLOBINOPATHIES

The discovery that natural variations in DNA sequences occur randomly throughout the genome has led to another major approach to the prenatal diagnosis of the haemoglobinopathies and in principle, for the detection of any genetic disorder whether the basic biochemical defect is known or not. The approach depends on demonstrating linkage of a DNA polymorphism to the mutant gene under study and requires the production of a gene specific probe and the discovery of a DNA polymorphism which is very close to the mutant gene, otherwise the linkage is not tight enough due to the increased possibility of DNA recombination between the gene and the DNA polymorphism. DNA polymorphisms occur because variations in DNA sequence result in the loss of an existing recognition site or the acquisition of a new one. A polymorphic restriction site will produce DNA fragments of different lengths in different people and the fragments can be identified by their different positions in a Southern blot. The polymorphic fragments are inherited in a simple Mendelian manner and can be used as markers for chromosomes carrying either normal or abnormal genes. Such DNA polymorphisms are referred to as restriction fragment length polymorphisms (RFLPs).

More than 17 different polymorphic restriction sites have been discovered in the β-globin gene cluster and many of these have proved very useful for the detection of the β-thalassaemias, Hb S, Hb E and Hb C. Most of the polymorphic sites, however, occur with similar frequencies in linkage to both normal and abnormal globin genes and therefore although the study of these polymorphic sites has proved very useful for determining the number, origin and spread of the different types of β-globin mutations, their use for prenatal diagnosis requires the establishment of linkage to a particular β-globin gene mutation by carrying out a family study beforehand. Such studies require the couple at risk to have a previously born child (either normal or affected) or if not, the study of both sets of grandparents. Hence RFLP linkage analysis cannot be used for prenatal diagnosis in many cases for several reasons: either the assignment of linkage is not possible because of an incomplete pedigree, or often in cases where the pedigree is complete, the couple at risk do not have any heterozygous β-globin RFLPs to use as markers. Studies on the feasibility of using RFLPs in most populations at risk for β-thalassaemia have shown that providing linkage can be assigned, prenatal diagnosis is possible for 70–80% of families. In addition, for a majority of the remaining families, a diagnosis is possible in 50% of the cases. This latter situation occurs when only one parent has a heterozygous RFLP and therefore a fetal diagnosis of normal or β-thalassaemia trait (a successful diagnosis) will occur statistically in half the cases studied. For those families which cannot be helped by RFLP analysis the alternatives are either a diagnosis by oligonucleotide analysis of fetal DNA or a diagnosis by fetal blood analysis.

27.5 FIRST TRIMESTER DIAGNOSIS

Since 1982 when the first cases were reported (Old *et al.*, 1982), many thalassaemia centres around the world have begun a programme of first trimester diagnosis of the haemoglobinopathies. A wide variety of haemoglobinopathies have been diagnosed including Hb S (Goossens *et al.*, 1983) and β°-thalassaemia by oligonucleotide analysis (Rosatelli *et al.*, 1985). Table 27.2 shows the various types diagnosed at Oxford at the National Haemoglobinopathy Reference Centre, John Radcliffe Hospital. The cases of sickle cell anaemia have all been done by Mst II analysis and the

Table 27.2 Summary of the first trimester diagnosis for haemoglobinopathies carried out at Oxford

Disorder	*Number*	*Normal*	*Heterozygous*	*Homozygous*
Sickle-cell anaemia	30	4	17	11
β-thalassaemia	57	6	24	16
α°-thalassaemia	5	0	4	1
Hb Lepore	1	1	0	0
Hb S/Hb C	1	0	1	0
Hb S/β-thalassaemia	1	0	0	1

Note: 11/57 cases of β-thalassaemia had only a 50% chance of a successful prenatal diagnosis by RFLP analysis. The results of these are: normal or heterozygous, 7; heterozygous or homozygous, 4.

β-thalassaemias have either been detected directly in the case of the Indian β° deletion type or by RFLP analysis.

Chorionic villi are an excellent source of DNA for prenatal diagnosis. On average it is possible to obtain 30 μg of DNA from a chorionic villus sample, enough for five to six different restriction enzyme digestions. Studies of the presence of maternal DNA polymorphisms in chorionic villi DNA have shown that maternal contamination is not a serious problem for DNA analysis methods provided that the chorionic villi are carefully dissected out from any contaminating maternal debris with the aid of a phase-contrast microscope. The only difficulties which have been encountered to date in the Oxford first trimester programme are: a case in which a bizarre RFLP inheritance pattern turned out to be due to non-paternity, although it was still possible to determine the genotype of the fetus; one family in which a crossover has arisen within the β-globin gene complex; and one instance of a misdiagnosis due to plasmid contamination, which generated a false α-globin gene band in DNA from a fetus that turned out to be an α°-thalassaemia homozygote.

Chorion villus sampling offers many advantages to couples at risk for the haemoglobinopathies compared to the other methods of prenatal diagnosis by fetal blood sampling or by analysis of DNA from amniotic fluid cells. There is now considerable experience of prenatal diagnosis of the haemoglobin disorders using chorionic villi DNA and provided that fetal loss rate (the most recent information suggests 4–5%) is proved acceptable, prenatal diagnosis by one of the many DNA methods in the first trimester of pregnancy will replace fetal blood sampling as the main approach to the control of the haemoglobinopathies.

REFERENCES

Alter, B. P. (1984) Advances in prenatal diagnosis of hematologic disease. *Blood*, **64**, 329–40.

Goossens, M., Dumez, Y., Kaplan, L., Luper, M., Chabret, C., Henrion, R. and Rosa, J. (1983) Prenatal diagnosis of sickle-cell anemia in the first trimester of pregnancy. *New Engl. J. Med.*, **309**, 831–3.

Higgs, D. R. and Weatherall, D. J. (1983) Alpha thalassaemias. In *Current Topics in Haematology* vol. 4. (eds S. Piomelli, S. Yachin,), Alan R. Liss, New York. pp. 37–97.

Kan, Y. W., Golbus, M. S. and Dozy, A. M. (1976) Prenatal diagnosis of α-thalassaemia. Clinical application of molecular hybridisation. *New Engl. J. Med.*, **295**, 1165.

Lawn, R. M., Fritsch, E. F., Parker, R. C., Blake, G. and Maniatis, T. (1978) The isolation and characterisation of linked δ and β-globin genes from a cloned library of human DNA. *Cell*, **15**, 1157–74.

Old, J. M. (1984) First trimester diagnosis of haemoglobinopathies by DNA analysis of chorionic villi. In *Prenatal Diagnosis* (eds C. H. Rodeck and K. H. Nicolaides), Royal College of Obstetricians and Gynaecologists, London, pp. 105–20.

Old, J. M., Ward, R. H. T., Petrou, M., Karagozlu, F., Modell, B. and Weatherall, D. J. (1982) First trimester diagnosis for haemoglobinopathies: a report of three cases. *Lancet*, ii, 1413–16.

Orkin, S. H., Antonarakis, S. E. and Kazazian, H. H. (1983) Polymorphism and molecular pathology of the human β-globin gene. *Prog. Hematol.*, **13**, 49–73.

Orkin, S. H. and Kazazian, H. H. (1984) The mutation and polymorphism of the human β-globin gene and its surrounding DNA. *Ann. Rev. Genetics*, **18**, 131–71.

Rosatelli, C., Falchi, A. M., Tuveri, T., Scalas M. T., DiTucci, A., Monni, G. and Cao, A. (1985) Prenatal diagnosis of beta-thalassaemia with the synthetic-oligomer technique. *Lancet*, i, 241–3.

Southern, E. M. (1975) Detection of specific sequences among DNA fragments separated by gel electophoresis. *J. Mol. Biol.*, **98**, 503–17.

Thein, S. L., Wainscoat, J. S., Lynch, J. R., Wetherall, D. J., Sampietro, M. and Fiorelli, G. (1985) Direct detection of β°39 thalassaemic mutation with Mae 1. *Lancet*, i, 1095.

Weatherall, D. J. and Clegg, J. B. (1981) *The Thalassaemia Syndromes*, 3rd edn, Blackwell Scientific Publications, Oxford.

Wilson, J. T., Wilson, L. B., DeRiel, J. K., Villa-Komoroff, L., Efstratiadis, A., Forget, B. G. and Weissman, S. M. (1978) Insertion of synthetic copies of human genes into bacterial plasmids. *Nucleic Acid Res.*, **5**, 563–81.

28

Extraction of DNA from chorionic villi

—— R. Quaife and D. T. Y. Liu ——

28.1 INTRODUCTION

Antenatal diagnosis by DNA analysis is almost ten years old (Kan *et al.*, 1976; Orkin *et al.*, 1978; Kan and Dozy, 1978). These analyses used cultured amniocytes as the source of fetal DNA. Cultures are established at about the sixteenth week of pregnancy and some two to three weeks are needed to allow the cells to replicate so that there are sufficient to enable DNA to be extracted in usable quantities. The analysis of the DNA obtained in this way takes perhaps a week (although this may be reduced, Law *et al.*, 1984). If everything goes well a result should be available at about 19–20 weeks gestation. Such a time-scale serves to demonstrate the special advantage of chorion villus sampling (CVS) because using such tissue fetal DNA (and chromosomes) can be obtained and analysed within the first trimester.

Chorionic material at this stage in pregnancy represents most of the tissue of zygotic origin. It is a rapidly growing tissue and as such is obviously ideal for DNA extraction. Of course, in initially obtaining the tissue clinical expertise and instrumentation used in the sampling procedures are of the utmost importance. Modell (1985) has discussed relative risks to pregnancies as a result of such sampling, and it is worthwhile noting that possible contamination by maternal tissue will inevitably also present some additional risk. Elles *et al.* (1983) have concluded that in their study maternal DNA contamination was not detectable, although Liu *et al.* (1984) have related increased syringe capacity used in villus aspiration to increased maternal cell contamination. Obviously such risks can be considerably reduced by starting with tissue that demonstrates large numbers of buds on typical branching villus 'fronds' free of contaminants such as blood cells.

Extraction of DNA from chorionic villi is similar in methodology to that used for blood and other tissues. In general it is a process of cell lysis and protein degradation followed by repeated purification of the subsequently liberated DNA. Modifications upon this general principle are made by various workers, and some of these will be discussed.

28.2 METHODS AND NOTES

The protocol we follow is essentially that of Williamson *et al.* (1981) who modified the method used by Kan and Dozy (1978). Since some of the specimen may be needed for chromosome analysis, it is initially washed in sterile Hams F10 medium (Gibco). If this is not available sterile isotonic saline may be used. For transportation purposes the villi to be used for DNA analysis may be 'blotted' relatively dry and then frozen. They can then be packed in dry ice and thawed at the destination. Frozen specimens (as in the case for whole blood) will yield as much DNA as fresh ones, and indeed it may be that such a single freeze-thaw cycle may aid subsequent DNA extraction. Transportation in medium or saline will also be satisfactory for the short term.

Normally we attempt to estimate the weight of the villi obtained. Of course such wet weight measurements will be somewhat inaccurate. None the less, we 'blot' the specimen on a dry surface such as a sterile petri dish and then transfer it to a pre-weighed 1.5 ml sterile screw-cap micro-centrifuge tube (Sarstedt). (Screw-cap tubes are less liable to leak, and this advantage becomes more important when using noxious substances such as phenol.)

In a series of seventy-five patients from whom we obtained chorionic villi samples (this being an initial study used to determine parameters for future DNA work) we found wet weights varied from 2.1 mg up to 73.9 mg with a mean of 27.97 mg. A more detailed discussion of parameters is given below, but for the moment it should be said that whatever the wet weight of tissue, it was dealt with in the same way using the same quantities and concentrations of reagents.

The protocol for the preparation of DNA from chorionic villi is as follows:

1. 400 μl of 10 mM Tris pH 10.5, 1 mM EDTA, 0.15 M NaCl is added to the 1.5 ml tube containing the specimen.
2. 20 μl of 10% SDS are then added, together with 5 μl of a 20 mg/ml stock solution of proteinase K (BRL). The tube is then incubated at 37°C for 16 hours.
3. After this period 400 μl of Tris saturated phenol/chloroform (1:1) is added (see below) and the suspension is then gently mixed by rotation for 10 min.
4. This is then centrifuged for 1 min at low speed on an MSE Micro-Centaur centrifuge.

5. The supernatant is then removed into a fresh tube using a Gilsen pipette with a yellow tip, and 400 µl of chloroform/octanol (24:1) added.
6. Again the solution is gently mixed for 10 min, followed by a 1 min centrifugation at low speed.
7. This supernatant is removed into another fresh tube and 40 µl of 3 M sodium acetate added. This is then thoroughly combined and 800 µl of ice-cold ethanol added with gentle mixing. A precipitate should be observed at this stage which can be pelleted by centrifugation at low speed for 2 min.
8. The ethanol is then pipetted away and the tube inverted to drain. The pellet can then be washed with 70% ethanol to dissolve any remaining salt.
9. The supernatant is then removed (after a further centrifuge step if necessary) and the pellet rinsed with 100% ethanol.
10. Once again the supernatant is removed and the pellet then lyophilized for 10 min.
11. It can then be dissolved in 100 µl of 10 mM Tris, 1 mM EDTA pH 8.0 overnight at 4°C.
12. The solution is warmed to 37°C for one hour prior to reading the optical density at 260 and 280 nm. To conserve the extracted DNA we use a semi-micro cuvette cell with a 1.5 ml capacity, but still sacrifice 10% of the DNA in measurement. The concentration of the DNA solution is calculated as a solution of DNA at 1 mg/ml being equivalent to 20 OD units. The readings at 260/280 should be 1.8. Contamination by phenol or protein will depress this figure, and such contamination can be refractory to restriction endonuclease digestion. Under these circumstances re-extraction with chloroform/octanol with the prior addition of 1/10th volume of 3M sodium acetate will normally cure the problem.

At this stage, some mention should be made of Proteinase K. This is a powerful endoprotease and will actively hydrolyse protein, glycoproteins and peptides as well as esters and amides. The use of Proteinase K in DNA extraction will result in glycopeptides from the glycoproteins co-purifying with the DNA and again these may be refractory to restriction digests. For this reason some workers omit a Proteinase K step in their protocols, relying on phenol and chloroform to remove proteins. Other sorts of DNA contamination resulting in poor restriction digests, can sometimes also be resolved by adding spermidine (Sigma) to the actual digest. Again some laboratories will do this routinely. While discussing contamination, it is worth pointing out some 'rules' that most laboratories engaged in DNA analysis will normally observe:

1. The use of 'Analar' or equivalent grade reagents will be considered mandatory.

2. As will the use of sterile disposable tips, tubes and transfer pipettes and whenever possible the wearing of sterile gloves.
3. Reagents used for patient DNA extraction will be separated from those used for other purposes such as plasmid extraction, if these two processes are carried out in the same laboratory. Plasmid contamination in particular can give spurious results when using sensitive autoradiographic techniques.

Finally, in our extractions we use phenol (obtained from BDH) of a grade specially prepared for chromatography. This is not redistilled but is prepared as described in Maniatis *et al.* (1982). Once the phenol is equilibrated with Tris (containing 0.2% β-mercaptoethenol) it is removed and a 1:1 solution made with chloroform/isoamyl alcohol 24:1. This solution is stable and can be stored at 4° for some months.

28.3 PARAMETERS AND OBSERVATIONS

In an attempt to rationalize our approach to chorionic villus sampling, with special regard to DNA analysis, we initially collected data from a group of 75 patients who had elected for termination of pregnancy. All of these samples were delivered to the laboratory fresh and were weighed in the manner described previously. They were then frozen at −20°C until we were ready to extract the DNA. All the samples in this group were treated with the same batch of reagents. They were all collected by one of us (DTYL) and all were extracted by one of us (RQ). Table 28.1 gives an idea of the distribution of measurements that we have found.

Table 28.1 Amount and proportion of DNA extracted from studied chorionic villi (wet weight)

	Min	*Max*	*Mean*	*Standard deviation*
Wet weight (mg)	2.1	73.9	28.5	17.56
DNA weight (μg)	2.8	203.9	43.02	40.36
Proportion DNA/wet weight	0.3	3.3	1.62	0.76

A linear relationship between DNA yield and wet weight of biopsy material has been determined (Weatherall *et al.*, 1985). We have extended this idea, so that if the DNA yield (in micrograms) is considered to be dependent upon the wet weight (in milligrams) of villi obtained and this is considered as an independent variable, then a simple linear regression analysis can be applied to give a more precise picture of any relationship. The results of such an analysis using this sample of 75 individuals can be seen in Fig. 28.1. The slope of the regression line gives an indication of the DNA yield to be expected from

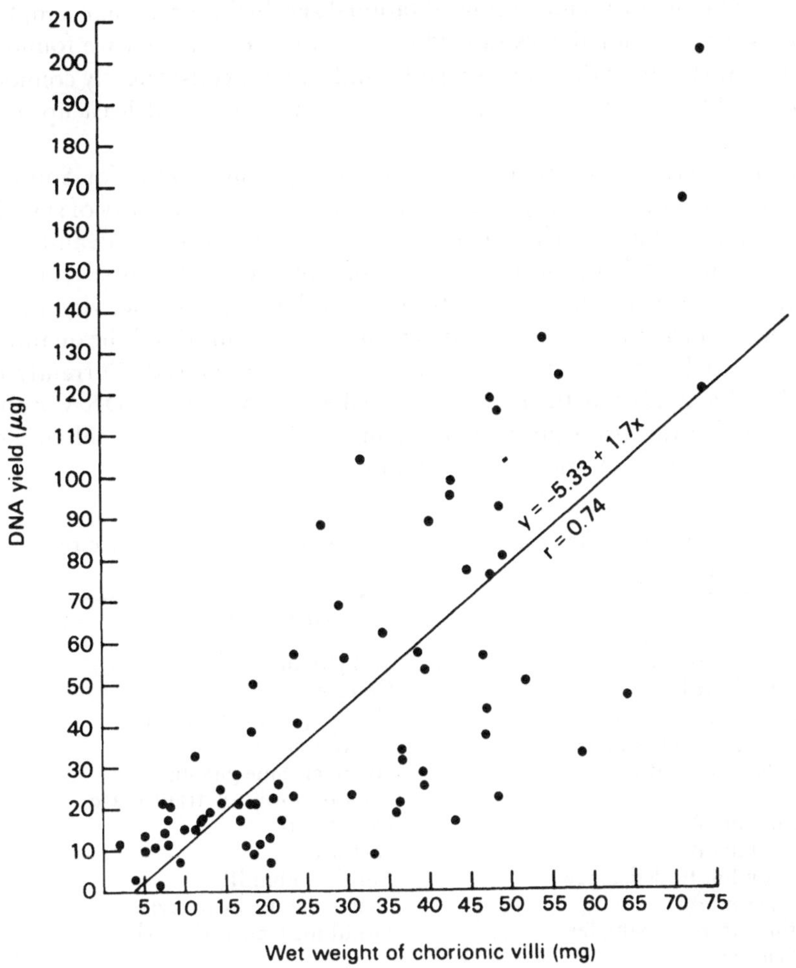

Figure 28.1 Line of regression for predicting DNA yield (Y) from wet weight of chorionic villus (X).

particular amounts of villi, i.e. for each milligram of villus we would expect a yield of 1.7 μg of DNA. Realizing that we may need between 5 and 10 μg of DNA for a diagnosis (and perhaps 5 μg as a back-up) we aim to sample 10 mg of wet weight villi. The analysis of our data suggests the relationship between wet weight tissue and DNA yield, that we have derived, will be correct in about 70% of cases. Our second consideration in attempting to further define our parameters concerned gestational age and the proportion DNA yield to milligram of villus tissue. We reasoned that since the most actively proliferating trophoblast region is the chorion frondosum but that sampling may be from progressively degenerating chorion laeve, there was a possibility of the

DNA yield falling with increasing gestational age. In this particular sample of patients the gestational ages ranged from 6–14 weeks. In fact we found no relationship between these two variables and we were consequently confident of our yield expectations irrespective of gestational age, at least up to 14 weeks.

In summary, chorion tissue can be used to produce DNA for Southern analysis and, within reason, the expected yields from any quantity of sampled tissue can be predicted. The use of this tissue presents distinct advantages in allowing antenatal diagnosis results to be obtained in the first trimester. Furthermore, by using probes labelled to a high specific activity by the oligodeoxynucleotide method (Feinberg and Vogelstein, 1984) the quantities of DNA used and the time-scales involved may be reduced. Currently the listed (Table 28.2) genetic diseases can be diagnosed by use of DNA probes. The length of this list is growing at an impressive rate and will enhance the potential worth of chorion villus sampling.

Table 28.2 Current list of genetic diseases diagnosed by DNA probes (courtesy of Dr J. Old, Oxford)

Diseases	*Gene probe*
Haemoglobinopathies	α, β-globin
Collagen disorders	Collagen
Growth hormone deficiency	Human growth hormone
αl-Antitrypsin deficiency	α-l Antitrypsin
Lesch–Nyhan syndrome	Hypoxanthine guanine phosphoribosyl transferase
Haemophilia A	Factor VIII
Haemophilia B	Factor IX
Antithrombin III deficiency	Antithrombin III
Phenylketonuria	Phenylalanine hydroxylase
Ornithine transcarbamylase deficiency	Ornithine transcarbamylase
Duchenne muscular dystrophy	Linked RFLPs
Becker muscular dystrophy	Linked RFLPs
Huntington's chorea	Linked RFLPs
Adult polycystic kidney disease	Linked RFLPs
Cystic fibrosis	Linked RFLPs

REFERENCES

Elles, R. G., Williamson, R., Niazi, M., Coleman, D. V. and Horwell, D. (1983) Absence of maternal contamination of chorionic villi used for fetal-gene analysis. *New Engl. J. Med.*, **308**, 1433–5.

Feinberg, A. P. and Vogelstein, B. (1984) A technique for radiolabelling DNA restriction endonuclease fragments to high specific activity. *Anal. Biochem.*, **137**, 266–7.

Kan, Y. W. and Dozy, A. M. Antenatal diagnosis of sickle cell anaemia by DNA analysis of amniotic fluid cells. *Lancet*, **ii**, 910–12.

Kan, Y. W., Golbus, M. S. and Dozy, A. M. (1976) Prenatal diagnosis of thalassemia: clinical application of molecular hybridisation. *New Engl. J. Med.*, **295**, 1165–7.

Law, D. J., Frossard, P. M. and Rucknagel, D. L. (1984) Highly sensitive and rapid gene mapping using miniaturised blot hybridisation: application to prenatal diagnosis. *Gene* **28**, 153–8.

Liu, D. T. Y., Slater, E. and Norman, S. (1984) Aspiration as a technique for biopsy of chorionic villi. *J. Obstet. Gynae.*, **5**, 75–7.

Maniatis, T., Fritsch, E. F. and Sambrook, J. (1982) *Molecular cloning: a laboratory manual.* Cold Spring Harbor Laboratory, New York.

Modell, B. (1985) Chorionic villus sampling, evaluating safety and efficiency. *Lancet*, **i**, 737–40.

Orkin, S. H., Alter, B. P., Altay, C., Mahoney, M. H., Lazarus, H., Hobbins, J. C. and Nathan, D. G. (1978) Application of endonuclease mapping to the analysis and prenatal diagnosis of thalassemias caused by globin gene deletion. *New Engl. J. Med.*, **299**, 166–72.

Weatherall, D. J., Old, J. M., Thein, S. L., Wainscoat, J. S. and Clegg, J. B. (1985) Prenatal diagnosis of the common haemoglobin disorders. *J. Med. Genet.*, **22**, 422–30.

Williamson, R., Eskdale, J., Coleman, D. V., Niazi, M., Loeffler, F. R. and Modell, B. M. (1981) Direct gene analysis of chorionic villi: a possible technique for first trimester antenatal diagnosis of haemoglobinopathies. *Lancet*, **ii**, 1125–7.

Section V

GENETIC COUNSELLING

29

Counselling in prenatal diagnosis

—— *J. S. Fitzsimmons* ——

29.1 COUNSELLING IN PRENATAL DIAGNOSIS

Chorion villus sampling is the most recent of the various technical procedures available for the prenatal diagnosis of genetic disease. More information is still needed about its risks to the fetus and the pregnancy but the advantages are such that it has already proved useful and has been welcomed by many couples. Unfortunately there continues to be considerable parental anxiety associated with all types of prenatal diagnosis and chorion villus sampling will do little to lessen this or to reduce the concern about the social consequences. Termination of pregnancy for whatever reason remains a controversial issue and has already generated a fair amount of public criticism, some of which has been levelled at the profession. While there is probably little we can do to resolve the conflict of values surrounding the abortion debate it is important that we ensure that our patients are seen to have been adequately counselled and have freedom of choice. This is essential not only for optimum patient care but hopefully to minimize the risk of malpractice suits, an increasing hazard for those involved in this work.

There is wide variation in people's concept of what constitutes counselling but the definition proposed by an *ad hoc* committee of the American Society of Human Genetics is comprehensive and remains useful. They defined conselling as an attempt by one or more appropriately trained persons to help an individual or family:

Comprehend the medical facts including the diagnosis, the probable cause of the disorder and the available management; appreciate the way heredity contributes to the disorder and the risk of recurrence in specified individuals and relatives; understand the options for dealing with the risk of recurrence; choose the course of action which seems appropriate to them in view of their risk and their family's goal and act in accordance with that decision; make the best possible adjustment to the disorder in an affected family member and/or to the risk of a recurrence of that disorder.

This definition underlines the importance of effective communication between the counsellor and those counselled and serves to emphasize the non-directive nature of this process. Individuals concerned are not told what they should do but are given the opportunity of discussing the various options available to them and of making an informed choice. However, to be really successful, the counsellor must also be sensitive to the difficulties of imparting medical information and must be aware of the psychological consequences of genetic disease (Hof Op't and Kopinsky, 1982). As experience has accumulated the emphasis has tended to switch from counselling with the main emphasis on content to that more tailored to meet individual needs. This person-oriented counselling (Kessler, 1979) is particularly important when prenatal diagnosis is under consideration. The genetic risk in these circumstances may become secondary to the concern about the interruption of a pregnancy and the emotional, social, religious or ethical price to be paid for this. The counsellor has to attempt an assessment of such concerns and to help those involved come to terms with them. The decision to terminate a pregnancy is anything but emotionally neutral (Emery and Pullen, 1984) and attention to the psychological aspects becomes of equal or even greater importance than the giving of factual information. This makes it essential that adequate time is made available if these various aspects are to be explored and discussed. This will often require more than one counselling session and it would be difficult to offer counselling at this level in the usual busy antenatal clinic. Patients will usually be sensitive to the limits on the doctor's time and to the needs of other waiting individuals. Even the most sympathetic and communicative of doctors is unlikely to have the time to encourage the sort of questions that are necessary or to deal with the emotional or social issues which may arise. Furthermore some couples trying to decide about prenatal diagnosis may be unhappy mixing with other patients having apparently anxiety-free pregnancies and may find the presence of medical students or other observers inhibiting. Many of them have conflicting emotional responses, particularly if they have already had an affected infant, and this may surface as anger or aggression; responses which can seriously jeopardize effective communication (Smith and Antley, 1979). For all these reasons it is important to have a non-clinical and reasonably relaxed atmosphere in the counselling room which should be away from a busy out-patient area. It is also clear that counselling patients in the way suggested demands a different technique from that usually employed in standard clinical practice. Clinicians are normally expected to maintain a positive and optimistic approach to patients' problems, whereas the counselling role is concerned with the giving of accurate information even when this may be very depressing. It would be difficult therefore for a busy obstetrician to switch from the usual therapeutic role to that of counsellor and there are dangers in assuming the giving of a risk figure to be all that is necessary. Despite this, many of us will have experience of an anxious telephone call from a busy colleague wanting a quick risk estimation for a couple sitting in the consulting room. This is rarely appropriate even in the most straightforward situations and could, in some circumstances, particularly with an unexpected outcome, devalue the public view of the service.

The facilities and expertise appropriate for counselling in prenatal diagnosis should normally be provided by established genetic counselling services. They usually have support staff such as genetic nurses or genetic associates who will be able to reinforce the information that has been given and to visit the patients in their homes when this is appropriate. They will also be able to contribute to a more in-depth assessment of the patient's social and personal goals. Many couples in the security of their homes will reveal private concerns that they may be unwilling to discuss in the more formal and threatening clinic atmosphere. It is now appreciated that many patients have real difficulty in deciding about pregnancy termination by consideration only of probability or risk figures. A number of studies have confirmed that reproductive decision making is more clearly related to the parents' responses to uncertainty than to any specific risk that they may face (Lippman-Hand and Fraser, 1979). Coming to terms with this uncertainty requires the patients to attempt an analysis of how they would cope with various outcomes and to review their coping ability from previous pregnancy or personal experiences (Pauker and Pauker, 1979). Obstetricians offering prenatal diagnosis need to be aware of the importance of these previously underestimated issues and this applies equally to their nursing and junior medical colleagues. A team approach is essential and all involved staff need to be familiar with the genetic problems in individual cases, the difficulties involved in decision making and the dangers of ill-advised directive advice, however well meaning. This team will also be responsible for the constant evaluation of the techniques currently in use and their attendant risks and advantages. They will have to ensure that they have a high level of support laboratory services and that everything possible is done to minimize false positive and false negative test results. Both obstetric and genetic staff will need to make patients aware of the impossibility of absolute guarantees about the outcome of prenatal diagnosis and their consent to any procedure must be on this basis.

Whether or not they should be asked to sign a consent form is of less importance than an awareness on everyone's part that consent means patient participation in decision making. It is a continuous process and in this respect differs very significantly from consent obtained for a more straightforward surgical procedure (Editorial, *Lancet*, 1985).

Despite increasing experience of its use some ethical and social consequences of prenatal diagnosis continue to be controversial. Many doctors are aware that in most cases their medical training failed to address these sorts of issues and they find themselves concerned and distressed at public condemnation of their work. In these circumstances guidelines are obviously welcomed particularly if these express the views not only of the profession but of a wide section of informed public opinion. Such guidelines have been proffered by the Genetics Research Group of The Hastings Centre, USA, Institute of Society, Ethics and Life Sciences (Powledge and Fletcher, 1979) with members from various backgrounds including medicine, law, philosophy, biology, theology, social services and genetics. They examined some of the wider issues raised by prenatal diagnosis and concluded that despite the many difficulties involved, prenatal diagnosis was here to stay, was of undoubted benefit to many families and would be increasingly requested. Their eventual recommendations were issued primarily to help professionals provide the most favourable circumstances for informed decision-making by parents and to help plan future developments. These continue to be useful guidelines for those involved in this field and some of them are listed in Table 29.1 which has been adapted from their report. Effective communication with the parents is seen as paramount and comprehensive and experienced counselling essential. In the course of their investigations of existing services on offer in the United States they found grounds for criticism of this and other aspects and they rightly stress the value of communication as an aid to good doctor–patient relations. They further commented on the need for a much more comprehensive follow-up service and the need for further counselling and support; something which might become even more important with the earlier termination made possible by chorion villus sampling. The relevance

Table 29.1 Recommendations for patient management and developments in prenatal diagnosis

Prenatal diagnosis
1. Patients should be well informed before and adequately counselled after.
2. Counselling should be non-directive and options clear.
3. Comprehensive follow-up and evaluation essential.
4. A full clinical/genetic evaluation is essential.
5. Prenatal diagnosis should be undertaken only where high quality support services available.
6. Programmes should be directed at and reach well defined at-risk groups.
7. Findings should not be withheld even when of disputed importance.
8. Privacy should be protected.
9. Balance between service and research should be made clear.
10. Education of public and professionals should be encouraged.

Note: Adapted from the guidelines for the ethical, social and legal issues in pre-natal diagnosis. Genetics Research Group of The Hastings Centre, USA, 1979.

of this recommendation was confirmed by a recent report from the United Kingdom (Lloyd and Laurence, 1985) which revealed that couples who had elected for termination of pregnancy on genetic grounds had less than adequate follow-up support from existing services. Of the 48 women who had a genetic termination, 77% experienced an acute grief reaction after the index pregnancy was terminated. The reaction was considered similar to that documented after stillbirth or neonatal death. Forty-six per cent of the women remained symptomatic six months after the pregnancy had ended and some required psychiatric support. Obstetric and genetic services need to investigate ways of dealing with this problem and innovations such as a parents' self-help group is one of a number of possible solutions. Such a scheme is in existence in the author's own service area and appears to be helpful.

The Hastings Group further recommended that the findings on prenatal testing should not be withheld even when of disputed importance. This is most likely to apply in advanced maternal age when the fetal karyotype is unexpectedly found to be that of the Turner or Kleinfelter syndrome. Some professionals might decide to withhold such information in the belief that the patient is better off without it. However this could be interpreted as the doctor deciding what is best for the patient in a situation where such an attitude would be considered inappropriate. Any information found on prenatal testing is deemed to belong to the patient and this particular aspect of patient management has been the basis of several malpractice suits in the United States (Wright and Shaw, 1981). The other recommendations listed in Table 29.1 are of obvious relevance, particularly the importance of differentiating between research and service aspects of the work. The encouraging central theme of the report is the Group's acceptance of, and encouragement for, prenatal diagnostic services provided these are properly conducted.

No such national body has offered opinion or advice of this sort as yet in the United Kingdom where there has been little or no public debate about genetic terminations. Presentation of the associated social and ethical issues by the media, particularly television, may be over-dramatized and is not always free from bias. Technical innovations such as chorion villus sampling tend to be presented as another major breakthrough and this encourages non-realistic expectations by many patients. The British public in general is misinformed about the limitations of technology and few are familiar with simple facts relating to probability or the relevance of recent advances in genetics for their health; findings which apply also to North America (McInerney *et al.*, 1978). Since counselling is more likely to be effective when it is a two-way process a better informed public should be more able to understand and contribute to the management of their own problems. Ways of achieving this are being explored and their does appear to be a genuine desire by the public to play more of a part in their own health care. In view of this welcome development obstetric and genetic services need to co-operate in public education campaigns to advertise prenatal diagnosis and to encourage patients to present themselves earlier to hospital particularly now with the advent of chorion villus sampling. This could obviously result in an increased need for more preconception counselling clinics, an inevitable development which could ensure earlier identification and registration of at-risk pregnancies. None of these objectives should require a massive capital investment and at a local level the author's service has combined very usefully with the school teachers and the Department of Health Education to ensure that adolescents are made more aware of birth defects and their prevention (Fitzsimmons, 1985).

The pace of developments in prenatal diagnosis and molecular genetics gives limited time for assessment and adaptation by the profession. New technical procedures such as chorion villus sampling will continue to attract their share of criticism and medico-legal problems. However it seems that the latter when they do arise are just as likely to result from lack of communication, real or imagined, as with faulty technique. With this in mind, now is probably a useful time for reflection on current practice and the effectiveness of communication between doctor and patient. There is good evidence that properly conducted counselling, in sufficient depth, by experienced personnel and in the right environment, should go some way to resolve at least some of the difficulties we are likely to encounter (Seller, 1982).

REFERENCES

Ad Hoc Committee on Genetic Counselling (1975) Genetic Counselling. *Am. J. Hum. Genet.*, **27**, 240–2.

Editorial (1985) If only you had told me. *Lancet*, **i**, 1022.

Emery, A. E. H. and Pullen, I. (1984) *Psychological Aspects of Genetic Counselling*, Academic Press, London.

Fitzsimmons, J. S. (1983) The Teaching of Human Genetics in Schools. *J. Med. Genet.*, **20**(4), 244–8.

Hof Op't J. and Kopinsky, S. M. (1982) Communication in Genetic Counselling. *SA Med. J.*, **62**, 758–64.

Kessler, S. (ed) (1979) The psychological foundations of genetic counselling. In *Genetic Counselling*, Academic Press, New York, pp. 17–33.

Lippman-Hand, A. and Fraser, F. C. (1979) Genetic counselling: parents' responses to uncertainty. *Risk, Communication, and Decision Making in Genetic Counselling, Birth Defects*: Original Article Series, vol. XV, no. 5C, 325–39.

Lloyd, J. and Laurence, K. M. (1985) Sequelae and Support after termination of pregnancy for fetal malformation. *Br. Med. J.*, **290**, 907–9.

McInerney, J. D., Hickman, F. M. and Kennedy, M. H. (1978) Human Genetics: A Context for Health Education. *Health Education*, **9**, 33.

Pauker, S. P. and Pauker, S. G. (1979) The Amniocentesis Decision: An Explicit Guide for Parents. *Risk, Communication and Decision Making in Genetic Counselling, Birth Defects*: Original Article Series, vol. XV, no. 5C, 289–324.

Powledge, T. M. and Fletcher, J. (1979) Guidelines for the ethical, social and legal issues in pre-natal diagnosis. *New Engl. J. Med.*, **300**, 168–72.

Seller, M. J. (1982) Ethical aspects of genetic counselling. *J. Med. Eth.*, **8**, 185–8.

Smith, R. W. and Antley, R. M. (1979) Anger: A Significant Obstacle to Informed Decision Making in Genetic Counselling. *Risk, Communication, and Decision Making in Genetic Counselling, Birth Defects*: Original Article Series, vol. XV, no. 5C, 257–60.

Wright, E. E. and Shaw, M. W. (1981) Legal Liability in Genetic Screening, Genetic Counselling, and Pre-natal Diagnosis. *Clin. Obstet. Gynaecol.*, **24**(4), 1133–49.

30

Chorion villus sampling in X-linked genetic disorders

Peter S. Harper, M. Upadhyaya
A. Roberts and H. Williams

More than 200 X-linked disorders are now recognized in man (McKusick, 1983); while many are extremely rare, some are both serious in effects and relatively frequent. The X-linked muscular dystrophies, the haemophilias, X-linked mental retardation due to 'fragile X' and the X-linked mucopolysaccharidosis type II (Hunter syndrome) are all important examples. The mode of inheritance creates particular problems in genetic counselling: numerous female relatives may be at risk of transmitting the disorder, techniques of carrier detection are commonly imperfect, some heterozygous females may themselves be clinically affected, while specific methods of prenatal diagnosis only exist for a small proportion of the disorders.

Recently, the isolation of DNA probes on the X chromosome in increasing numbers has made it possible to use these as genetic markers for those X-linked disorders closely linked to them, even when nothing is known about the disorder itself (Botstein *et al.*, 1980). Uncertainty of the likely error rate due to recombination has so far limited the prenatal application of these linked probes, but the rapid evolution of the X chromosome gene map now means that close markers are potentially available for almost all X-linked disorders (Davies, 1985). For some X-linked conditions the gene itself has been isolated and can be used as a specific probe without risk of error from recombination. Table 30.1 shows some of the disorders where DNA prediction is now feasible.

The validity of using DNA isolated from chorion samples in early prenatal diagnosis has been well documented in both experimental and clinical situations (Williamson *et al.*, 1981; Old *et al.*, 1982; Upadhyaya *et al.*, 1984); X-chromosome probes are no different in this respect from those on other chromosomes. Careful dissection of samples removes significant maternal

Table 30.1 X-linked disorders for which prediction is feasible in first trimester material

Adrenal hypoplasia (X-linked)	DNA (linked)
Albinism (ocular)	DNA (linked)
Fabry's disease	Enzyme assay; specific DNA probe
Fragile X syndrome	Cytogenetic defect
Glucose 6 phosphate dehydrogenase deficiency	Cytogenetic defect; specific DNA probe
Chronic granulomatous disease	DNA (linked); also fetal blood sampling
Haemophilia A	DNA (linked and specific); also fetal blood sampling
Haemophilia B	Specific DNA probe; also fetal blood sampling
Lesch–Nyhan syndrome	Enzyme assay; specific DNA probe
Menkes syndrome	Enzyme assay
Mucopolysaccharidosis II (Hunter)	Enzyme assay
Muscular dystrophy, Duchenne	DNA (linked); some gene deletions
Muscular dystrophy, Becker	DNA (linked)
Norrie's disease	DNA (linked); some gene deletions
Ornithine trancarbamylase deficiency	Enzyme assay; specific DNA probe (some deletions)
Retinitis pigmentosa (X-linked type)	DNA (linked)

contamination, while culture is unnecessary since adequate amounts of DNA (1–2 μg per mg wet weight) can be obtained from the uncultured sample. We have shown no effect of site of sampling on the DNA yield or typing (Upadhyaya *et al.*, in press).

Enzyme studies are currently feasible on chorion sample material in only a few X-linked disorders, and require careful documentation on normal tissue before diagnostic use, since normal ranges in chorionic villi may differ considerably from those of cultured amniotic fluid cells or fibroblasts. We have documented this for Hunter syndrome, where the deficiency is that of the lysosomal enzyme iduronate sulphate sulphatase (Upadhyaya *et al.*, 1984).

30.1 SPECIFIC X-LINKED DISORDERS

30.1.1 Duchenne muscular dystrophy (DMD) (Harper, 1985)

This is the most frequent and most serious of the muscular dystrophies; the primary defect is unknown and until now only fetal sexing has been possible prenatally. The identification of linked probes allows more accurate prediction of carriers (Williams *et al.*, 1986) and can, in selected cases, now allow accurate prenatal prediction (Bakker *et al.* 1985). Very rarely a visible chromosomal deletion may cause DMD (Francke *et al.*, 1985); we have recently identified such a family in which the boy and his mother showed both chromosomal loss and deletion of DNA probes (Clarke *et al.*, 1986); the sister, presenting at eight weeks of pregnancy and scheduled for chorion sampling and fetal sexing, was shown to be normal by both approaches, so that prenatal testing could be cancelled. An exciting development has been the use of a similar patient to isolate probes from the region of the deletion (Kunkel, *et al.*, 1985) leading to the finding that 5–10% of DMD boys have a chromosomally invisible gene deletion in this region (Monaco *et al.*, 1985). In these families specific prenatal diagnosis can now be offered; in one such family identified by us, a carrier sister had previously had termination of a male fetus following chorion sampling; retrospective study of stored material showed no deletion present, indicating that the male fetus would have been normal (Thomas *et al.*, 1986).

30.2 OTHER X-LINKED MYOPATHIES

The later onset Becker muscular dystrophy has been shown to be closely linked or allelic to DMD (Kingston *et al.*, 1984), though no cases have yet been convincingly shown to be the result of gene deletion. The same linked probes are applicable in both carrier detection and prenatal diagnosis. The very rare Emery–Dreifuss muscular dystrophy may possibly be on the long arm of the X chromosome (Hodson *et al.*, 1986), so only fetal sexing can be offered here at present. Yet another X-linked muscle disorder is the lethal X-linked myotubular myopathy, resulting in stillborn or neonatal death in most affected males (Van Wijngaarden *et al.*, 1969). In one such family studied by us, a carrier female lost six successive male pregnancies before delivering a healthy girl. Interestingly, this mother declined chorion sampling in favour of amniocentesis because of the possible risk of miscarrying with a female pregnancy; her sister, also a carrier, may prefer chorion sampling. No specific early prenatal diagnosis is yet feasible.

30.3 THE HAEMOPHILIAS

Specific gene probes are now available for both factor VIII (Gitschier *et al.*, 1985) and factor IX (Gianelli *et al.*, 1984); occasionally haemophilia patients results from gene deletions, but most do not, so diagnosis must be based on the pattern of transmission in the family of a polymorphism for the probe. These developments are likely to allow the later approach of fetal blood sampling to be avoided in most cases, though it remains an option in difficult situations. Thus a haemophilia-carrier patient studied by us proved to be carrying twins and preferred the greater experience of fetal blood sampling in twin pregnancy. DNA analysis is greatly increasing the accuracy of carrier detection in the haemophilias, so carrier status must always be established as accurately as possible before chorion sampling is undertaken (preferably before pregnancy is embarked on).

30.4 HUNTER'S SYNDROME

There is evidence to suggest that the gene is linked to markers on the distal long arm of the X chromosome (Upadhyaya *et al.*, 1985), but this is not firm enough to use clinically; a gene-specific probe may be available before long. Enzyme studies appear to be accurate on chorion sampling material (Upadhyaya *et al.*, 1984). It is important to combine these with fetal sexing, since some female carriers may have low enzyme levels that could be compared with those of an affected male.

30.5 FRAGILE X SYNDROME

This is now recognized to be one of the commonest causes of moderate to severe mental retardation in males, and of mild retardation in females. The fragile site is not uniformly expressed in cultured amniotic fluid cells, so diagnosis has relied on fetal blood sampling; recent studies suggest that it can be detected in chorion sampling material (Mikkelsen, 1985) but experience is limited; certainly such samples should only be studied in an expert centre. No DNA probes show close enough linkage to be useful prenatally.

30.6 RETINITIS PIGMENTOSA

This is commonly X-linked, and is located on the X chromosome short arm (Bhattacharya *et al.*, 1984). The linked probes are not very close, and in one large family studied personally, most members did not wish for prenatal diagnosis, though they did wish to have their carrier status determined as accurately as possible with the new markers.

A number of other serious eye disorders are located on the X chromosome, for some of which linked DNA probes exist (see Table 20.1). In one disorder, *Norrie's disease*, a gene deletion has been proved in some cases and has been used for prenatal diagnosis by chorion sampling (Chapelle *et al.*, 1985).

30.7 IMMUNE DEFICIENCIES

Again several forms exist on the X chromosome, including chronic granulomatous disease, severe combined immunodeficiency and Bruton's agammaglobulinaemia; none can yet be detected in the first trimester.

30.8 FETAL SEXING AND CHORION SAMPLING

Since a specific first trimester diagnosis is still impossible for most X-linked disorders, fetal sexing remains of major importance in this group of conditions. The greater acceptability of chorion sampling compared with amniocentesis is particularly apparent here, since the late termination of a male pregnancy that is likely to be normal in at least half the cases is a distressing outcome for all women and unacceptable for some. Fetal sexing on chorionic villus material may be achieved by chromosomal study on direct or cultured material (Brambati *et al.*, 1985). It can also be undertaken by DNA techniques relying on either Y chromosome repetitive DNA sequences (Gosden *et al.*, 1984) (Fig. 30.1) or on an XY homologous probe that gives a specific band for the Y chromosome (Page *et al.*, 1982) (Fig. 30.2).

Our diagnostic series of chorion samples, partly reported previously

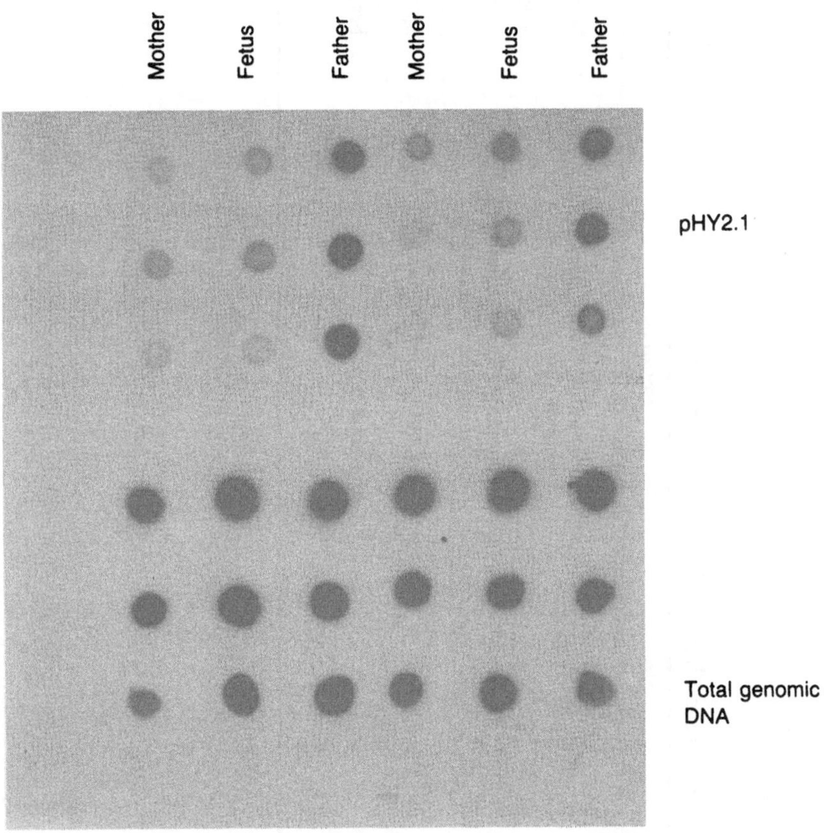

Figure 30.1 Dot blot method using probe HY2.1. Samples of DNA from chorionic villi and from both parents, with three dilutions of each sample containing approximately 1, 0.5 and 0.25 μg DNA. Aliquots of each sample in duplicate were applied to nitrocellulose paper. One half of the filter was hybridized with probe HY2.1 and the other half with total genomic DNA, which has highly repeated sequences represented equally in male and female. The signal generated by male DNA is 20–100 times stronger than for female DNA.

Table 30.2 Diagnostic chorion sampling for X-linked disorders (Cardiff series)

Disorder	*No.*	*Result*	*Special points*
Muscular dystrophy			
Duchenne	13	delivered (3), miscarriages (2) therapeutic abortions (3) continuing (5)	Some genes result from gene deletion; linked probes also available
Becker	2	miscarriage (1), continuing (1)	Linked DNA probes available
Emery–Dreifuss	1	therapeutic abortion (1)	No firm localization or other specific test
Hunter syndrome	5	delivered (3)	Specific Enzyme diagnosis (normal) made in addition to sexing
Fragile X syndrome	1	delivered (1)	Fragile site may be detectable
Total	22		

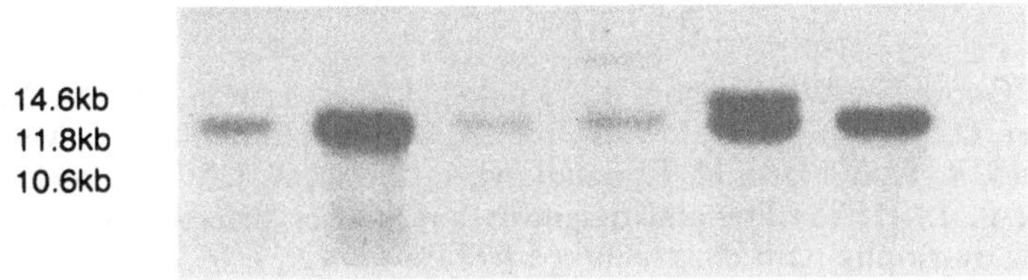

Figure 30.2 Autoradiogram of chorionic villus DNA digested to completion with restriction endonuclease TAQ1 and hybridized with probe DXYS1 detecting 14.6 kb (Y specific), 11.8 and 10.6 kb (X specific) bands.

(Upadhyaya *et al.*, 1985), includes twenty-two cases referred for fetal sexing. Details of these are summarized in Table 30.2. We have used a combination of DNA and cytogenetic techniques, which have been particularly useful in the event of culture failure and which have shown no disagreement in this or in more extensive experimental material.

30.9 GENETIC COUNSELLING

Genetic counselling has been discussed elsewhere in relation to prenatal diagnosis in general, but there are several points in relation to chorion sampling that are particularly relevant.

Perhaps the most important in our own experience is the necessity for a planned approach, with the major decisions and relevant investigations completed before a pregnancy is embarked upon. The advantage of this is seen clearly in our own DMD population in Wales, where we have had a policy of systematic genetic counselling and carrier detection for all girls in known families, following on a total population study of the disorder. This means that potential carriers are already divided into those that are definite or at high risk, who will in general wish for prenatal testing, and those at low risk, who in general will not.

All women at risk for a child with DMD in our series from Wales requesting chorion sampling had been fully studied in advance, making a striking contrast with referrals and enquiries from other regions, in whom the carrier status was often uncertain and where study of multiple family members in a hurried manner would have often been necessary. The advantage of such a planned approach is as great in other X-linked disorders, and demonstrates the need for genetic counselling to be achieved as far in advance as possible before pregnancy (Harper, 1983). A genetic register for X-linked disorders is also of great value in ensuring that girls at risk are appropriately counselled and tested as they enter the reproductive age group.

REFERENCES

Bakker, E., Goor, N., Wrogemann, K., Kunkel, L. M., Fenton, W. A., Majoor-Krakauer, D., Jahoda, M. G. J., van Ommen, G. J. B., Hofker, M. H., Mandel, J. L., Davies, K. E., Willard, H. F., Sandkuyl, L., Essen, A. J. V., Sachs, E. S. and Pearson, P. L. (1985) Prenatal diagnosis and carrier detection of Duchenne muscular dystrophy with closely linked RFLPs. *Lancet*, i, 655–8.

Bhattacharya, S. S., Wright, F. P., Clayton, J. F., Price, W. H., Phillips, C. I., McKeown, C. M. E., Jayel, M., Bird, A. C., Pearson, P. L., Southern, E. M. and Evans H. J. (1984) Close genetic linkage between X linked retinitis pigmentosa and a restriction fragment length polymorphism identified by recombinant DNA probe L1.28. *Nature*, **309**, 253–5.

Botstein, D., White, R. I., Skolnick M. and Davis R. W. (1980) Construction of a genetic linkage map in man using restriction fragment length polymorphisms. *Am. J. Hum. Genet.*, **32**, 314–31.

Brambati, B., Simoni, G., Danesino, C., Oldrini, A., Ferrazzi, E., Romitti, L., Terzoli, G., Rossela, F., Ferrari, M. and Fraccaro, M. (1985) First trimester fetal diagnosis of genetic disorders: clinical evaluation of 250 cases. *J. Med. Genet.*, **22**, 92–9.

Chapelle, A. De la, Sankila, E-M., Lindlof, M., Aula, P. and Norio, R. (1985) Norrie disease caused by a gene deletion allowing carrier detection and prenatal diagnosis. *Clin. Genet.*, **28**, 317–20.

Clarke, A., Thomas, N. S. T., Roberts, S. H., Whitfield, A. and Williams, J. (1986) Duchenne muscular dystrophy with adrenal insufficiency and glycerol kinase deficiency: high resolution cytogenetic analysis with molecular, biochemical and clinical studies. *J. Med. Genet.*, in press.

Davies, K. E. (1985) Molecular Genetics of the human X chromosome. *J. Med. Genet.*, **22**, 243–9.

Francke, U., Ochs, H. D., de Martinville, B., Giacalone, J., Lindgren, V., Disteche, C., Pagon, R. A., Hofker, M. H., van Omman, G-J. B., Pearson, P. L. and Wedgwood, R. J. (1985) *Am. J. Hum. Genet.*, **37**, 250–67.

Gianelli, F., Anson, D. S., Choo, K. H., Rees, D. J. G., Winship, P. R., Ferrari, N., Rizza, C. R. and Brownlee, G. (1984) Characterisation and use of an intragenic polymorphic marker for detection of carriers of haemophilia B (factor IX deficiency). *Lancet*, 239–43.

Gitschier, J., Wood, W. I., Tuddenham, E. G. D., Shuman, M. A., Goralka, T. M., Chen, E. Y. and Lawn, R. M. (1985). Detection and sequence of mutations in the factor VIII gene of haemophiliacs. *Nature*, **315**, 427–30.

Gosden, J. R., Gosden, C. M., Christie, S., Cooke, H. J., Morsman, J. M. and Rodeck, C. H. (1984) The use of cloned Y chromosome-specific DNA probes for fetal sex determination in first trimester prenatal diagnosis. *Hum. Genet.*, **66**, 347–751.

Harper, P. S. (1983) Genetic counselling and prenatal diagnosis. *Br. Med. Bull.*, **39**, 302–9.

Harper, P. S. (1985) The genetics of muscular dystrophies. In *Progress in Medical Genetics* (ed. A. Bearn), Praeger Scientific, Philadelphia. pp. 53–90.

Hodgson, S. V., Boswinkel, E., Walker, A., Bobrow, M., Davies, K., Dubowitz, V., Granata, G. and Merlini, L. (1986) Linkage analysis using nine DNA polymorphisms along the length of the X chromosome locates the gene for Emery–Dreifus muscular dystrophy to distal Xq. *J. Med. Genet.*, **23**, 169–70.

Kingston, H. M., Sarfarazi, M., Thomas, N. S. T. and Harper, P. S. (1984) Localisation of the Becker muscular dystrophy gene on the short arm of the X chromosome by linkage to cloned DNA sequences. *Hum. Genet.*, **67**, 6–17.

Kunkel, L. M., Monaco, A. P., Middlesworth, W., Ochs, H. D. and Latt, S. A. (1985) Specific cloning of DNA fragments absent from the DNA of a male patient with an X chromosome deletion. *Proc. Natl. Acad. Sci. USA.*, **82,** 4778–82.

McKusick, V. A. (1983) *Mendelian inheritance in Man.* 6th edn, Johns Hopkins University Press, Baltimore.

Mikkelsen, M. (1985) *Cytogenetic findings in first trimester chorionic villi biopsies: A collaborative study – in first trimester fetal diagnosis* (ed. Fraccaro M., Simoni G. and Brambati B), Springer-Verlag, Berlin.

Monaco, A. P., Bertelson, C. J., Middlesworth, W., Colletti C-A., Aldridge, J., Fischbeck, K. H., Bartlett, R., Pericak-Vance, M. A., Roses, A. D. and Kunkel, L. M. (1985) Detection of deletions spanning the Duchenne muscular dystrophy locus using a tightly linked DNA segment. *Nature*, **316,** 842–5.

Old, J. M., Ward, R. H. T., Petrou, M. *et al.* (1982) First-trimester fetal diagnosis for haemoglobinopathies: three cases. *Lancet*, **ii,** 1413–16.

Page, D., De Martinville, B., Barker, D., Wyman, A., White, R., Francke, U. and Botstein, D. (1982) Single copy sequence hybridises to polymorphic and homologous loci on human X and Y chromsomes. *Proc. Natl. Acad. Sci. USA.*, **79,** 5352–6.

Thomas, N. S. T., Williams, H., Harper, P. S. and Kunkel, L. M. (1986) Gene deletion in Duchenne muscular dystrophy. *J. Med. Genet.*, in press.

Upadhyaya, M., Archer, I. M., Harper, P. S., Jasani, B., Roberts, A., Shaw, D. J., Thomas, N. S. T. and Williams, H. (1984) DNA and enzyme studies on chorionic villi for use in antenatal diagnosis. *Clin. Chim. Acta*, **140,** 39–46.

Upadhyaya, M., Bamforth, S., Young, I., Thomas, N., Sarfarazi, M., Davies, K. and Harper, P. S. (1985) Hunter's syndrome: evidence supporting a location on the distal part of the X chromosome long arm. *J. Med. Genet.*, **22,** 394–5.

Upadhyaya, M., Harper, P. S., Williams, H. and Roberts, A. (1985) DNA polymorphisms and fetal sexing for X-linked disorders with chorionic biopsy. In: *First trimester fetal diagnosis* (ed. M. Fraccaro, G. Simoni, B. Brambati), Springer-Verlag, Berlin.

Upadhyaya, M., Jasani, B., Little, E., Roberts, A., Rees, D. (1986) Lack of sampling site variation in chorionic villus biopsy used for antenatal diagnosis. *Prenat. Diag.*, in press.

Van Wijngaarden, G. K., Fleury, P., Bethlem, J. and Meijer, A. E. F. H. (1969) Familial 'myotubular' myopathy. *Neurol.*, **19,** 901–8.

Williams, H., Sarfarazi, M., Brown, C., Thomas, N. and Harper, P. S. (1986) The use of flanking markers in prediction for Duchenne muscular dystrophy. *Arch. Dis. Child.*, **61,** 218–22.

Williamson, R., Eskdale, J., Coleman, D. V. *et al.* (1981) Direct gene analysis of chorionic villi: a possible technique for first trimester antenatal diagnosis of haemoglobinopathies. *Lancet*, **ii,** 1125–7.

Index

Page numbers in italics refer to illustrations.